MOSBY'S

PEDIATRIC NURSING REFERENCE

MOSBY'S
PEDIATRIC NURSING REFERENCE

SECOND EDITION

Cecily Lynn Betz, RN, PhD
Nursing Training Coordinator,
University Affiliated Program,
UCLA Neuropsychiatric Institute,
Los Angeles, California

Elizabeth C. Poster, RN, PhD
Director, Nursing Research and Education,
UCLA Neuropsychiatric Institute,
Los Angeles, California

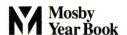

**Mosby
Year Book**

St. Louis   Baltimore   Boston   Chicago   London   Philadelphia   Sydney   Toronto

Mosby
Year Book
Dedicated to Publishing Excellence

Senior Editor: Linda L. Duncan
Developmental Editor: Teri Merchant
Project Manager: Karen Edwards
Production Editor: Jim Russell
Designer: Jeanne Wolfgeher
Cover Illustration: John Dyess

SECOND EDITION
Copyright © 1992 by Mosby–Year Book
A Mosby imprint of Mosby–Year Book, Inc.

Previous edition copyrighted 1989

A NOTE TO THE READER
The authors and publisher have made every attempt to check dosages and nursing content for accuracy. Because the science of pharmacology is continually advancing, our knowledge base continues to expand. Therefore, we recommend that the reader always check product information for changes in dosage or administration before administering any medication. This is particularly important with new or rarely used drugs.

Printed in the United States of America

Mosby–Year Book, Inc.
11830 Westline Industrial Drive   St. Louis, MO 63146

Library of Congress Cataloging-in-Publication Data

Betz, Cecily Lynn.
  Mosby's pediatric nursing reference / Cecily Lynn Betz, Elizabeth
C. Poster.—2nd ed.
    p. cm.
  Includes bibliographical references and index.
  ISBN 0-8016-0613-6
  1. Pediatric nursing—Handbooks, manuals, etc. I. Poster,
Elizabeth C. II. Title. III. Title: Pediatric nursing reference.
  [DNLM: 1. Pediatric Nursing—handbooks. 2. Pediatrics—handbooks.
WY 39 B565m]
RJ245.B47 1992
610.73'62—dc20
DNLM/DLC
for the Library of Congress   91-45991
                                                              CIP

92 93 94 95 96 GW/DC 9 8 7 6 5 4 3 2 1

Reviewers

Jane W. Ball, RN, PNP, DrPH
Trauma Services, Children's Hospital,
Washington, DC

Mary Ellen Brown, RNC, MN
Nursing Instructor,
Florence-Darlington Technical College,
Florence, South Carolina

Karen A. Dadich, RN, MN
Associate Professor Clinical Nursing,
Texas Tech University Health Sciences Center,
School of Nursing, Lubbock, Texas

Diana Fendya, RN, MSN
Surgical Clinical Specialist,
Cardinal Glennon Children's Hospital,
St. Louis, Missouri

Bernadette Frager, RN, MN
Nursing Consultant,
Los Gatos, California

Jean M. Francis, RN, MSN
Clinical Director, Pediatric Nursing Division,
The University of Iowa, Iowa City, Iowa

Jeannie Frank, RN
Pediatric Nurse Practitioner,
Department of Neurology,
Childrens Hospital, Los Angeles, California

Jody Harris, RN, MN, CCRN
Clinical Nurse Specialist
Gladstone, Oregon

Mary Fran Hazinski, RN, MSN, FAAN
Division of Trauma,
Department of Surgery and Pediatrics,
Vanderbilt University,
Nashville, Tennessee

Marilyn Hockenberry-Eaton, RN, MSN, CPNP
Assistant Professor, Graduate Pediatric Oncology
  Program,
Emory University School of Nursing,
Atlanta, Georgia

Patricia Killam, MS, PNP
Pediatric Nurse Practitioner,
Department of Neurology,
Childrens Hospital, Los Angeles, California

Sally Valentine Kimpel, RN, MN
Clinical Nurse Specialist,
Kaiser Hospital,
San Diego, California

Corrine McCarthy, MSN, RN, CPN
Pediatric Outreach Coordinator
Children's Hospital–San Diego
San Diego, California

Kristie S. Nix, RN, EdD
Associate Professor, University of Tulsa School
of Nursing, Tulsa, Oklahoma

Linda Sowden, RN, MN
Nurse Manager,
All Children's Hospital,
St. Petersburg, Florida

Judith A. Vinson, MSN, RN
Nursing Education Coordinator,
Center of Nursing Excellence,
Children's Hospital,
Washington University Medical Center,
St. Louis, Missouri

Ronda Wood, RN, MN
Clinical Nurse Specialist,
Children's Hospital, Los Angeles, California

Cynthia J. Wright, MSN, RNC
Trauma Center, Children's Hospital National
   Medical Center,
Washington, DC

Preface

Mosby's Pediatric Nursing Reference is designed to serve nurses and nursing students who provide care to ill children and their families. Its small size and concise format were purposefully created for the nurse who wants an easily accessible reference. This book is divided into two parts. Part I contains information about the most frequently encountered medical and surgical conditions in the pediatric population. Part II presents diagnostic procedures and tests. For the user's convenience, the chapters in each part are listed in alphabetical order. In the appendixes, the nurse will find valuable information about growth and development, immunization schedules, commonly used antibiotics, laboratory values, and guidelines for taking blood pressure measurement. Guidelines for conducting complete nursing assessments for each body system are also in the appendixes.

The organization of the care-planning guidelines reflects our philosophical orientation — a family-centered approach. The needs of the child and family are addressed from a biopsychosocial perspective. The care-planning guidelines reflect a holistic approach to the child's and the family's short-term and long-term needs.

It is our hope that this compact yet powerful tool will prove a useful resource in the delivery of high-quality bedside care for children and the associated care required by their families.

Cecily Lynn Betz
Elizabeth C. Poster

A Note on Pediatric Drug Dosages

Since children vary widely in weight, age, body surface area, and their ability to absorb, metabolize, and excrete medications, extreme caution should be used when determining the proper dosage for a particular patient. Although the physician is responsible for writing the order correctly, the nurse is responsible for administering medications, always being careful to determine whether the dosage is correct. The nurse is urged to use the body surface method for calculating dosages (see Appendix H, *West Nomogram*).

The authors of this reference have endeavored to provide pediatric dosages consistent with safe practice. The nurse is advised, however, to rely on her own calculations, experience, judgment, and authoritative pharmacologic sources when administering drugs to specific patients.

Contents

PART TWO

Pediatric Diagnostic Tests and Procedures

APPENDIXES

PART ONE

Pediatric
Medical
and
Surgical
Conditions

1 ❖ Acquired Immunodeficiency Syndrome

PATHOPHYSIOLOGY

Since 1981, more than 179,136 cases of this severe form of acquired immune deficiency, known as acquired immuno-deficiency syndrome (AIDS), have been reported nationally to the Centers for Disease Control (CDC). Of this number, 2192 cases occurred in children under 13 years of age. As of February 1988, 80% of children diagnosed with AIDS were younger than 3 years old. Diagnosis of infants is difficult because their signs and symptoms can lead to only a presumptive diagnosis.

Research findings strongly support the theory that the cause of AIDS is a retrovirus termed human HIV. Only two retroviruses are known to infect humans, and they are implicated in malignancies of the thymus-derived lymphocytes and a T cell variant of hairy-cell leukemia. The retrovirus believed to cause AIDS infects the helper T lymphocytes, which are responsible for cellular immunity.

The routes of transmission for adults and adolescents include sexual contact and parenteral exposure to needles or blood transfusions. The major risk factor associated with the occurrence of AIDS in early childhood is birth to an AIDS-infected mother who is a member of a high-risk group or who has a sexual partner who is a member of a high-risk group. In young children, another route of transmission is through blood or the administration of blood products. The five high-risk groups for AIDS (95% of the adult and adolescent cases have occurred in individuals in these five groups) include the following:

1. Homosexual or bisexual men
2. Intravenous drug abusers
3. Hemophiliacs
4. People receiving blood or blood products
5. Sexual partners of infected persons

The actual route of transmission in children born to high-risk mothers remains unknown, although it is suspected that the AIDS virus is acquired in utero. There is no evidence that the virus is transmitted through casual person-to-person contact.

The diagnosis of AIDS is currently based on the clinical signs and symptoms defined by the CDC (see box on p. 4). These symptoms include an opportunistic infection or malignancy, indicating an underlying cellular immunodeficiency. No diagnosis of AIDS is definitive without the presence of *Pneumocystis carinii*. The diagnosis of AIDS-related complex is made when some signs and symptoms are evident but before opportunistic infections or malignancies have developed. The signs and symptoms of the AIDS-related complex are as follows:

1. Generalized lymphadenopathy
2. Chronic diarrhea
3. Failure to thrive
4. Weight loss
5. Recurrent infections
6. Interstitial pneumonia
7. Hepatosplenomegaly
8. Persistent oral candidiasis

Incubation periods vary between perinatally acquired and transfusion-acquired cases, with the incubation period for transfusion-acquired AIDS longer than for perinatally acquired AIDS. The mean age for perinatally acquired AIDS is 17 months (ranges from 1 to 86 months) compared to 24.4 months (ranges from 4 to 82 months) for transfusion-acquired AIDS (Rogers et al, 1987).

INCIDENCE

1. Eighty percent of children diagnosed with AIDS are younger than 6 years of age.

Diseases Accepted by CDC as Indicative of Underlying Cellular Immunodeficiency

Protozoal and Helminthic Infections

Cryptosporidiosis — duration >1 month
Pneumocystis carinii pneumonia
Strongyloidosis*
Toxoplasmosis*

Viral Infections

Cytomegalovirus — disseminated infection with onset at >6 months of age
Herpes simplex virus — chronic or disseminated infection with onset at >1 month of age
Progressive multifocal leukoencephalopathy

Fungal Infections

Candidiasis — esophageal
Cryptococcosis — central nervous system or disseminated infection

Bacterial Infections

Mycobacterium avium — disseminated infection

Cancer

Kaposi's sarcoma
Lymphoma limited to the brain

*Pulmonary, central nervous system, or disseminated infection.

2. Ethnic distribution is 54% black, 19% Hispanic, and 27% white.
3. Majority of children with AIDS (79%) live in New York, New Jersey, Florida, or California.
4. Gender prevalence is 61% male and 39% female.

CLINICAL MANIFESTATIONS
Infants
The clinical findings and evolution of the disease in infants are similar to those in older children and adults.

The prodromal stage includes the following signs and symptoms:

Low birth weight
Failure to thrive
Generalized lymphadenopathy
Hepatosplenomegaly
Interstitial pneumonia (unidentified cause)
Parotitis
Chronic diarrhea
Recurrent bacterial and viral infections
Persistent Epstein-Barr virus infection
Oropharyngeal thrush
Thrombocytopenia

The number of infants progressing to the full syndrome remains unknown.

Infants infected during the neonatal period demonstrate the following characteristics before 1 year of age:

Failure to thrive
Persistent or recurrent oral candidiasis (thrush)
Chronic or recurrent diarrhea
Bacterial infections such as meningitis
Hepatosplenomegaly
Chronic interstitial pneumonia

Adolescents

The following signs and symptoms are experienced by adolescents for weeks to months before the development of opportunistic infections and malignancies:

Fever
Malaise
Fatigue
Night sweats
Insidious onset of weight loss
Recurrent or chronic diarrhea
Generalized lymphadenopathy
Oral candidiasis
Arthralgias and myalgias

The long-term effects of this syndrome include an opportunistic infection (*Pneumocystis carinii* pneumonia, which occurs in 70% of cases) and malignancies (Kaposi's sarcoma, which occurs in 5% of cases, and non-Hodgkin's lymphomas).

LABORATORY/DIAGNOSTIC TESTS

1. HIV — serologic test for measuring antibody to AIDS virus; positive results indicate exposure but do not mean individual will be diagnosed with AIDS. Asymptomatic seropositive individuals have been identified, suggesting that they are carriers of AIDS.
2. The following abnormalities characterize AIDS:
   a. Lymphopenia (decreased helper T lymphocytes)
   b. Poor response to skin tests
   c. Serum immunoglobulin levels normal or increased

NURSING ASSESSMENT

Refer to "Respiratory Assessment" and "Gastrointestinal Assessment" in Appendix A.

NURSING DIAGNOSES

High risk for infection
High risk for fluid volume deficit
High risk for injury
Altered family processes
Anticipatory grieving
Altered growth and development
Impaired social interactions

NURSING INTERVENTIONS

1. Protect infant, child, or adolescent from infectious contacts (see box on p. 7).
   a. Although casual person-to-person contact does not transmit the AIDS virus, a number of recommendations have been made for children with AIDS.
   b. Providers in foster homes are educated on precautions regarding blood exposure, saliva contamination, and infection protection.
   c. Day care attendance is evaluated on an individual basis.
   d. They should attend school if health, neurologic development, behavior, and immune status is appropriate.
2. Other general measures to prevent the transmission of

Preventive Measures

Preventive efforts are of vital importance in dealing with AIDS. Reducing the number of sexual partners, especially those in high-risk groups, would decrease the incidence of this disease in the adolescent population, as would involvement in drug rehabilitation programs and avoidance of nonsterile needles. Also, sexual abuse of adolescents contributes to AIDS risk.

Prevention of AIDS in the adult population would result in the greatest decrease of this disease in children. In addition, elimination of infected blood and blood products would decrease the likelihood of transmission to children. Blood and blood products are now screened for the antibody HIV, thereby eliminating 95% of infected blood from the market.

Research indicates that hepatitis B vaccine is safe from AIDS virus contamination. An HIV-positive mother should not breastfeed, since transmission via breast milk is supported but not proven.

AIDS include the following:
a. Clean spills of blood or other body fluids with bleach solution (10:1 ratio of water to bleach).
b. Wear rubber gloves when cleaning blood or contacting body fluids.
c. Carefully wash or dispose of all materials that contact the blood or body fluids of AIDS patients.
d. Avoid recapping needles; this practice has been the cause of most accidental needlestick wounds and of contamination with infectious material.

Acute Care

Nursing care is directed to the symptomatic relief of clinical manifestations. The symptoms the child demonstrates vary considerably. The following interventions provide *general guidelines* for care.
1. Protect child from infectious contacts when he or she is immunocompromised.

    a. Screen for infections.
    b. Provide reverse isolation.
    c. Use gloves when handling secretions.
    d. Double bag specimens and linens.
2. Provide age-appropriate, stimulating activities (see Appendix B, *Growth and Development*).
3. Provide emotional support to child and parents during acute care and home care.
    a. Encourage ventilation of feelings.
    b. Encourage family interactions and communications.
    c. Refer to social service and/or psychologist.
    d. Refer to AIDS support group as needed.
4. Support child and family with grieving process.
    a. Encourage ventilation of feelings.
    b. Refer to clergy for spiritual support.
    c. Discuss likelihood of child's death with parents and child.
    d. Encourage family members to discuss with each other, relatives, and friends the likelihood of the child's death.
5. Encourage discussion of feelings related to the stigma of AIDS.
    a. Discuss adolescent's concerns about disclosure of sexual preferences and resultant family and peer reactions.
    b. Discuss public misconceptions associated with AIDS.
6. Provide information about AIDS and its mode of transmission to family, friends, relatives, and community members.
    a. Contact school nurse and discuss child's condition.
    b. Encourage use of support network of family and friends.

BIBLIOGRAPHY

American Academy of Pediatrics: *American Academy of Pediatrics report of the committee of infectious diseases*, Elk Grove Village, 1991, AAP.

Centers for Disease Control: The HIV/AIDS epidemic: the first 10 years, MMWR 40(22), 1991.

Centers for Disease Control: Update: Acquired immunodeficiency syndrome—United States, 1981-1988, *MMWR* 38(14):229-235, 1989.

Cohen D: Similarities between the nursing care needs of children with human immunodeficiency virus infection, *J Pediatr Oncol Nurs* 7(4):149-153, 1990.

Klein RS et al: Oral candidiasis in high risk patients as the initial manifestations of the acquired immunodeficiency syndrome, *N Engl J Med* 311:354, 1984.

Klug R: Children with AIDS, *Am J Nurs* 86(10):1126, 1986.

Pizzo P, Wilfert C: *Pediatric AIDS: the challenge of HIV infection in infants, children, and adolescents,* Baltimore, 1991, Williams & Wilkins.

Rogers M: AIDS in children: a review of the clinical, epidemiologic and public health aspects, *Pediatr Infect Dis* 4(3):230, 1985.

Rogers M: Transmission of human immunodeficiency virus infection in the United States. In Silverman BK, Waddell A, editors: *Report of the surgeon general's workshop on children with HIV infection and their families (April 6-9, 1987),* Rockville, Md, 1987, US Department of Health and Human Services.

Rubenstein A: Acquired immunodeficiency syndrome in infants, *Am J Dis Child* 137:825, 1983.

Scott GB et al: Mothers and infants with acquired immunodeficiency syndrome (AIDS): evidence for both symptomatic and asymptomatic carriers, *JAMA* 253:363, 1985.

Scott G: Natural history of HIV infection in children. In Silverman BK, Waddell A, editors: *Report of the surgeon general's workshop on children with HIV infection and their families (April 6-9, 1987),* Rockville, Md, 1987, US Department of Health and Human Services.

2 ❖ Aplastic Anemia

PATHOPHYSIOLOGY

Aplastic anemia is a disorder of bone marrow failure resulting in the depletion of all marrow elements. The production of blood cells is decreased or lacking. The normal
cellular elements are replaced by fat. Pancytopenia and
hypocellularity of the marrow occur. The manifestation of
symptoms is dependent on the extent of the thrombocytopenia (hemorrhagic symptoms), neutropenia (bacterial
infections, fever), and anemia (pallor, fatigue, congestive
heart failure, and tachycardia). Severe aplastic anemia is
characterized by a granulocyte count less than 500 mm^3, a
platelet count less than 20,000 per mm^3, and a reticulocyte
count of less than 1%. Aplastic anemia can be acquired or
inherited. Acquired forms can be caused by drugs (chloramphenicol), chemicals (benzene), radiation, viral hepatitis,
and, in rare instances, paroxysmal nocturnal hemoglobinuria. Fanconi's anemia is the most common inherited type.
Prognosis is grave. Fifty percent of patients die within the
first 6 months of diagnosis. With more than 70% nonhe-
matopoietic cells, the patient's prognosis is poor.

Incidence

1. May occur at any age.
2. Affects 5000 individuals annually in the United States.

3. Fifty percent of cases are idiopathic.
4. Three-year survival rate with bone marrow transplant (BMT) from histocompatible donors is 50% to 70%.
5. Acquired aplastic anemia's prevalence is one in one million, its male-to-female ratio is 1:1, and it may occur at any age.
6. Fanconi's anemia has been reported in 7200 patients; its male-female ratio is 1.4:1; and its age of onset is 5 to 10 years.

CLINICAL MANIFESTATIONS

1. Petechiae
2. Ecchymosis
3. Epistaxis
4. Signs and symptoms of bacterial infection (depend on site)
5. Occasional fever
6. Pallor
7. Fatigue
8. Tachycardia
9. Congestive heart failure
10. Anemia
11. Bleeding

Fanconi's anemia includes the following: café-au-lait spots, melanin-like hyperpigmentation, and absent thumbs.

COMPLICATIONS

1. Sepsis
2. Sensitization to cross-reacting donor antigens resulting in uncontrollable bleeding
3. Graft vs. host disease (occurs after bone marrow transplantation)
4. Failure of marrow graft (occurs after bone marrow transplantation)
5. Acute myelogenous leukemia (AML) — associated with Fanconi's anemia

LABORATORY/DIAGNOSTIC TESTS

1. Complete blood count (CBC) (macrocyctic anemia)
2. Platelet count (decreases but maintains normal morphology)

3. Reticulocyte count (reticulocytopenia <1%)
4. Sugar water test—to detect paroxysmal nocturnal hemoglobinuria
5. Ham's test—to detect paroxysmal nocturnal hemoglobinuria
6. Serum folate
7. Serum B_{12}
8. Plasma iron (measures marrow erythroid activity)
9. Bone scan—to detect skeletal abnormalities
10. Bone marrow aspiration (BMA) and bone marrow biopsy (hypocellular)
11. Hemoglobin electrophoresis—to assess level of electropoiesis
12. Red cell i antigen titer—to assess level of electropoiesis
13. Acid lysis smear—to assess level of electropoiesis
14. Type and crossmatch—for transfusion treatment
15. Human lymphocyte antigens (HLA) typing—to determine type-specific platelets
16. Blood cultures
17. Immunologic function tests—IgG, IgE, IgA, IgD, and IgM
18. Antibody titers for isohemagglutinin A and B, *Candida*, adenovirus, mumps, measles, influenza A, herpes simplex, cytomegalovirus, typhoid O and H, and antistreptolysin O
19. T cells in peripheral blood
20. Delayed hypersensitivity

MEDICATIONS/TREATMENT

1. BMT is treatment of choice when histocompatible donor available
2. Androgen therapy
3. Immunosuppressive agents
   a. Cyclophosphamide (Cytoxan)—interferes with DNA synthesis and T cell function
   b. Procarbazine—interferes with DNA synthesis and T cell function
4. Antibiotics—used to aggressively treat infection
5. Antithymocyte globulin (ATG)—inactivates T lymphocytes

BLOOD PRODUCTS

1. Packed red blood cells — to maintain hematocrit (Hct) at 30%. For long-term therapy, use deferoxamine as chelating agent to prevent complications of iron overload. Use single donor to decrease number of human lymphocyte antigens (HLA) to which patient is exposed.
2. Platelets — to maintain platelet count > 20,000 mm. Granulocytes — to transfuse patient who has gram-negative sepsis.

NURSING ASSESSMENT

1. Refer to "Hematologic Assessment" in Appendix A.
2. Assess for sites of bleeding and for hemorrhagic symptoms.

NURSING DIAGNOSES

High risk for injury
Altered tissue perfusion
Activity intolerance
High risk for infection
Decreased cardiac output
Fatigue
Altered growth and development
Anxiety

NURSING INTERVENTIONS

1. Monitor for signs and symptoms of hemorrhage.
   a. Vital signs (increased apical pulse, thready pulse, decreased blood pressure)
   b. Bleeding sites
   c. Skin color (pallor) and signs of diaphoresis
   d. Weakness
   e. Level of consciousness
2. Monitor for and protect from infection.
   a. Limit contact with potential source of infection.
   b. Use strict isolation precautions (refer to institution's policies and procedures).
   c. Maintain laminar airflow (refer to institution's policies and procedures).
   d. Monitor for signs of infection.

3. Administer and monitor child's response to infusion of blood products (after bone marrow transplant to avoid sensitization to donor transplantation antigen).
    a. Observe for side effects or untoward response (transfusion reaction).
    b. Observe for signs of fluid overload.
    c. Monitor vital signs 15 minutes before infusion; monitor q15 min during first hour and then q½ hr during infusion.
4. Monitor child's therapeutic and untoward response to medications; monitor the action and side effects of administered medications.
5. Monitor for signs of bone marrow transplant complications (see "Complications").
6. Protect from further trauma.
    a. Do not administer aspirin.
    b. Avoid use of IM injection and suppositories.
    c. Use contraceptive to decrease excessive menstruation.
7. Prepare child and family for bone marrow transplant.
8. Provide age-appropriate diversional and recreational activities (see Appendix B, *Growth and Development*).
9. Provide emotional support to parents.
    a. Encourage ventilation of feelings.
    b. Encourage use of preexisting support systems.
    c. Provide and reinforce information about child's condition and treatment.
    d. Provide physical comforts (e.g., sleeping arrangements and hygiene needs).
10. Provide age-appropriate explanation before procedures.

Home Care

1. Instruct parents to monitor for signs of complications (see "Complications").
2. Instruct parents about the administration of medication.
    a. Monitor child's therapeutic response.
    b. Monitor for untoward responses.
3. Instruct parents about measures to protect child from infection.
    a. Limit contact with infectious contacts.

b. Instruct about signs and symptoms of infection.
c. Advise about appropriate dress for climate changes.
4. Provide child and family with information about community support systems for long-term adaptation.
   a. School reintegration
   b. Parent groups
   c. Children and sibling groups
   d. Financial advice

BIBLIOGRAPHY

Alter B: Bone marrow failure in children, *Pediatr Ann* 8(7):53, 1979.

Antibiotic-associated blood dyscrasias, *Nurses Drug Alert* 13(8): 58-59, 1989.

Bhamb Hani K: Seasonal clustering to transient erythroblastopenia of childhood, *Am J Dis Child* 142(2):175, 1988.

Corcoran-Buchsel P: Long-term complications of allogeneic bone marrow transplantation: nursing implications, *Oncol Nurs Forum* 13(6):61-70, 1986.

Gastearena J et al: Fanconi's anemia: clinical study of six cases, *Am J Pediatr Hematol Oncol* 8(3):173, 1986.

Lipton J, Nathan D: Aplastic and hypoplastic anemia, *Pediatr Clin North Am* 27(2):217, 1980.

Neuwissen H et al: Successful retransplantation of bone marrow following failure of initial engraftment in a patient with aplastic anemia, *J Pediatr* 89(4):58, 1976.

3 ❖ Appendicitis/Appendectomy

PATHOPHYSIOLOGY

Appendicitis is the most common disease that requires surgical intervention during childhood. Appendicitis is the result of inflammation of the vermiform appendix or blind sac at the end of the cecum. It may lead to necrosis and perforation of the appendiceal wall, resulting in peritonitis.

Causes for obstruction of the lumen are many, including hyperplasia of the submucosal lymphoid tissue, fibrotic stenosis caused by inflammation, and appendiceal fecaliths. The prognosis is excellent, especially when surgery is performed before perforation occurs.

INCIDENCE

1. Perforation is associated with age—it occurs more frequently in younger children.
2. Noninflamed appendix is found in 15% of cases.
3. Incidence is slightly greater in males.
4. Incidence is highest in teens and young adults.
5. Occurrence is unusual in children less than 2 years of age and is rare in children less than 1 year old.
6. Appendectomies are performed in four out of 1000 people annually.
7. Prevalence is highest during spring and autumn.

CLINICAL MANIFESTATIONS

1. Pain—cramping located in periumbilical area
2. Abdominal rigidity (boardlike abdomen)

3. Vomiting (common early sign; less common in older children)
4. Nausea
5. Fever — low-grade early in disease; can rise sharply with peritonitis
6. Rebound tenderness
7. Decreased or absent bowel sounds
8. Constipation
9. Anorexia
10. Right lower quadrant tenderness
11. Diarrhea
12. Dysuria
13. Pallor
14. Flushing
15. Tachycardia
16. Irritability
17. Symptoms progress rapidly; may be diagnosed within 4 to 6 hours after initial occurrence of symptoms
18. Infants — irritability; lie with hips flexed to guard abdomen (posturing)
19. Children — pain when walking or flexing legs

COMPLICATIONS (IF NOT DIAGNOSED)

1. Perforation (abdominal distention)
2. Peritonitis

LABORATORY/DIAGNOSTIC TESTS

1. Complete blood count (CBC) — leukocytosis, neutrophilia, absence of eosinophils
2. Urinalysis — pyuria
3. Chest x-ray (preoperative procedure)
4. Abdominal x-ray examination
5. Barium enema — reveals nonfilling of appendix and perineal inflammation

MEDICATIONS

1. Generally no medications are given for pain preoperatively because rebound tenderness and location of pain are important symptoms.
2. Narcotic/analgesic medications are used postoperatively.

NURSING ASSESSMENT

1. Refer to "Gastrointestinal Assessment" in Appendix A.
2. Monitor for rapid progression in severity of symptoms.

NURSING DIAGNOSES

High risk for infection
High risk for fluid volume deficit
Acute pain
Anxiety
Knowledge deficit

NURSING INTERVENTIONS

Preoperative Care

1. Monitor child's status for progression of symptoms and complications.
   a. Shock—decreased blood pressure, decreased respiratory rate, pallor, diaphoresis, rapid thready pulse
   b. Perforation/peritonitis—absent bowel sounds, increased apical pulse, increased temperature, increased respiratory rate, abdominal splinting, diffuse abdominal pain followed by sudden relief from pain
   c. Intestinal obstruction—decreased or absent bowel sounds, abdominal distention, pain, vomiting, no stools
2. Maintain fluid and electrolyte balance.
   a. Monitor infusion of intravenous saline solution at maintenance rate.
   b. Monitor and record output of vomitus, urine, stool, and nasogastric drainage.
3. Provide pain relief and comfort measures.
   a. Position of comfort
   b. Avoidance of unnecessary movements and unnecessary palpation of abdomen
   c. Pain medications if ordered
4. Prepare child physically for surgery.
   a. Give nothing by mouth.
   b. Collect specimens for analysis preoperatively.
   c. Prepare for and support during radiographic tests.
   d. Prepare for and explain use of procedures and treatments (e.g., insertion of nasogastric tube, obtaining vital signs).

5. Prepare parents and child emotionally for surgery to alleviate preoperative stress.
   a. Provide age-appropriate explanations about surgery and surgical procedure.
   b. Provide age-appropriate explanations about postoperative care.

Postoperative Care

1. Assess child's postoperative status.
   a. Auscultate abdomen for peristalsis.
   b. Observe for stools and record if any.
   c. Monitor vital signs; report deviations.
2. Prevent and monitor for abdominal distention.
   a. Provide nothing by mouth.
   b. Maintain patency of nasogastric tube.
   c. Monitor for presence of bowel sounds.
3. Prevent spread of infection.
   a. Monitor child's response to medications.
   b. Perform wound care and appropriate disposal of dressings.
   c. Universal isolation.
4. Monitor for signs of infection.
   a. Monitor vital signs as ordered.
   b. Observe wound for signs of infection—warmth, drainage, pain, swelling, and redness.
   c. Administer antibiotics; monitor child's response.
   d. Monitor IV site.
5. Promote wound healing.
   a. Perform wound care—maintain site, keeping it clean and dry.
      (1) Use Penrose drain.
      (2) Position child in semi-Fowler's position to promote drainage.
   b. Report signs of infection.
   c. Monitor wound response to topical antibiotic, if used.
6. Support child and parents to help them deal with emotional stresses of hospitalization and surgery.
   a. Provide age-appropriate information before procedures.
   b. Encourage use of recreational and diversional activities.

c. Promote contacts and visits with peers.
d. Incorporate child's home routine into daily activities.
7. Assess and provide pain relief measures as needed.
a. Administer analgesics as needed.
b. Use distraction to alleviate pain.
c. Use comfort measures such as massage, positioning.

Home Care

1. Instruct parents about follow-up support and management.
a. Name and phone number of private medical doctor
b. Phone number of clinic
c. Name and phone number of clinical nurse specialist and primary nurse
2. Instruct parents to observe child's response to medications.
3. Instruct parents to observe for and report signs of complications.
a. Infection
b. Obstruction

BIBLIOGRAPHY

Bellet P: *The diagnostic approach to common symptoms and signs in infants, children, and adolescents,* Philadelphia, 1989, Lea & Febiger.
Crain E, Gershel J: *A clinical manual of emergency pediatrics,* East Norwalk, Conn, 1986, Appleton-Century-Crofts.
Edwinson M, Arnbjornsson E, Ekman R: Psychologic preparation program for children undergoing acute appendectomy, *Pediatrics* 82:30-36, 1988.
Elmore J et al: The treatment of complicated appendicitis. What is the gold standard? *Arch Surg* 122(4):424, 1987.
Savrin R et al: Appendiceal rupture: a continuing diagnostic problem, *Pediatrics* 63(1):36, 1979.
Shandling B et al: Perforating appendicitis and antibiotics, *J Pediatr Surg* 9:79, 1974.

4 ❖ Asthma

PATHOPHYSIOLOGY

Asthma is a condition in which widespread narrowing of the bronchi and bronchioles occurs, resulting in airway obstruction and hyperinflation of the lung. An asthma attack may be precipitated by specific allergens (e.g., pollen, mold, animal dander, dust, or food) or other causes such as psychogenic factors, vigorous exercise, weather changes, or respiratory infections. The following anatomic, biochemical, and physiologic alterations occur when an asthma attack occurs:

Spasm of bronchiolar smooth muscle
Edema of bronchiolar mucosa
Increased production of mucus
Increased viscosity of mucus
Increased airway resistance
Hyperactivity of large and small airways
Air trapping, which causes prolonged expiration and less effective ventilatory exchange
Insufficient oxygenation of blood as a result of decreased carbon dioxide and oxygen exchange in alveoli
Air hunger responses, resulting in anxious behavior

INCIDENCE

1. Condition affects 5% to 10% of all children
2. Seventy-five percent of children with asthma have immediate family members with asthma.

3. Asthma accounts for 25% of school absences caused by chronic illness (leading cause of absenteeism).
4. Approximately 8000 deaths per year occur from asthma.
5. Seventy-five percent experience first attack before 4 to 5 years of age.

CLINICAL MANIFESTATIONS

1. Onset of attack may be gradual or acute.
2. Abrupt onset often occurs at night.
   a. Audible wheezing during expiration
   b. Diaphoresis (prominent as attack progresses)
   c. Uncontrollable cough
   d. Anxiety, apprehension, restlessness
3. Asthma includes the following symptoms:
   a. Dyspnea with prolonged expiration
   b. Tenacious mucous secretions
   c. Fine and coarse rales
   d. Nasal flaring
   e. Substernal, suprasternal, and intercostal retractions
   f. Circumoral cyanosis of lips and cyanosis of nailbeds
   g. Increased AP and increased respiratory rate
   h. Abdominal pain
   i. A drop in P_{CO_2} is initially due to hyperventilation; then, P_{CO_2} rises as obstructive process worsens

COMPLICATIONS

1. Status asthmaticus
2. Chronic persistent bronchitis, bronchiolitis, pneumonia
3. Chronic emphysema
4. Cor pulmonale with failure of right side of heart
5. Drug dependency
6. Family dysfunction
7. Side effects from medication
8. Psychosocial problems
9. Atelectasis
10. Pneumothorax
11. Collapsed lung
12. Death

LABORATORY/DIAGNOSTIC TESTS

1. Arterial blood gases: initially—increased pH, decreased partial pressure of oxygen (P_{O_2}), and decreased partial

pressure of carbon dioxide (P_{CO_2}); subsequently—decreased pH, decreased P_{O_2}, and increased P_{CO_2}
2. Increased eosinophil count (in blood, sputum, and nasal discharge)
3. Chest x-ray film (hyperinflation, peribronchial thickening, pulmonary infiltrates, atelectasis)
4. White blood count (increased with infection)
5. Pulmonary function tests (decreased tidal volume, decreased vital capacity, decreased maximal breathing capacity)
6. Skin testing

MEDICATIONS

1. Adrenergics—cause bronchial muscle relaxation; used for temporary relief of bronchospasm and acute asthmatic attacks
   a. Epinephrine (short-acting)—0.01 mg/kg dose subcutaneously of 1:1000 solution, up to six times
   b. Epinephrine hydrochloride (Sus-Phrine)—0.005 ml/kg subcutaneously of 1:200 suspension, q8 to 12 hr; 0.008 ml/kg subcutaneously of 1:400 suspension, q8 to 12 hr
   c. Isoproterenol (Isuprel)—1:400, 1:200, and 1:100 solutions in nebulizer (pressurized mist)
2. Bronchodilators act as a smooth muscle relaxant; used to prevent and relieve symptoms of bronchial asthma
   a. Aminophylline/theophylline preparations—12-30 mg/kg/day to achieve therapeutic levels of 10-20 µg/ml
3. Corticosteroids—modifies immune response, resulting in suppressed hypersensitivity reactions; used to suppress inflammatory process
   a. Prednisone—2 mg/kg during 24-hour period, then reduce to lowest effective maintenance dose po
   b. Solu-Medrol—less than half of adult dose, administered intravenously (IV), and related to severity of condition
   c. Hydrocortisone sodium succinate (Solu-Cortef)—dosage, administered IV, dependent on severity of condition
4. Antibiotics—drug of choice dependent on results of culture

5. Sedation — used to alleviate anxiety as an indirect way to improve respiratory function
6. Antiasthmatic (prophylactic) — inhibits release of bronchoconstrictors (e.g., histamine and slow-reacting substance of anaphylaxis), resulting in suppression of allergic response; used prophylactically as adjunct in management of severe chronic asthma — is not useful during acute asthmatic attack. Cromolyn sodium (for patients 5 years and older) — one capsule inhaled (using specially designed turbo-inhaler) four times per day at regular intervals
7. Expectorants — aid in the expectoration of excessive mucous secretions that occur during acute asthmatic attacks

Adverse Effects

1. Adrenergics — nervousness, anxiety, dizziness, diaphoresis, hypertension, tachycardia, bronchial and pulmonary edema, altered state of perception and thought
2. Bronchodilators — irritability, restlessness, vomiting of blood, convulsions, coma
3. Corticosteroids — extensive number of possible adverse side effects; refer directly to pediatric drug resource
4. Antibiotics — observed side effects dependent on medication administered
5. Cromolyn sodium — generally well tolerated; cough, bronchospasm, wheezing, dry mouth, nausea, vomiting, erythema, urticaria, fever, anemia, joint pain

NURSING ASSESSMENT

Refer to "Respiratory Assessment" in Appendix A.

NURSING DIAGNOSES

Ineffective airway clearance
Impaired gas exchange
Activity intolerance
High risk for fluid volume deficit
Anxiety
Knowledge deficit
Noncompliance

NURSING INTERVENTIONS

Acute Care

1. Monitor respiratory status (including vital signs).
2. Observe and report signs of increased respiratory distress and changes in respiratory status.
3. Monitor child for therapeutic response and untoward effects to medications (see "Adverse Effects").
4. Monitor child's response to oxygen therapy (continuous oxygen therapy/intermittent positive pressure breathing [IPPB]).
   a. Therapeutic response—decreased respiratory rate, less labored breathing, improved color, improved blood gas values, decreased wheezing
   b. Signs of oxygen toxicity—increased P_{CO_2} levels, increased hypoventilation, decreased level of consciousness
5. Assess and monitor child's hydration status.
   a. Monitor intake and output.
   b. Assess for signs of dehydration.
   c. Monitor urine output—volume, frequency, and specific gravity.
   d. Monitor infusion of IV fluids; observe for signs of fluid overload.
6. Promote respiratory function.
   a. Administer aerosol treatment with bronchodilators.
   b. Perform postural drainage and percussion; initially be careful because procedure can aggravate problem.
   c. Elevate head of bed (high-Fowler's position) to promote increased lung expansion.
7. Promote use of age-appropriate diversional play.
8. Alleviate or minimize child's and parents' anxiety during hospitalization.
   a. Provide age-appropriate explanations before procedures.
   b. Encourage use of play therapy.
   c. Explain to parents the rationale or basis for the child's responses to hospitalization.
   d. Encourage use of familiar objects from home (e.g., favorite stuffed animal, blanket).

  e. Provide parents with information to help them deal
     with anxiety about unknowns.
  f. Encourage parents to ventilate concerns.

Home Care

1. Instruct parents about the implementation of environmental control.
   a. Frequent vacuuming and dusting
   b. Removal of pollen
   c. No adoption of cats and dogs
   d. Temperature modulations to avoid extremes
2. Instruct parents and reinforce information about child's
   nutritional needs and special problems.
   a. Refer to nutritionist.
   b. Reinforce nutritionist's plan of care to parents.
   c. Assess parents' and child's abilities to comply with
      medical regimen.
3. Refer to medical doctor or pediatric nurse practitioner
   for hyposensitization.
4. Provide anticipatory guidance.
   a. Use child-rearing practices that avoid labeling child's
      behavior as deviant, a practice that may have a self-
      fulfilling result.
   b. Use "time out" discipline (NOTE: Parents must ac-
      quire additional training to do this).
   c. Encourage interactions with peers.
   d. Encourage growth and development behaviors and
      activities (see Appendix B, *Growth and Development*).

BIBLIOGRAPHY

The American Academy of Allergy and Immunology: Forty-fourth
annual meeting (abstracts), *J Allergy Clin Immunol* 81(1):167, 1988.

Baxmann R et al: Asthma home education self-management program for school-aged children, *J Home Health Care Pract*
1(2):55-62, 1989.

Brim S: A quick guide for home use of inhalant medications, *Pediatr
Nurs* 15(1):87-88, 1989.

Ghory J: The ABC's of educating the patient with chronic bronchial
asthma, *Clin Pediatr* 16(10):879, 1977.

Hill M: Asthmatic child or asthma expert, *Pediatr Nurs* 3(2):25, 1977.

Janson-Bjerklie S: Status asthmaticus, *Am J Nurs* 90(9):53-55, 1990.

Leeks H: Appraisals of cromolyn sodium and corticosteroids in the treatment of asthmatic children, *Clin Pediatr* 16(10):861, 1977.

Murray A et al: Passive smoking and the seasonal difference of severity of asthma in children, *Chest* 94(4):701-708, 1988.

Psychological effects of theophylline in children, *Nurses Drug Alert* 13(7):51, 1990.

Rew L: Children with asthma: the relationship between illness behaviors and health locus of control, *West J Nurs Res* 9(4):465, 1987.

Silver R, Ginsburg C: Early prediction of the need for hospitalization in children with acute asthma, *Clin Pediatr* 23(2):81, 1984.

Zahr L et al: Assessment and management of the child with asthma, *Pediatr Nurs* 15(2):109-114, 1989.

Zimo D et al: The efficacy and safety of home nebulizer therapy for children with asthma, *Am J Dis Child* 143(2):208-211, 1989.

5 ❖ Botulism (Infant)

PATHOPHYSIOLOGY

Botulism in infants is a systemic infectious disease caused by *Clostridium botulinum.* Toxins are produced in the infant's intestinal tract after the ingestion of spores from honey, soil, or house dust. A wide spectrum of symptoms are manifested, ranging from fulminating to mild disease. Characteristically, the infant exhibits a descending pattern of flaccid paralysis that is preceded by constipation. In severe cases, both respiratory failure that requires mechanical ventilation and loss of neurologic function that progresses to hypotonia may ensue.

INCIDENCE

1. Highest incidence occurs in western and middle-Atlantic states.
2. Unusually high incidence rate occurs in Pennsylvania, Utah, and Arizona.
3. Type A botulism occurs predominantly in the West.
4. Type B botulism occurs predominantly in the East.
5. High rate occurs in high socioeconomic status groups.
6. High rate is associated with infants who have been fed honey.
7. Actual incidence is unknown.

CLINICAL MANIFESTATIONS
(INCUBATION 12-36 HOURS)

1. Nausea and vomiting
2. Progressive hypotonia ("floppy infant")
3. Weak cry
4. Decreased sucking, difficulty feeding
5. Drooling
6. Absent gag reflex
7. Weakened or absent deep-tendon reflexes
8. Decreased facial movements
9. Pronounced head lag (no head control)
10. Bilateral ptosis
11. Urinary retention
12. Irritability, listlessness
13. Described by parent as "not being himself"
14. Lethargy
15. Collection of food and secretions in posterior pharynx
16. Green, foul-smelling stool

COMPLICATIONS

1. Nosocomial infection
2. Respiratory insufficiency or aspiration
3. Upper airway obstruction or suffocation
4. Tension pneumothorax
5. Respiratory arrest

LABORATORY/DIAGNOSTIC TESTS

1. Complete blood count (CBC)
2. Urine toxicology (diagnostic)
3. Stool specimen
4. Type A or Type B toxin
5. Electromyography (less than normal value — brief duration, small amplitude, overly abundant motor-unit action)

MEDICATIONS

1. Antibiotics
2. Curare (used during mechanical ventilation)
3. Stool softener (used during recovery period until normal bowel action returns)

NURSING ASSESSMENT

1. Refer to "Neurologic Assessment" in Appendix A.
2. Document extent and presence of muscle weakness.

NURSING DIAGNOSES

Ineffective airway clearance
Ineffective breathing pattern
Altered nutrition: less than body requirements
Anxiety
Knowledge deficit

NURSING INTERVENTIONS

1. Monitor child's clinical status.
   a. Progression of neuromuscular weakness
   b. Absence of gag reflex or sucking reflex
   c. Bowel motility
   d. Level of activity
   e. Respiratory insufficiency/failure
2. Prevent pulmonary complications (infection or atelectasis).
   a. Perform pulmonary toilet.
   b. Monitor for signs of infection (increased temperature, congestion, increased respiratory rate, increased apical pulse).
3. Provide ventilator care to promote maximal therapeutic outcomes.
4. Maintain adequate nutritional intake and fluid intake.
   a. Assess infant's need to feed.
   b. Gavage feed as needed.
   c. Monitor IV infusion.
   d. Assess hydration status.
5. Monitor child's untoward and therapeutic response to medications—may exacerbate growth of *C. botulinum* in intestine.
6. Provide emotional support to parents during infant's hospitalization.
   a. Encourage ventilation of feelings (guilt, helplessness, blame).
   b. Provide information before procedures.
   c. Reinforce information given about disease and treatment.

d. Encourage parents' use of social supports.
7. Promote sense of trust and security during hospitalization.
   a. Primary nursing
   b. Rooming-in
   c. Infant stimulation

Home Care and Discharge Planning

1. Assess parents' ability to comply with treatment regimen.
2. Instruct parents about administration of medications and monitoring for therapeutic and untoward effects.
3. Instruct parents about identifying symptoms that indicate a worsening condition.
4. Instruct not to push feedings because infant tires easily until full strength is regained.
5. Instruct about careful diaper disposal and hand washing.
6. Instruct not to use honey or corn syrup.

BIBLIOGRAPHY

Binder H, Bidell A, Dykstra D, Easton J, Matthews D, Molnar G, Noll S, Perrin J: Pediatric rehabilitation: disorders of the motor unit, part 4, *Archives of Medicine Rehabilitation — Supplement* 70(5-5): Study Guide Issue: S175-178, 1989.

Carriere B, Broski L: Infant botulism: diagnosis and treatment, *Clin Manag Physic Therapy* 9(1):20-23, 1989.

Hatheway C et al: Examination of feces and serum for diagnosis of infant botulism in 336 patients, *J Clin Microbiol* 25(12):2334, 1987.

Kunkel D: Botulism: an old new tale in two chapters: clinical aspects, part 2, *Emerg Med* 18(3):205, 1986.

Lancaster M: Botulism: north to Alaska, *Am J Nurs* 90(1):60-62, 1990.

L'Hommedieu C, Polin R: Progression of clinical signs in severe infant botulism, *Clin Pediatr* 20(2):90, 1981.

Morris J et al: Infant botulism in the United States: an epidemiologic study of cases occurring outside of California, *Am J Public Health* 73(17):1385, 1983.

Pickett J et al: Syndrome of botulism in infancy: clinical and electrophysiologic study, *N Engl J Med* 295(14):770, 1976.

Turick-Gibson T: Infant botulism, *Pediatr Nurs* 14(4):280-283, 347, 1988.

Wilkinson W, Close E: Infant botulism: a dilemma for nursing, *J Pediatr Nurs* 3(3):164, 1988.

6 ❖ Bronchiolitis

PATHOPHYSIOLOGY

Bronchiolitis is a respiratory viral illness characterized by inflammation of the smaller bronchioles. Edema of the mucous membranes lining the walls of the bronchioles plus cellular infiltrates result in obstruction. The obstruction causes hyperinflation of the affected areas as expired air is trapped distally, causing hypoxemia. The obstructions do not occur uniformly throughout the lung. Symptoms are more severe in infants because the diameter of their bronchiole lumina is smaller. The infection is most commonly caused by the respiratory syncytial virus (RSV). Other causative agents include adenovirus, parainfluenza, and rhinovirus. RSV is transmitted by way of droplets. Prognosis is generally good.

INCIDENCE

1. Bronchiolitis is one of the most frequent reasons for hospitalization of infants less than 1 year old.
2. Its mortality is 1% to 7%, occurring most often in infants 1 to 12 months old (peak age at 6 months); the rate is higher if RSV is present.
3. Occurs most frequently in winter and early spring.

CLINICAL MANIFESTATIONS

1. Upper respiratory infection for 1 to 4 days; then acute phase for 2 to 3 days; resolves in 7 to 14 days

2. Labored respirations (rapid and shallow with nasal flaring and retractions)
3. Expiratory wheezing of acute onset
4. Anorexia or difficult to feed
5. Coryza, otitis media
6. Hacky, harsh paroxysmal cough
7. Cyanosis
8. Audible and palpable rhonchi
9. Temperature range: normal to as high as 41° C
10. Malaise
11. Increased mucus production
12. Irritability
13. Tachycardia (greater than 60/min)

COMPLICATIONS

1. Atelectasis
2. Apnea
3. Hypoxemia
4. Lobar collapse (cause unknown but may be related to hypoxia and obstruction)

LABORATORY/DIAGNOSTIC TESTS

1. Chest x-ray (hyperinflation with air trapping, atelectasis, slight perihilar infiltrate) — widely varied diagnostic criteria
2. Immunoassay — used to diagnose RSV

MEDICATIONS

1. Acetaminophen (Tylenol) — used for antipyretic effect
2. Expectorants (potassium iodide [SSKI]) — used to bring up or remove secretions
3. Chloral hydrate — to alleviate anxiety if necessary (avoid sedatives that depress respiration)
4. Bronchodilators — used with nebulization depending on severity
5. Ribavirin — antiviral agent used against respiratory syncytial virus (RSV)

NURSING ASSESSMENT

Refer to "Respiratory Assessment" in Appendix A.

NURSING DIAGNOSES

Ineffective airway clearance
Activity intolerance
Altered nutrition: less than body requirements
Anxiety
Knowledge deficit

NURSING INTERVENTIONS

1. Monitor respiratory status (including vital signs).
   a. Monitor vital signs initially q2 hr until stable, then q4 hr.
   b. Observe frequently for and report signs of increased respiratory distress and changes in respiratory status.
   c. Apnea monitoring may be indicated in acute phase.
2. Monitor child's response to oxygen therapy and humidified oxygen through hood, tent, or nasal catheter.
   a. Therapeutic response—improving respiratory status
   b. Signs of oxygen toxicity—increase in P_{CO_2} levels, increase in hypoventilation, decrease in level of consciousness
   c. Monitor oxygen status with noninvasive method.
3. Promote respiratory function.
   a. Raise head of bed to semi- or high-Fowler's position; use infant seat, neck extended.
   b. Perform pulmonary toilet—postural drainage and percussion, suctioning, and intermittent positive pressure breathing (IPPB).
4. Monitor hydration status.
   a. Monitor intake and output and urine specific gravity.
   b. Assess for signs of dehydration or fluid overload.
   c. Monitor urine output—volume, frequency, and specific gravity.
5. Monitor child for untoward therapeutic response to medications.
   a. Acetaminophen
   b. Potassium iodide
   c. Bronchodilators (e.g., epinephrine)
6. Encourage intake of diet high in calories and protein.
   a. Serve favorite foods if possible.
   b. Arrange food attractively on tray.

c. Encourage use of routine feeding practices (e.g., usual mealtimes, presence of parents, or favorite cup).
7. Encourage age-appropriate quiet play (see Appendix B, *Growth and Development*).
8. Alleviate or minimize the child's and parents' anxiety during hospitalization.
   a. Provide age-appropriate explanations before procedures.
   b. Encourage use of play therapy.
   c. Provide explanations to parents about rationale or basis for the child's responses to hospitalization.
   d. Encourage use of familiar objects from home (e.g., favorite stuffed animal).
   e. Encourage parents to ventilate concerns.
9. Provide consistent nursing care to promote trust and to alleviate anxiety.

Critical Care Management

1. Mechanical ventilation may be necessary at beginning of illness.
   a. Pressure limited ventilator (positive end-expiratory pressure [PEEP])
   b. Slow ventilator rate and long expiratory interval — to allow adequate time for expiration
2. Administer intravenous (IV) therapy.
   a. Maintain fluid and electrolyte balance.
   b. Provide route for administration of medications.

Home Care

Instruct parents about the following for home care of the child:
1. Use of humidifiers (may use moisture from hot shower) — cold vs. warm mists
2. Rationale for treatments (medication administration)
3. Signs of secondary infection
4. Infection control and prevention measures

BIBLIOGRAPHY

Guerra I, Kemp J, Shearer W: Bronchiolitis. In Oski F et al, eds: *Principles and practice of pediatrics*, Philadelphia, 1990, JB Lippincott.

Hartsell M: Chest physiotherapy and mechanical vibration, *J Pediatr Nurs* 2(2):135, 1987.

Lepon M, Hethington S: Respiratory tract infections. In Green M, Haggerty R: *Ambulatory pediatrics,* Philadelphia, 1990, WB Saunders.

Nelson D: Bronchitis and bronchiolitis. In Gillis S, Kagan E: *Current pediatric therapy,* Philadelphia, 1990, WB Saunders.

Wagener S: Respiratory distress: exploring the causes in young children, *Consultant* 26(1):23, 1986.

7 ❖ Bronchopulmonary Dysplasia

PATHOPHYSIOLOGY

Bronchopulmonary dysplasia (respiratory lung syndrome) is a significant complication that results from providing extended mechanical ventilation to neonates. It is a form of chronic lung disease that affects the lung parenchyma and airways (long-term survivors have a near-normal resolution of pulmonary function within 1 to 3 years). The disease is characterized by hypoxia, hypercapnia, oxygen dependence, abnormal chest x-ray results, and abnormal chest physical examination.

Factors contributing to bronchopulmonary dysplasia are (1) prolonged exposure to an elevated inspired oxygen concentration, (2) endotracheal intubation and mechanical ventilation, (3) severity of underlying primary lung disease, (4) patent ductus arteriosus, (5) degree of prematurity, (6) intraventricular and subarachnoid hemorrhage, (7) disseminated intravascular coagulation, (8) necrotizing enterocolitis, and (9) prolonged use of fluid therapy. Bronchopulmonary dysplasia has been characterized by the following progressive stages:

Stage I—respiratory distress (tachypnea, grunting, retractions, and cyanosis), abnormal chest x-ray results, and atelectasis; ventilation is required.

Stage IIa — improving respiratory status; is weaned from ventilator.

Stage IIb — respiration worsens; increasingly difficult to ventilate; increased oxygen required; pulmonary interstitial emphysema; "whiteout" visible on chest x-ray film, pneumonia is present.

Stage III — stabilizing, slowly improving respiratory status.

Stage IV (chronic or improving) — scattered areas of atelectasis with hyperexpansion; amount of healing tissue greater than necrotic or damaged tissue.

Stage V (terminal) — progressive respiratory failure; failure of right side of heart, fluid retention; pulmonary hypertension.

The effects of increased inspired concentrations of oxygen are as follows: (1) edema of the intravascular spaces with vascular engorgement; (2) atelectasis, causing decreased lung compliance; (3) increased airway resistance with air trapping; (4) epithelial necrosis and hemorrhage; and (5) formation of hyaline membrane.

INCIDENCE

1. No sex difference is evident in incidence.
2. Males have greater risk of dying than females.
3. Higher incidence is associated with a second-born twin.
4. Increased incidence is associated with diabetic mothers.
5. The disease affects 5% to 30% of preterm infants who have respiratory distress syndrome.
6. Mortality is 25% to 39% during first 6 months of initial hospitalization (infants with severe hyaline membrane disease and birth weight less than 1000 g).

CLINICAL MANIFESTATIONS

1. Recurrent ventilator dependency
2. Increased oxygen dependency
3. Tachypnea
4. Retractions
5. Crepitus
6. Wheezing during bronchopneumonia
7. Cyanosis
8. Hypoxic during feedings

9. Poor feeder
10. Decreased weight gain
11. Hypotonia or hypertonia
12. Asymmetry of movement

COMPLICATIONS

1. Failure of right side of heart (cor pulmonale)
2. Pulmonary failure
3. Bronchiolitis
4. Atelectasis
5. Sepsis
6. Central nervous system hemorrhage
7. Pulmonary hypertension
8. Fractures (decreased calcium and decreased vitamin D as a result of effects of chronic furosemide [Lasix] administration)

Long-Term Signs and Symptoms

1. Recurrent wheezing
2. Recurrent respiratory infections
3. Respiratory rate of 60 to 80/min
4. Retractions
5. Bilateral rales
6. Need for continuous supplemental oxygen
7. Barrel chest
8. Cardiomegaly, hepatomegaly, bounding pulses
9. Increased hospitalizations for pulmonary disorders (pneumonia, bronchiolitis, bronchitis)
10. Chronic hypoxemia
11. Chest x-ray results lag several weeks to months behind clinical status
12. Most severe pulmonary symptoms persisting for 1 year
13. Normal clinical findings by second or third year
14. Delayed motor development
15. Increased exercise tolerance
16. Increased weight gain
17. Growth retardation (5th to 25th percentile)

LABORATORY/DIAGNOSTIC TESTS

1. White blood count (WBC) and tracheal specimens for culture and sensitivities

2. Arterial blood gas values and venous blood gas values
3. Pulmonary function tests (decreased inflating pressures and prolonged inspiratory/expiratory ratio)
4. Serial ECG to document right-axis deviation and right-ventricular hypertrophy and to monitor right-ventricular failure
5. Electrolytes (increased bicarbonate with chronic respiratory failure)
6. Chest x-ray examination
   a. Initial (first 24 hours) — no findings documented
   b. 5 to 8 days — streaky bilateral infiltrates around perihilar region
   c. 8 to 15 days — coarser bilateral infiltrates
   d. 15 to 18 days — focal areas of hyperaeration; cystic changes prominent at base of lungs
   e. Long-term results — interstitial emphysema (unilateral or bilateral) with coarse interstitial markings; "whiteout" of lungs; signs of patent ductus arteriosus, with increased left-to-right shunt

MEDICATIONS

1. Digitalis — used if right-ventricular failure or pulmonary hypertension is present
2. Diuretics (furosemide [Lasix])
3. Bronchodilators (aminophylline) — decrease obstruction and increase ventilation
4. Corticosteroids — to increase pulmonary function (controversial)
5. Antibiotics — to treat infections; use of antibiotic dependent on culture and sensitivity
6. Surfactant replacement therapy — increases lung compliance
7. Antioxidants (vitamin E and acetylcysteine) to reduce oxygen toxicity
8. Pancuronium — to sedate infant and to provide improved oxygenation while on a ventilator
9. Routine immunizations (refer to Appendix C, *Immunizations*)

NURSING ASSESSMENT

Refer to "Respiratory Assessment" in Appendix A.

NURSING DIAGNOSES

Impaired gas exchange
Decreased cardiac output
Activity intolerance
Fluid volume excess
Altered family processes
Knowledge deficit

NURSING INTERVENTIONS

1. Observe and monitor respiratory status for changes or distress.
2. Observe and monitor patient's response to mechanical ventilation.
3. Administer and monitor patient response (respiratory status) after postural drainage, percussion, and suctioning.
4. Position in semi-Fowler's position to increase chest expansion.
5. Monitor action and side effects of medications.
6. Promote adequate caloric balance through nasojejunal feedings and peripheral hyperalimentation.
7. Monitor intake and output; maintain urine output at 40 to 100 cc/kg/day.
8. Monitor hydration status (fluid restriction and diuretics to prevent overload).
9. Monitor patient response to administered blood products (hemoglobin [Hb] 13 g and higher).
10. Provide developmentally appropriate visual, auditory, tactile stimulation.
11. Promote infant-parent bonding.
12. Evaluate client and family's readiness for discharge.
    a. Adequacy of feeding behaviors
    b. Frequency of feedings
    c. Medications required
    d. Requirements for percussion and suction
    e. Percent oxygen required (transcutaneous oxygenation at 55 torr or oxygen at no more than 1 L/min through a cannula)
    f. Social support at home
    g. Environmental control measures (no smoking)
    h. Need for monitoring respiratory distress

Home Care

1. Instruct parents about the following:
   a. Monitoring signs of respiratory distress
   b. Maintaining continuous administration of supplemental oxygen
   c. Performing suctioning, postural drainage, and percussion
   d. Administering and monitoring the effects of medications
   e. Performing dietary management (120 cal/kg to maintain growth)
2. Facilitate compliance with long-term management (through chest x-ray examination every 2 months and monitoring pulmonary function).
3. Refer to ongoing support network.

BIBLIOGRAPHY

Berry D: Neonatology in the 1990's: surfactant replacement therapy becomes a reality, *Clin Pediatr* 30(3): 167, 1991.

Edwards D: Radiographic aspects of bronchopulmonary dysplasia, *J Pediatr* 95(5):823, 1979.

Fox W: Bronchopulmonary dysplasia (respiratory lung syndrome): clinical course and outpatient therapy, *Pediatr Ann* 7(1):75, 1978.

Jackson D: Nursing care plan: home management of children with BPD, *Pediatr Nurs* 12:342, 1986.

Koops B, Abman S, Accurso F: Outpatient management and follow-up of bronchopulmonary dysplasia, *Clin Perinatol* 11(1): 101, 1984.

Lund C, editor: *Bronchopulmonary dysplasia: strategies for total patient care*, Petaluma, Calif, 1990, Neonatal Network Publishing.

Phelan P, Landau L, Olinsky A: *Respiratory illness in children*, Oxford, 1982, Blackwell Scientific Publications, Ltd.

Pridham K et al: Parental issues in feeding young children with bronchopulmonary dysplasia, *J Pediatr Nurs* 4(3):177, 1989.

Sauve R, Singhal N: Long term morbidity of infants with bronchopulmonary dysplasia, *Pediatrics* 76:725, 1985.

8 ❖ Burns

PATHOPHYSIOLOGY

Burns refer to the tissue damage that results from contact with thermal, chemical, radioactive, or electrical agents. The severity of the burn is assessed by determining (1) the type of burn (flame, liquid, chemical, electrical, or radiation); (2) the duration of contact, which affects the depth of burn injury (first, second, or third degree); (3) the areas affected, including both the body surface and the location (vital anatomic areas); (4) related injuries; and (5) any pre-existing illness or condition. See the box on p. 44 and Figure 1 for further descriptions of burn severity. The types of burns usually sustained during childhood and adolescence are age-related. The predominant types of burns that are sustained from 0 to 2 years of age, in descending order, are scald, contact, chemical, and flame. For children ages 3 to 8 years, flame and scald burns predominate. From 9 to 12 years of age, children are most commonly burned by thermal agents. Flame and chemical burns are the most commonly occurring burns in 13 to 19 year olds. Prognosis is dependent on the severity of the burn that is sustained.

Hospitalization is indicated for individuals with burns on approximately 10% of body surface.

INCIDENCE

1. Burns are the second leading cause of accidental injury and death in children under 14 years of age.
2. More than 50% of burns occur in children 5 years old and younger.
3. Burns caused by thermal agents are the most common.

CLINICAL MANIFESTATIONS (INITIAL) FOR MODERATE-TO-SEVERE BURN

1. Tachycardia
2. Decreased blood pressure
3. Cold extremities
4. Change in level of consciousness
5. Dehydration (decreased skin turgor, decreased urinary output, dry tongue and skin)
6. Increased rate of respirations
7. Pale (not present with second- and third-degree burn)

COMPLICATIONS

1. Renal failure
2. Metabolic acidosis

Burn Classification According to Depth

First Degree (Partial Thickness)

Superficial; involves only superficial epidermis. Symptoms — pain, redness, no tissue or nerve damage (e.g., sunburn).

Second Degree (Partial Thickness)

Superficial to deep dermal; involves entire epidermis and varying amounts of dermis. Symptoms — pain, red edematous skin, vesicles (e.g., scald).

Third Degree (Full Thickness)

Epidermis and dermis destroyed; involves subcutaneous adipose tissue, fascia, muscle, and bone. Symptoms — no pain, white, red, or black skin, edematous (e.g., fire).

3. Hyperkalemia
4. Hypokalemia
5. Hyponatremia
6. Hypocalcemia
7. Pulmonary problems
   a. Pulmonary edema
   b. Pulmonary insufficiency
   c. Pulmonary embolus
   d. Bacterial pneumonia
8. Wound sepsis
9. Curling's ulcer

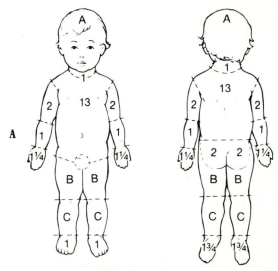

RELATIVE PERCENTAGES OF AREAS AFFECTED BY GROWTH

AREA	BIRTH	AGE 1 YR	AGE 5 YR
A = ½ of head	9½	8½	6½
B = ½ of one thigh	2¾	3¼	4
C = ½ of one leg	2½	2½	2¾

Figure 1. Estimated distribution of burns in children. **A,** Children from birth to age 5 years.

Continued.

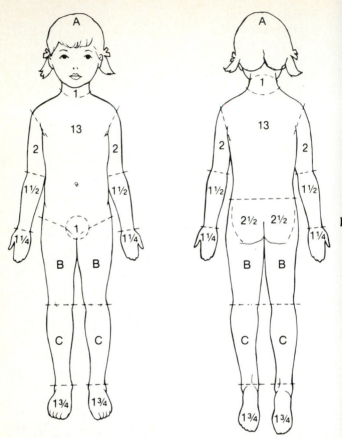

RELATIVE PERCENTAGES OF AREAS AFFECTED BY GROWTH

AREA	AGE 10 YR	AGE 15 YR	ADULT
A = ½ of head	5½	4½	3½
B = ½ of one thigh	4½	4½	4¾
C = ½ of one leg	3	3¼	3½

Figure 1, cont'd. B, Older children. From Whaley LF and Wong DL: *Nursing care of infants and children*, ed 4, St Louis, 1991, Mosby–Year Book.

10. Encephalopathy
11. Hypertension

MEDICAL TREATMENT FOR BURNS

1. Open method—burn is exposed to air. Topical medication that is applied includes the following:
   a. Mafenide cream (Sulfamylon Cream)
   b. Silver sulfadiazine (Silvadene)
   c. Neosporin ointment
2. Closed method—burn is covered with topical medication (e.g., mafenide cream or silver sulfadiazine) and fine mesh gauze; also includes biologic dressings
3. Surgery
   a. Excision of burned tissue
   b. Debridement of wound; hydrotherapy
   c. Grafting
   d. Cosmetic surgery

LABORATORY/DIAGNOSTIC TESTS

1. Complete blood count (CBC)—decreased
2. Arterial blood gas values—metabolic acidosis (decreased pH, increased partial pressure of carbon dioxide [P_{CO_2}], and decreased partial pressure of oxygen [P_{O_2}])
3. Blood urea nitrogen (BUN)—increased because of tissue breakdown and oliguria
4. Serum glucose—increased because of stress-invoked glycogen breakdown or glyconeogenesis
5. Hematocrit (Hct)—decreased
6. Serum electrolytes—decreased because of loss to traumatized areas and interstitial spaces
7. Creatinine—increased because of tissue breakdown and oliguria
8. Serum protein levels—decreased because of protein breakdown for massive energy needs
9. Hemoglobin (Hb)—decreased because of loss of red blood cells (RBCs) and bleeding

NURSING ASSESSMENT

1. Observe and monitor for signs and symptoms of the following:
   a. Shock

   b. Dehydration
   c. Electrolyte imbalances (see box below)
   d. Respiratory distress
2. Assess extent and depth of burns.
3. Assess for presence of pain.
4. Determine cause of burn (accidental or result of abuse).
5. Determine type of burn (scald, flame, chemical, or electrical).

NURSING DIAGNOSES

Ineffective airway clearance
Fluid volume deficit

Electrolyte Imbalances

Hyperkalemia

    Oliguria or anuria
    Diarrhea
    Muscle weakness
    Arrhythmias
    Intestinal colic

Hypokalemia

    Muscle cramping
    Muscle weakness
    Arrhythmias
    Respiratory arrest or apnea

Hyponatremia

    Apprehension
    Abdominal cramps
    Fear of impending doom
    Diarrhea

Hypocalcemia

    Tingling in fingers
    Muscle cramps
    Tetany
    Convulsions

High risk for infection
Impaired skin integrity
High risk for injury
Altered nutrition: less than body requirements
High risk for disuse syndrome
Anxiety
Altered growth and development
Altered family processes

NURSING INTERVENTIONS
First Aid/Emergency Care
Prevent further injury.
1. Scald burn—douse with water; remove clothing.
2. Flame burn—drop and roll to extinguish; douse with cool liquid; remove nonadherent clothing.
3. Chemical burn—flush eyes and skin for 20 minutes with water.
4. Electrical burn—turn off power sources; initiate cardio-pulmonary resuscitation.

Hospitalization
1. Maintain patent airway
   a. Monitor and report signs of respiratory distress (dyspnea, increased respiratory rate, air hunger, nasal flaring).
   b. Perform pulmonary toilet.
   c. Monitor use of respirator and oxygen as ordered.
   d. Provide tracheostomy care as ordered.
2. Monitor child for signs and symptoms of hypovolemic shock.
   a. Monitor vital signs q1 hr or more frequently until stable.
   b. Monitor input and output q1 hr (output—20 to 30 ml/hr >2 years; 10 to 20 ml/hr <2 years).
3. Monitor child for signs and symptoms of electrolyte imbalances (see box on p. 48).
4. Monitor child for signs and symptoms of hemorrhage.
   a. Vital signs (q1 hr or more frequently when first admitted [during critical period], then q2 hr until stable, then q4 hr)
   b. Bleeding

    c. Decreased blood pressure

    d. Decreased temperature

    e. Rapid, thready pulse

5. Provide pain relief measures to alleviate or control child's pain.

    a. Use comfort measures (pillow, bed, cradle).

    b. Position for comfort.

    c. Use distraction, guided imagery, hypnosis.

    d. Monitor child's therapeutic response to medications.

6. Protect child from potential infections.

    a. Administer tetanus booster as ordered.

    b. Monitor child's therapeutic and untoward response to antibiotics.

    c. Maintain and monitor use of reverse isolation.

    d. Use sterile technique during wound care.

    e. Monitor for wound infections (offensive odor, redness at site, increased temperature, warmth, purulent drainage).

7. Promote adequate nutritional intake to counteract nitrogen loss and potential gastrointestinal complications.

    a. Provide diet high in calories and protein (total caloric requirement equals 60 calories times weight in kilograms plus calories times percent of burn).

    b. Monitor for signs of Curling's ulcer (decreased hemoglobin, decreased red blood count [anemia], coffee-ground emesis, abdominal distention).

    c. Administer antacids as needed.

    d. Monitor bowel sounds for ileus.

8. Promote optimal healing of wounds (see "Medical Treatment").

    a. Use sterile technique when dressing wound.

    b. Observe for cellulitus or area that is trapping pus.

9. Promote maximal function of joints.

    a. Use splints appropriately to prevent contractures.

    b. Check splints q4 hr for pressure sores.

    c. Perform range of motion exercises and passive range of motion exercises for extremities.

    d. Encourage ambulation when patient is able.

    e. Encourage participation in self-care activities.

10. Encourage verbalization of feelings regarding altered body image.

    a. Depression (associated with injury and pain)

    b. Anxiety (associated with treatments)

    c. Shame (associated with appearance)

11. Provide for child's developmental needs during hospitalization.

    a. Encourage use of age-appropriate toys (see Appendix B, *Growth and Development*); modify according to child's condition (e.g., use passive coloring—child directs nurse in coloring pictures).

    b. Encourage contact with peers (as appropriate).

    c. Provide age-appropriate roommate as dictated by condition.

    d. Encourage academic pursuits.

12. Provide emotional support to family.

    a. Encourage ventilation of concerns.

    b. Refer to social service as necessary.

    c. Refer to other appropriate parents in comparable situation.

    d. Provide for physical comforts (e.g., place to sleep and bathe).

    e. Refer to support group (e.g., parent, religious) as needed.

BIBLIOGRAPHY

Artz C, Moucrief J, Pruitt J: *Burns: a team approach,* Philadelphia, 1979, WB Saunders.

Baker M, Chiaviello C: Household electrical injuries in children, *Am J Dis Child* 143:59-62, 1989.

Cockington R: Ambulatory management of burns in children, *Burns* 15:271-273, 1989.

Mikhail J: Acute burn care: an update, *J Emerg Nurs* 14(1):9-18, 1988.

Poteet G et al: Care of the burned patient with herpes simplex, *J Pediatr Nurs* 1(6):376, 1986.

Rollens J: Danger—children and lighters, *Pediatr Nurs* 14(1):64, 1988.

Sato R: Burns. In Levin D, ed: *A practical guide to pediatric intensive care,* St. Louis, 1984, Mosby–Year Book.

Slater S et al: Burned children: a socioeconomic profile for focused prevention programs, *J Burn Care Rehab* 8(6):566, 1987.

Surveyer J, Halpern J: Age and related burn injuries and their prevention, *Pediatrics* 65:29, Sept/Oct 1981.

Sutherland S: Burned adolescents' descriptions of their coping strategies, *Heart Lung* 17(2):150, 1988.

9 ❖ Cellulitis

PATHOPHYSIOLOGY

Cellulitis is an infection that affects the skin and subcutaneous tissue. Sites of involvement may include the scalp, head, and neck (particularly the cheek and periorbital region [see box on p. 53]), the extremities, and the cervical lymph glands. In many instances, a nonspecific upper respiratory infection precedes the onset of cellulitis. Organisms causing cellulitis include *Haemophilus influenzae* type b, *Streptococcus pneumoniae*, group A beta-hemolytic streptococci, *Staphylococcus aureus*, and *Escherichia coli*. The site of infection is characterized by a swelling with indistinct margins that are tender and warm. Infection may extend systemically with the following symptoms and signs: a red streak along the lymphatic drainage path, enlarged lymph nodes, malaise, and elevated temperature. Outcome is excellent with treatment.

INCIDENCE

1. Five percent to 14% of cellulitis in children is caused by *H. influenzae* type b.
2. Over 85% of children with *H. influenzae* type b cellulitis are under 2 years of age.

CLINICAL MANIFESTATIONS

Local Reaction

1. Indistinct margins
2. Usually red, warm, and painful
3. Warm
4. Indurated
5. Febrile

For orbital and periorbital reactions, see box.

Systemic Reaction

1. Red streak along lymphatic drainage path
2. Malaise
3. Elevated temperature
4. Enlarged and painful lymph glands

COMPLICATIONS

1. Loss of visual acuity (periorbital cellulitis)
2. Systemic involvement

Orbital/Periorbital Symptoms

Orbital Cellulitis

Infection easily spreads from sinuses because orbit shares common wall with ethmoid, maxillary, and frontal sinuses (caused by group A streptococci, *S. aureus*, and *E. coli*).

Symptoms: exophthalmos, ophthalmoplegia, and loss of visual acuity.

Periorbital Cellulitis

Caused by infection (varicella), trauma, or insect bite.

Symptoms: rapid onset of fever and swelling; area is warm, indurated, and tender.

Idiopathic Periorbital Cellulitis

Caused by *H. influenzae* type b and *S. pneumoniae*.

Symptoms: preceded 1 to 5 days by mild upper respiratory infection; rapid onset of fever and swelling.

---

3. Meningitis
4. Arthritis
5. Potential for brain abscess and periorbital cellulitis

LABORATORY/DIAGNOSTIC TESTS

1. Blood cultures (positive)
2. Tissue aspirate culture (positive)
3. Sinus radiographs (opacification of sinuses)
4. Computerized tomographic scan of orbit and paranasal sinus

MEDICATIONS

1. Antibiotics—used to treat infection
2. Acetaminophen as antipyretic or analgesic
   <1 year—60 mg by mouth (po) as needed
   1 to 3 years—60-120 mg po or per rectum
   3 to 6 years—120 mg (not to exceed 480 mg/day)
   6 to 12 years—150-325 mg (not to exceed 1.2 g/day)

NURSING ASSESSMENT

Assess for local and systemic reactions.

NURSING DIAGNOSES

Impaired tissue integrity
High risk for fluid volume deficit
Pain
Impaired physical mobility

NURSING INTERVENTIONS

1. Assess skin locally for changes, minimize palpation because of pain
2. Prevent and monitor for further signs of infection.
   a. Assess for systemic reactions.
   b. Immobilize affected extremity.
   c. Provide bed rest.
3. Monitor child's therapeutic and untoward response to parenteral antibiotics; administer antibiotics up to 1 week after symptoms have subsided.
4. Maintain fluid and electrolyte balance.
   a. Record accurate intake and output.

    b. Monitor hydration status (skin turgor, moist mucous membranes).
5. Encourage age-appropriate play and recreational activities (see Appendix B, *Growth and Development*).
6. Provide emotional support to child and family.
    a. Provide age-appropriate explanations before procedures.
    b. Incorporate home routine into care.
    c. Encourage parental ventilation of concerns.
    d. Refer to social service as needed.

BIBLIOGRAPHY

Bateman J et al: *Aeromonas hydrophila* cellulitis and wound infections caused by waterborne organisms, *Heart Lung* 17(1):99-102, 1988.

Ellett M: Anusitis associated with group A beta-hemolytic streptococci, *Gastroenterol Nurs* 12(1):53-54, 1989.

Gillady H, Shulman S, Ayoub E: Periorbital and orbital cellulitis in children, *Pediatrics* 61:272, 1978.

Shapiro E, Wald E, Bronzanski B: Periorbital cellulitis and paranasal sinusitis: a reappraisal, *Pediatr Infect Dis* 1(2):91, 1982.

Smith T, O'Day D, Wright P: Clinical implications of preseptal (periorbital) cellulitis in childhood, *Pediatrics* 62:1006, 1978.

10 ❖ Cleft Lip, Cleft Palate, and Repair

PATHOPHYSIOLOGY

Cleft lip and cleft palate are the outcomes of the failure of the soft tissue and/or bony structure to fuse during embryonic development. They may occur on one or both sides of the palate's midline and may occur separately or together. Several factors—drugs (e.g., cortisone, anticonvulsants, chlorcyclizine), vitamin deficiencies, and chronic systemic disease—have been associated as causes of these defects. Other factors include irradiation and the rubella virus, which causes German measles. The child initially seen with cleft lip and/or cleft palate defects must also be assessed for other anomalies, including spina bifida, anencephalic hydrocephalus, and cardiac abnormalities. These children should also be examined for chromosomal abnormalities. Cleft lip can be repaired immediately after birth, although the general consensus recommends performing surgery when the infant is 2 to 3 months of age. Cleft palate is repaired when the child is 18 to 24 months old. After cleft lip repair, children usually require two additional surgeries, including scar revision, correction of vermilion, correction of nasolabial fistula, and correction of lip deformity.

INCIDENCE

1. Condition occurs once in 700 births.
2. Condition occurs once in 2500 white births.
3. Condition occurs most frequently in the white and Japanese populations and is rare among blacks in the United States.
4. Genetic factors account for 10% of cases.
5. Of those born with a cleft lip, 63% are male and 37% are female.
6. Occurrence of cleft palate predominates in females.
7. Highest prevalence associated with Asians; lowest in blacks.
8. Incidence is not associated with socioeconomic status.

CLINICAL MANIFESTATIONS

1. Apparent at birth
   a. Unilateral usually left sided
   b. Bilateral usually associated with cleft palate
2. The following symptoms are secondary to cleft lip and palate
   a. Feeding problems
   b. Hearing problems
   c. Recurrent otitis media
   d. Eustachian tube dysfunction

COMPLICATIONS

1. Speech difficulties—hypernasality, compensatory articulation
2. Malocclusion—abnormal tooth eruption pattern
3. Hearing problems—caused by recurrent otitis media
4. Self-esteem and body image—affected by degree of disfigurement and scarring

LABORATORY/DIAGNOSTIC TESTS

1. Complete blood count—routine preoperative workup
2. Urinalysis—routine preoperative workup
3. Chest x-ray examination—routine preoperative workup
4. Viral studies for rubella and toxoplasmosis—performed if mother has history of infection
5. Intravenous pyelogram—performed if other anomalies exist

SURGICAL MANAGEMENT: CLEFT LIP AND CLEFT PALATE REPAIR

Cleft lip is repaired either immediately after birth or within 3 months. It has been suggested that early surgical repair facilitates parent-infant attachment because of the infant's resultant aesthetic appearance. Repairs are performed at 2 to 3 months of age if the infant demonstrates steady weight gain and a hemoglobin rate greater than 10 g/dl. Several types of surgery are performed to correct the cleft lip: (1) a straight line operation, (2) a lower one-third flap operation, (3) an upper one-third flap operation, and (4) a combined upper and lower one-third flap operation. In each of the surgeries, closure of the lip is usually performed with a Z-plasty procedure to avoid the risk of contracture and elevation of the lip.

Cleft palate surgery is usually performed when the child is 18 to 24 months of age. Palatoplasty involves closure of the mucous membrane and restoration of the anatomic structure. Several types of surgical procedures are used to repair the many different forms of cleft palates. Staged procedures may continue until patient is 4 to 5 years of age with a severe defect.

Patient Response to Surgery

Barring the development of surgical complications (see "Complications"), the infant's problems with feeding are relieved through surgery. Long-term consequences of cleft palate include speech difficulties (e.g., increased nasality and compensating articulation), malocclusion problems (abnormal pattern of tooth eruption), and hearing problems resulting from recurrent otitis media caused by eustachian tube dysfunction.

MEDICATIONS

Analgesics are administered to relieve postoperative pain.

NURSING ASSESSMENT

Refer to "Gastrointestinal Assessment" in Appendix A.

NURSING DIAGNOSES

High risk for injury
High risk for altered nutrition: less than body requirements

High risk for infection
Knowledge deficit

NURSING INTERVENTIONS

Preoperative Care

1. Facilitate parents' positive adjustment to an infant who is imperfect.
   a. Assist parents in dealing with phasic reactions — shock, denial, grief, and mourning.
   b. Encourage parents to discuss negative feelings about child (see "a") and themselves (guilt, blame, feelings of helplessness).
   c. Discuss surgery with parents and role play the behavioral strategies for coping with the reactions of family and friends.
   d. Provide information that instills hope and positive feelings for infant (e.g., comment on infant's positive features; note positive aspects of parent-child interactions).
2. Provide and reinforce information to parents about infant's prognosis and treatment.
   a. Stages of surgical intervention
   b. Feeding techniques
   c. Cause of cleft
3. Promote and maintain adequate fluid and nutritional intake.
   a. Feed with appropriate bottle and nipple — regular nipple with enlarged hole or Breck feeder (syringe adapted with 2-inch tubing).
   b. Direct fluids inside gums near tongue (Breck feeder).
   c. Hold in upright position with head tilted backward.
   d. Bubble frequently (after every ½ ounce) during feeding.
   e. Assess infant's response to feeding and proceed at rate suitable to needs.
4. Monitor child's clinical status — monitor vital signs (temperature, respiration, blood pressure, apical pulse) and report significant deviations.
5. Provide information to parents before procedures are performed to enhance understanding and to decrease anxiety about the surgical preparation and the surgery the child undergoes.

6. Prepare infant for surgery.
   a. Provide nothing by mouth after midnight (water may be given 3 to 4 hours before surgery).
   b. Refer to institutional regimen for preoperative procedure.
   c. Monitor reactions to preoperative medications (e.g., scopolamine, 0.1 mg).

Preoperative home care

1. Instruct parents about care and maintenance of presurgical orthodontic device (promotes alignment of maxilla and proper lateral arch position).
   a. Remove and clean every day.
   b. Replace after cleaning.
   c. Monitor for white pressure areas in palate.
   d. Apply elbow splints to child to prevent removal of plate.
2. Instruct parents about care of cleft lip and cleft palate.
   a. Cleanse lip and oral cavity with water before and after feedings.
   b. Cleanse affected nostril before and after meals.

Postoperative Care

1. Promote adequate nutritional fluid intake.
   a. Monitor intravenous (IV) infusion and its rate q1 hr (nothing by mouth for 24 hours).
   b. Offer sugar water (D_5W) q3 hr (when awake and bowel sounds heard) with Breck feeder.
   c. Advance to formula as tolerated.
   d. Bubble frequently during feeding (after every ½ ounce).
2. Promote healing and maintain integrity of child's incisional site.
   a. Dressing care: apply one-half strength hydrogen peroxide to incisional site and affected nostril for 3 days; then clean with soap and water.
   b. Apply warm compresses for 15 minutes QID to decrease swelling.
   c. Apply steroid cream to decrease inflammation.
   d. Apply antibiotic creams as prophylaxis.
   e. Rinse mouth with water before and after meals.

    f. Use no spoons, straws, or ice chips.
    g. Remove toys with pointed objects.
    h. Ensure Logan's bow is intact (lip guard is taped in place to prevent strain on suture site).
3. Prevent complications.
    a. Provide humidification to decrease dryness of mouth and throat mucosa.
    b. Change position q2 hr to prevent hydrostatic pneumonia and atelectasis.
    c. Use soft restraints on extremities to prevent child from injuring surgical site.
    d. Use elbow restraints to prevent child from injuring surgical site.
    e. Monitor for signs of infection—at surgical site, and systemically (pulmonary congestion and fever).

Postoperative home care

1. Instruct parents about care of surgical site.
2. Instruct parents about feeding practices.
3. Encourage parents to ventilate feelings of insecurity and concerns about caring for child at home, as well as about long-term management and prognosis.
4. Reinforce to parents the importance of long-term management to prevent development of speech and language and dentition problems.
5. Discuss with parents the possibility of long-term consequences and outcomes.
    a. Secondary lip deformity
    b. Excessive nasality
    c. Problems with articulation
    d. Crossbite
    e. Malocclusion
    f. Underdeveloped mandible

BIBLIOGRAPHY

Atkinson H: Care of the child with cleft lip and palate, *Am J Nurs* 67(9):1889, 1967.
Bardach J et al: Late results of multidisciplinary management of unilateral cleft lip and palate, *Ann Plast Surg* 12(3):235, 1984.
Curtin G: The infant with cleft lip or palate: more than a surgical problem, *J Perinatol Neonatal Nurs* 3(3):80-89, 1990.

Elkins S: Cranofacial anomalies in the neonate, *Plast Surg Nurs* 8(4):123-134, 1988.

Garcia-Valasco M et al: Surgical repair of the bilateral cleft of the primary palate, *Ann Plast Surg* 20(1):26, 1988.

Georgiade N: *Symposium on management of cleft lip and palate and associated deformities,* St. Louis, 1974, Mosby–Year Book.

Helms J et al: Effect of timing on long-term clinical success of alveolar cleft bone grafts, *Am J Orthodont Dentofac Orthop* 92(3):232, 1987.

Pate C: Care of the family following the birth of a child with cleft lip and/or palate, *Neonatal Network* 5(6):30, 1987.

Rutrick R, Black P, Jurlyewicz M: Bilateral cleft lip and palate: presurgical treatment, *Ann Plast Surg* 12(2):105, 1984.

Sauter S: Cleft lips and palate: types, repairs, nursing care, *J Assoc Oper Room Nurses* 50(4):813-815, 817-820, 822-824, 1989.

Scheuerle J et al: *Cleft Palate J* 21(3):110, 1984.

Wellman C, Coughlin S: Preoperative and postoperative nutritional management of the infant with cleft palate, *J Pediatr Nurs* 6(3):154-159, 1991.

11 ❖ Coarctation of the Aorta and Coarctectomy

PATHOPHYSIOLOGY

Coarctation of the aorta is a localized narrowing of the aortic lumen. This narrowing results in increased pressures in the ascending aorta, leading to higher pressures in the coronary arteries and great vessels arising from the aortic arch. There are three basic types of coarctation. They are (1) juxtaductal—narrowing at the level of the ductus arteriosus; (2) preductal—narrowing proximal to the ductus arteriosus; and (3) postductal—narrowing distal to the ductus arteriosus. Coarctation of the aorta is associated with several other defects, including anomalies of the left side of the heart, bicuspid aortic valve defect, and ventricular septal defect. Two thirds of children with this defect are a-symptomatic. Many cases are discovered during a physical examination when hypertension of the upper extremity is noted. Prognosis is excellent with surgical intervention.

INCIDENCE

1. Coarctation of the aorta accounts for 10% of congenital cardiac defects.
2. Electrocardiogram (ECG) is normal in 50% of cases.

CLINICAL MANIFESTATIONS

Infants

Most infants are asymptomatic. They may initially be seen with severe sudden onset of congestive heart failure.

Children

1. Absent or diminished lower-extremity pulses
2. Hypertension of upper extremities, with bounding pulses
3. Systolic or systolic and diastolic murmurs
4. Leg muscle cramps during exercise (tissue anoxia)
5. Headache
6. Epistaxis
7. Cool feet
8. Normal growth and development

COMPLICATIONS

1. Heart failure
2. Cardiovascular accident
3. Hypertensive encephalopathy
4. Dissecting aortic aneurysm
5. Bacterial endocarditis

LABORATORY/DIAGNOSTIC TESTS

1. ECG—normal or may reveal left-ventricular hypertrophy and ST and T wave abnormalities
2. Chest x-ray examination—in infants, consistent with clinical findings; in older patient, normal
3. Cardiac catheterization—to diagnose associated defects and abnormal gradient pressure
4. Echocardiogram—examines size, shape and motion of heart structures

SURGICAL TREATMENT: COARCTECTOMY

Repair of a coarctation may be accomplished through several methods, depending on the age of the child and the degree of constriction. Performing elective repair after the child is older is generally preferred; however, for infants with congestive heart failure that does not respond to medical treatment, surgery cannot wait. The left subclavian artery may be ligated distally, then is sutured over an opening in the aorta to provide for a patch enlargement of the aorta. This subclavian flap aortoplasty reduces the number of cases of restenosis because the natural tissue will grow with the child, causing less tension than an end-to-end anastomosis, and it requires less time than cross clamping. By age 4 to 8 years, the child's aorta is near adult size, and hypertension is still reversible; some physicians believe performing the procedure in 1- to 4-year-olds has results that are just as good and with fewer later complications. Postoperative complications increase if surgery is delayed until the child is more than 8 to 10 years old.

The area of coarctation is patched with Teflon material, leaving some natural material to grow with the child. Some surgeons excise the area of coarctation, but that procedure may lead to repeat coarctation. Entry to the thoracic cavity for both age groups is performed through a left posterolateral thoracotomy incision. Bypass is not necessary, although adequate flow to the lower extremities must be maintained through collateral circulation, hypothermia, a temporary shunt or grafts connecting the ascending and descending aorta, or a partial cardiopulmonary bypass.

Patient Response to Surgery

The child's response to surgery should be normal hemodynamic status and prevention of later hypertension. The prognosis is best for asymptomatic older children.

Complications

1. Chylothorax as a result of injury to thoracic duct or lymphatics
2. Congestive heart failure
3. Hemothorax caused by bleeding from the collateral network or aortic anastomosis
4. Mesenteric arteritis caused by paradoxical hypertension, which may lead to bowel infarctions
5. Paradoxical hypertension possibly caused by high plasma renin activity, the baroreceptors' reduced ability to regulate blood pressure, or preoperative damage to the proximal aortic wall
6. Paraplegia caused by inadequate circulation to the spinal cord during surgery

7. Repeat coarctation, especially in infants
8. Vomiting resulting from increased circulation to the gastrointestinal tract
9. No blood pressure in the left arm if the subclavian artery is used for surgery
10. An increased incidence of cardiovascular disease 11 to 25 years after surgery
11. Mortality rate ranging from 4% to 25%, depending on the age of the child, degree of constriction, other associated defects, and the medical center used for the surgery

MEDICATIONS: ANTIHYPERTENSIVES

1. Sodium nitroprusside (Nipride) — used to treat postoperative hypertension; acts on the smooth muscle to produce peripheral vasodilation, causing decreased arterial pressures; continuous infusion intravenously (IV), 2-8 mcg/kg/min
2. Propranolol (Inderal) — used to treat postoperative hypertension; acts as a beta blocker of cardiac and bronchial adrenoreceptors, resulting in decreasing heart rate and myocardial irritability and potentiating contraction and conduction pathway; 0.5 mg/kg/day IV
3. Reserpine — used to treat postoperative hypertension; acts as a sympathetic inhibitor, resulting in decreased blood pressure and cardiac output; 0.02 mg/kg/day intramuscularly (IM)
4. Captopril (Capoten) — used to treat postoperative hypertension; works on the renin-angiotensin system for afterload reduction; 0.5 mg/kg/day in divided doses, with dosage individualized (increased) to achieve desired effect

NURSING ASSESSMENT

1. Refer to "Cardiovascular Assessment" in Appendix A.
2. Assess for paradoxical hypertension.
3. No blood pressure is present in left arm.
4. Perform frequent assessment for bowel sounds, abdominal tenderness, distention, and vomiting; notify physician immediately if any changes occur.

NURSING DIAGNOSES

Activity intolerance
Decreased cardiac output
High risk for injury
High risk for fluid volume deficit
High risk for impaired gas exchange
Altered family processes
Knowledge deficit

NURSING INTERVENTIONS

Preoperative Care

1. Assess infant's or child's cardiac status.
   a. Color of mucous membranes and nailbeds
   b. Quality and intensity of peripheral pulses
   c. Capillary refill time
   d. Temperatures of extremities
   e. Apical pulse
   f. Blood pressure
   g. Respiratory rate
2. Assist in collection of preoperative laboratory and diagnostic data.
   a. Complete blood count, urinalysis, serum, glucose, blood urea nitrogen
   b. Baseline electrolytes — sodium, potassium, chloride, carbon dioxide
   c. Blood coagulation studies — prothrombin time (PT), partial thromboplastin time (PTT), platelet count
   d. Type and cross match for six units of blood, with two units drawn first day of surgery
   e. Chest x-ray examination
   f. ECG (to detect cardiac arrhythmias)
3. Provide age-appropriate preoperative information to child or infant.
4. Provide and reinforce information given to parents regarding surgery and condition.

Postoperative Care

1. Assess infant's or child's cardiac status q1 hr for first 24 to 48 hr, then q2 to 4 hr.
   a. Apical pulse, respiratory rate, temperature

  b. Arterial blood pressure
  c. Capillary refill time
  d. Blood pressure — hypertension often present initially
  e. Cardiac arrhythmias
2. Monitor for signs and symptoms of hemorrhage.
  a. Measure chest tube output q1 hr — greater than 3 to 5 ml indicates problems.
  b. Assess for clot formation in tubing (increased output of blood followed by an abrupt decrease).
  c. Assess bowel sounds and monitor for abdominal distention.
  d. Assess for bleeding from other sites (e.g., nose, mouth, gastrointestinal tract).
  e. Record strict input and output.
3. Monitor infant's or child's hydration status.
  a. Mucous membranes
  b. Bulging or depressed fontanels
  c. Decreased tearing
  d. Poor skin turgor
  e. Specific gravity (urine will be concentrated immediately after surgery)
  f. Daily weights
  g. Input and output
  h. Monitor fluids — IV at 50% to 75% of maintenance fluids first 24 hours postoperatively
4. Promote optimal respiratory status.
  a. Turn, cough, and deep breathe.
  b. Perform chest physiotherapy.
  c. Humidify air.
  d. Monitor for chylothorax (assess breath sounds).
  e. Keep thoracotomy tray at bedside for emergency use.
  f. Monitor for patency to prevent pneumothorax.
  g. Keep two chest tube clamps at bedside to prevent pneumothorax if tubing separates
5. Monitor child's response to medications and blood products.
  a. See "Medications: Antihypertensives."
  b. Assist with collection of laboratory data — hematocrit, template bleeding time.

6. Use no cuff pressure or arterial punctures in left arm if left subclavian flap was performed since only collateral vessels are providing the arterial circulation.
7. Resume by-mouth feedings slowly.
8. Relieve hypertension through medications and anxiety relief measures.
9. Control postoperative pain because pain provides added stress to the suture lines.
10. Provide age-appropriate diversional activities (see Appendix B, *Growth and Development*).
11. Provide age-appropriate explanations before treatments and painful procedures.
12. Provide emotional support to parents.
    a. Encourage ventilation of feelings.
    b. Provide and reinforce information regarding condition and hospitalization.
    c. Provide for physical needs (e.g., sleeping arrangements and hygiene).
    d. Encourage use of preexisting support systems.

Home Care

Stress importance of follow-up care for indefinite time for residual or premature cardiovascular problems, including the development of calcific aortic stenosis.

BIBLIOGRAPHY

Berman L et al: Coarctation of the aorta in children: late results after surgery, *Am J Dis Child* 134:464, 1980.

Foldy S et al: Preoperative nursing care for congenital cardiac defects, *Crit Care Nurs Clin North Am* 1(2):289-295, 1989.

Gerraughty A: Caring for patients with lesions obstructing systemic blood flow, *Crit Care Nurs Clin North Am* 1(2):231-243, 1989.

Hellman G, Coaley D, Gutgsell H: *Surgical treatment of congenital heart disease,* Philadelphia, 1987, Lea & Febiger.

McCorraka M et al: Isthmus flap aortaplasty, a new approach to long-segment coarctation repair, *J Assoc Oper Room Nurses* 45(3):762, 1987.

Moller J, Neal W: *Heart disease in infancy,* New York, 1981, Appleton-Century-Crofts.

O'Brien P et al: Discharge planning for children with heart disease, *Crit Care Nurs Clin North Am* 1(2):297-305, 1989.

Park M: *Pediatric cardiology for practitioners,* St. Louis, 1984, Mosby–Year Book.

Trinquet F et al: Coarctation of the aorta in infants: which operation? *Ann Thorac Surg* 45(2):186, 1988.

Uzark K et al: Health education needs of adolescents with congenital heart disease, *J Pediatr Health Care* 3(3):137-143, 1989.

12 ❖ Congenital Dislocation of the Hip

PATHOPHYSIOLOGY

Congenital dislocation of the hip is an orthopedic deformity that is acquired immediately before or at birth.

The condition ranges from minimal lateral displacement to complete dislocation of the femoral head out of the acetabulum. Generally, it is the result of capsular stretching caused by malposition of the fetus. Secondary causes include cerebral palsy, arthritis, meningocele, and spastic neurologic conditions. In newborns, the condition is not evident because the deformity of both the femoral head and the acetabulum is minimal and the soft tissue is not contracted. Most dislocated hips in the newborn are minimally unstable; some spontaneously stabilize during the first few weeks of life. Infants more than 3 months of age are initially seen with a triad of symptoms: (1) asymmetric thigh folds; (2) shortened leg; and (3) limited abduction. Prognosis is excellent if treatment is initiated early in the newborn period.

Incidence

1. Female to male ratio is 8:1.
2. Incidence increases 10 times with breech delivery.

3. More than 60% of dislocated hips spontaneously stabilize.
4. Occurrence is 11.5 in every 1000 births in the United States.
5. Increased incidence is evident among siblings of affected children.
6. Left hip is affected more often than right hip.
7. Increased incidence occurs in Canadian Eskimos and certain American Indian groups that swaddle children in cradle boards during first few months of life.

CLINICAL MANIFESTATIONS
Infancy
1. Possibly no symptoms evident because infant may have minimal displacement of femur
2. Asymmetry of skin folds in inner side of thigh
3. Shortened leg
4. Limitation of abduction
5. Positive Galeazzi's sign (see box on p. 73)
6. Positive Barlow's maneuver (see box)
7. Positive Ortolani's maneuver (see box)
8. Palpable femoral head in buttocks
9. Elevated trochanter

Toddler and Older Child
1. Abnormal "duck-waddle" gait (waddling) caused by bilateral dislocation of the hip
2. Leans to side of body that bears weight
3. Increased lumbar lordosis during standing
4. Standing position — knee flexed in unaffected leg and on toes of affected side
5. Adolescence — increasingly painful
6. Adulthood — degenerative arthritis

COMPLICATIONS
1. Postoperative infection
2. Postoperative stiffness
3. Femoral epiphyseal deformity (5% to 15%)
4. Iatrogenic avascular necrosis

Assessment Criteria

Ortolani's Maneuver

Fingers are placed over greater trochanter as thigh is abducted and lifted toward acetabulum. A click is heard in infants less than 3 months of age, and a jerk is felt in children more than this age.

Barlow's Maneuver

Hand is placed over knee. Leg is adducted past midline and outward. Positive sign is a sensation of abnormal movement.

Galeazzi's Sign

Flexing both hips at 90 degrees results in one knee being below the level of the other.

LABORATORY/DIAGNOSTIC TESTS

Anteroposterior pelvic roentgenogram is obtained (assesses extent of femoral displacement or dislocation; not useful for infants less than 1 month old).

MEDICATIONS (NOT USUALLY NEEDED)

1. Analgesics — used to control pain
2. Stool softeners — to stimulate bowel movements

NURSING ASSESSMENT

1. Refer to "Neuromuscular Assessment" in Appendix A.
2. Refer to boxed material, "Assessment Criteria," above.

NURSING DIAGNOSES

Impaired physical mobility
Altered tissue perfusion
Altered nutrition: less than body requirements
Knowledge deficit
Altered growth and development

NURSING INTERVENTIONS

Instruct parent about the maintenance and care of traction apparatus.

1. Pavlik harness (maintains hip flexion)
   a. Maintaining harness (on continuously for 2 to 3 months)
   b. Performing skin care (lubricant and sponge bath)
   c. Turning q2 hr
2. Abduction brace (maintains hip in abducted and fixed position)
   a. Performing skin care
   b. Monitoring for signs of skin irritation
   c. Changing diapers frequently (to prevent skin breakdown and to maintain clean brace)

If conservative treatment is unsuccessful or if condition is diagnosed after infant is 3 months of age, he or she is treated with traction (4-6 months) followed by open/closed reduction (as indicated) and then a spica cast.

1. Monitor child's response to traction (2 to 3 weeks).
2. Monitor child's response to spica cast.

If open reduction performed, do the following:

1. Prepare child and parents for surgery.
   a. Provide information about presurgical routine.
   b. Reinforce information given about surgery and open reduction.
2. Monitor child's response postoperatively.
   a. Monitor vital signs q2 hr until stable, then q4 hr.
   b. Monitor for signs of drainage on cast.
   c. Perform circulation checks q1 hr during the immediate postoperative period, then q4 hr.
3. Provide pain relief measures as necessary.
   a. Provide tactile comfort and holding.
   b. Administer analgesics.

Home Care

1. Instruct parents about care of spica cast.
   a. Apply waterproof material to cast edges in perineal area; change diaper often.
   b. Keep skin clean and dry under cast everyday.
   c. Check for signs of infection and pressure (e.g., musty odor and reddened area).

    d. Monitor for small items placed in cast (e.g., food and small toys).
2. Instruct parents about appropriate feeding techniques.
    a. Feed infant in supine position.
    b. Child can be held in mother's arm or propped with pillows.
3. Instruct parents to provide age-appropriate stimulating activities (refer to Appendix B, *Growth and Development*).

BIBLIOGRAPHY

Corbett D: Information needs of parents of a child in a Pavlik harness, *Orthopaed Nurs*7(2):20, 1988.

Kadkhoda M, Chung S, Adebonojo F: Congenital dislocation of the hip — diagnostic screening and treatment, *Clin Pediatr* 15(3):239, 1976.

Melkoman G: Congenital hip dysplasia, *Orthop Nurse* 6(3):47, 1987.

Ramsey P: The changing signs of congenital hip dislocation, *J Pediatr Surg* 12(3):437, 1977.

Sherk H, Pasquariello P, Walters W: Congenital dislocation of the hip: a review, *Clin Pediatr* 20(8):513, 1981.

Skinner S: Congenital dislocation of the hip. In Rudolph A: *Rudolph's pediatrics*, ed 19, Norwalk, Conn, 1991, Appleton & Lange, 1929-1932.

Wilkes J: Screening for congenital dislocation of the hip: professional guidelines, *Midwives Chron* 98(1186):260, 1986.

13 ❖ Congestive Heart Failure

PATHOPHYSIOLOGY

Congestive heart failure (CHF) refers to the inability of the heart to deliver sufficient blood to the systemic circulation to meet the body needs. CHF is the result of a variety of congenital heart defects or is a secondary manifestation of systemic disease. CHF can be classified as failure of the right or left side of the heart. Causes of the failure are listed below.

CHF of Right Side of Heart

Pulmonary vascular obstructions

Pulmonary valvular obstructions

Tricuspid disease

Atrial septal defect

Pulmonary venous anomaly

CHF of Left Side of Heart

Severe systemic hypertension (renal disease)

Coarctation of the aorta

Aortic stenosis

Mitral obstruction

Patent ductus arteriosus

Failure of the right side of the heart results in systemic venous hypertension. The right side of the heart is unable to pump blood into the pulmonary artery, resulting in increased pressure in the right atrium and in systemic venous circulation. This condition can lead to hepatomegaly, impaired liver function, and jaundice. Puffiness of the face, ascites, and anasarca are late symptoms. Failure of the left side of the heart results in pulmonary venous hypertension. The left ventricle is unable to pump blood into systemic circulation, creating increased left-atrial and pulmonary pressures and pulmonary edema.

CHF activates the cardiac reserve, an adaptive mechanism for maintaining adequate circulation. The cardiac reserve mechanisms include the following: (1) *tachycardia,* which maintains cardiac output by increasing heart rate and is often very effective, (2) *increased ventricular end-diastolic pressure,* which is caused by failure, and (3) increased aldosterone and antidiuretic hormone (ADH) release, which causes water and sodium retention as a result of decreased renal blood flow, leading to edema. These three mechanisms enable the failing heart to compensate temporarily.

INCIDENCE

1. Ninety percent of infants with congenital heart defects develop CHF within the first year of life.
2. Majority of affected infants manifest symptoms within the first few months of life.
3. Eight out of 1000 full-term infants are born with congenital heart defects; the majority do not have a life-threatening cardiac anomaly.
4. A critical congenital defect is present in 2.6 of 1000 full-term infants.

CLINICAL MANIFESTATIONS
Infants
1. Tachypnea greater than 50
2. Retractions, grunting
3. Tachycardia with apical pulse greater than 160
4. Diaphoresis
5. Hepatomegaly

6. Edema (appears first in face and eyes)
7. Failure to gain weight
8. Difficulty feeding
9. Listless and apathetic
10. Cyanosis particularly during crying (occurs only if cyanotic CHD present)

Children

1. Tachypnea
2. Dyspnea
3. Retractions
4. Tachycardia
5. Cyanosis (occurs only if cyanotic CHD present)
6. Pallor
7. Rales, rhonchi, wheezing, pulmonary edema
8. Hepatomegaly
9. Peripheral edema
10. Ascites
11. Gallop rhythm
12. Pulsus alternans (caused by variation in strength of ventricular contraction)
13. Cardiac enlargement
14. Orthopnea
15. Paroxysmal noctural dyspnea
16. Hemoptysis
17. Distended neck veins (late sign)

LABORATORY/DIAGNOSTIC TESTS

1. Arterial blood gas values (decreased partial pressure of oxygen [Po_2], normal/increased partial pressure of carbon dioxide [Pco_2], decreased pH [acidosis; only if shock])
2. Chest x-ray examination — reveals cardiac enlargement and engorgement of pulmonary vessels
3. Electrocardiogram (ECG) — may reveal left/right ventricular hypertrophy or decreased systolic time intervals
4. Echocardiogram — a noninvasive procedure that produces a two-dimensional image of the heart. The heart structures (valves, septa, and chambers) are identified by ultrasound through sound wave images.

5. Cardiac catheterization—an invasive procedure used to detect cardiac abnormalities. A radiopaque dye is injected through a catheter that is inserted into a peripheral blood vessel. The catheter is advanced into heart chambers from which blood samples and pressures are taken for analysis through which a septal defect can be identified.
6. Complete blood count—with CHF, decreased hemoglobin and decreased hematocrit may be present.
7. Serum electrolytes—decreased potassium (after using diuretics), decreased chloride (after using diuretics)

MEDICATIONS

1. Digitalis
   a. Digitalization
      (1) Administer 50% digitalization dose immediately.
      (2) Administer remaining 50% in two divided doses at 6- to 12-hr intervals.
   b. Full-term infant
      (1) Digitalization—0.03 to 0.05 mg/kg (intravenously [IV dose two thirds of oral] or [IM])
      (2) Maintenance—one tenth to one fifth of digitalization dose (by mouth [po], IV, or IM)
   c. Child 2 weeks to 2 years old
      (1) Digitalization—0.04 to 0.06 mg/kg (IV or IM)
      (2) Maintenance—one tenth to one fifth of digitalization dose IV or IM and one fifth to one third of digitalization dose po
2. Diuretics (cause excretion of water and sodium)
   a. Furosemide (Lasix)—initial dose—2 mg/kg, then 1 mg/kg IM or IV q6-12 hr; check K^+ before IV administration
   b. Chlorothiazide (Diuril)—administered alone or with spironolactone (Aldactone) po 2 to 3 mg/kg/24 hr
3. Nitroglycerin—relaxes smooth muscle of blood vessel; decreases systemic and pulmonary venous pressures
   a. Individualized sublingual dose (pediatric dose not established)—0.15 to 0.6 mg (1/150 g to 1/100 g)
   b. IV dose—5 μg in D_5W or 0.9 normal saline
4. Hydralazine (Apresoline)—stimulates force of contraction and arteriolar vasodilation; decreases systemic

hypertension; initial dose—0.75 mg/kg/24 hr QID po; may increase up to 10 times over next 3 to 4 weeks to 1.7 to 3.5 mg/kg/24 hr IV q4-6 hr

5. Captopril (Capoten)—a hypotensive; inhibits angio-tensin-converting enzyme; dosage (pediatric doses have not been established)—25 mg TID po; can be increased to 50 mg TID

6. Sodium nitroprusside (Nipride)—a vasodilator; relaxes arterial and venous smooth muscle and decreases hypertension; average dose (individualized)—3 μg/kg/m (rarely exceeds 10 μg/kg/m in D_5W IV)

7. Morphine—reduces energy requirements; dose—1 mg/kg subcutaneously

NURSING ASSESSMENT

Refer to "Cardiovascular Assessment" in Appendix A.

NURSING DIAGNOSES

Decreased cardiac output
Ineffective breathing pattern
Activity intolerance
Fluid volume excess
Altered family processes
Knowledge deficit

NURSING INTERVENTIONS

1. Observe and monitor child's clinical status.
   a. Monitor vital signs q1 hr until stable.
   b. Maintain temperature at 36.5° C (resting) or 37° C (morning). Maintain neutral thermal environment for infant.
   c. Monitor weight q8 hr until stable.
2. Promote oxygenation of body tissues.
   a. Maintain in Fowler's position (use cardiac chair), which allows pooling of blood in dependent areas, thus decreasing volume overload of heart and pulmo-nary congestion and alleviating respiratory distress.
   b. Use suction as needed; be careful not to stimulate vagus nerve, causing bradycardia.
   c. Provide humidified, warm oxygen.

3. Promote and maintain child's fluid and electrolyte balance.
    a. Monitor potassium levels (potassium lost with diuretics increases effects of digitalis).
    b. Restrict fluids to 65 ml/kg/day.
    c. Decrease salt in diet to 1 to 2 mEq/kg/day.
    d. Record accurate input and output.
    e. Monitor weight q8 hr until stable; then monitor daily.
    f. Monitor edema.
4. Promote child's nutritional status.
    a. Provide small frequent feedings q2 hr (conserves energy).
    b. Provide increased protein and increased calorie diet (100 kcal/100 ml).
    c. Limit sodium intake (no added salt diet).
    d. Feed in upright position to reduce respiratory effort.
    e. Plan mealtimes carefully around rest periods.
5. Provide comfort measures.
    a. Provide oxygen therapy (tent).
    b. Provide cardiac chair.
    c. Schedule activities to provide extended rest periods.
6. Prevent or treat pulmonary edema.
    a. Administer digitalis and diuretics.
    b. Administer morphine sulfate intramuscularly.
    c. Provide cardiac chair.
    d. Administer oxygen therapy (positive pressure).
7. Provide emotional support to child and parents.
    a. Provide age-appropriate play activities; provide both visual and tactile stimulation because oxygen tent interferes with activities (see Appendix B, *Growth and Development*).
    b. Encourage parents' expression of feelings (e.g., anxiety, guilt).
    c. Provide and reinforce information given to parents regarding procedures, child's condition, hospitalization.
    d. Provide consistent one-to-one nursing care.
    e. Encourage rooming-in.
    f. Encourage parents' use of preexisting support systems.

Home Care

Provide instruction to parents about long-term mainte-nance.

1. Medications (diuretics and digitalis)—monitor child's therapeutic and untoward reactions.
2. Diet—instruct about no-added-salt diet.
3. Activity—schedule more frequent rest periods and feed infant slowly to decrease amount of exertion.
4. Community referral—inform about infant stimulation programs and parent support groups.

BIBLIOGRAPHY

Adams F, Emmanouilidis G, Riemenschneider T: *Moss' heart disease in infants, children, and adolescents,* ed 4, Baltimore, 1989, Williams & Wilkins.

Friedman W: Congenital heart disease in infancy and childhood. In Braunwald E: *A textbook of cardiovascular medicine,* Philadelphia, 1980, WB Saunders Co.

Friedman W, George B: New concepts and drugs in treatment of congestive heart failure, *Pediatr Clin North Am* 31(6):1197, 1984.

Kellerher R: Cardiac drugs: new isotopes, *Critic Care Nurs Clin North Am* 1(2):391-397, 1989.

Modicin M, Schorr J: An update of congestive heart failure in infants, *Issues Compr Pediatr Nurs* 3(7):5, 1979.

Moynihan P, King R: Caring for patients with lesions increasing pulmonary blood flow, *Critical Care Clinics of North America* 1(2):195-213, 1989.

Shor V: Congenital cardiac defects: assessment and case finding, *Am J Nurs* 78(2):256, 1978.

Smith K: Recognizing cardiac failure in neonates, *MCN* 4:98, March/April 1979.

14 ❖ Croup

PATHOPHYSIOLOGY

Croup, or acute laryngotracheobronchitis, is a viral infection that affects the larynx and the trachea. Subglottic edema with upper respiratory obstruction results, accompanied by thick secretions. Children are susceptible to airway obstruction because the diameter of the subglottic area is narrow. Croup is caused by any virus associated with upper respiratory infection. Causative agents include parainfluenza virus types 1, 2, and 3; respiratory syncytial virus (RSv); influenza virus types A_1, A_2, and B; adenovirus; and rhinovirus. Onset occurs after 12 to 72 hours of cough. Coryza is often accompanied by fever.

Spasmodic croup is a sudden attack of croup, which usually occurs during the night and is associated with an upper respiratory infection and fever. This type of attack is of a recurrent nature. Mortality rate is 1%.

INCIDENCE

1. Seasonal prevalence — winter months
2. More prevalent in boys
3. Age range — 3 months to 3 years; peak age — 9 to 18 months
4. Development of significant airway obstruction in one of 20 children
5. Geographic locations — areas with increased atmospheric pollution and/or rapid atmospheric changes in humidity

CLINICAL MANIFESTATIONS
Initial

1. Persistent, brassy, barking cough that worsens
2. A cold for 1 to 2 days
3. Rhinorrhea accompanied by low-grade fever
4. Stridor (progression of stridor is an indicator of the severity of the disease)
5. Hoarse cry

Acute

1. Stridor at rest
2. Retractions at rest
3. Tachypnea (respiratory rate greater than 60)
4. Cyanosis
5. Agitation and restlessness
6. Listlessness
7. Decrease in stridor and retractions without clinical improvement

COMPLICATION

Potential respiratory failure resulting from airway obstruction is the main complication of croup.

LABORATORY/DIAGNOSTIC TESTS

1. Arterial blood gas values (normal to decreased pH, decreased partial pressure of oxygen, increased partial pressure of carbon dioxide)
2. Throat culture *(Haemophilus influenzae)*
3. Chest x-ray examination
4. Lateral neck x-ray examination (to rule out epiglottitis and foreign bodies)
5. Complete blood count (normal)

MEDICATIONS

1. Antibiotics — used to treat infection; choice dependent on culture and sensitivity (see Appendix D, *Commonly Used Antibiotics*)
2. Bronchodilators — used for temporary relief of bronchospasm and for mucosal congestion; administer 1:100% solution through aerosol, nebulizer, or intermittent positive pressure breathing (IPPB) machine

3. Corticosteroid or glucocorticoid—has antiinflammatory effect; dexamethasone (Decadron)—(20 mg/m^2/24 hr) TID by mouth (po), or intramuscular (IM) dose one third to one half of oral dose

NURSING ASSESSMENT

Refer to "Respiratory Assessment" in Appendix A.

NURSING DIAGNOSES

High risk for suffocation
Ineffective airway clearance
Fluid volume deficit
Anxiety

NURSING INTERVENTIONS

1. Monitor respiratory status (vital signs—use of accessory muscles, position, arterial blood gas values, color).
2. Report signs of increased respiratory distress such as increased respiratory rate, labored breathing, wheezing, stridor, intercostal retractions, circumoral cyanosis.
3. Raise head of bed to facilitate breathing.
4. Monitor and observe effects of oxygen therapy (IPPB with racemic epinephrine, mist tent).
   a. Quality of respiratory effort (see number 2)
   b. Arterial blood gas values—within normal limits
5. Assess and maintain hydration status; observe for signs of dehydration—decreased skin turgor, decreased urinary output, decreased moistness of mucous membranes.
6. Monitor action and side effects of medications (use of antibiotics is controversial).
   a. Bronchodilators—(i.e., racemic epinephrine)
   b. Corticosteroids—for antiinflammatory properties
   c. Antibiotics—if a secondary bacterial infection is present
7. Provide age-appropriate quiet play and recreational activities (see Appendix B, *Growth and Development*).
8. Provide for child's developmental needs during hospitalization.
   a. Encourage contact with siblings and parents.
   b. Incorporate home routines into hospital stay (e.g., feeding practices, night routine).

9. Provide emotional support to family.
   a. Encourage ventilation of concerns.
   b. Refer to social service person.
   c. Provide for physical comforts (e.g., place to sleep, bathe).
   d. Provide explanations before performing procedures.

Respiratory Failure

1. Establish and maintain patent airway.
2. Monitor effects of ventilator assistance.
   a. Respiratory status
   b. Functioning of ventilator
   c. Complications (e.g., subglottic stenosis)

Home Care

Instruct parents about home management.
1. Use of humidifiers (including use of shower)
2. Signs of secondary infection (increased temperature, signs of a cold, respiratory infections)
3. Administration of medications (see "Medications")
4. Infection control
   a. Avoid large groups of people.
   b. Avoid cold temperatures.

BIBLIOGRAPHY

Battaglia J: Severe croup: the child with fever and upper airway obstruction, *Pediatr Rev* 7:227-233, 1986.

Lepow M, Hethington S: Respiratory tract infections. In Green M, Haggerty R, eds: *Ambulatory pediatrics,* Philadelphia, 1990, WB Saunders.

Simkins R: Croup and epiglottitis, *Am J Nurs* 81(3):519, 1981.

Stokes D: The croup syndrome. In Gellis S, Kagan E, eds: *Current pediatric therapy,* Philadelphia, 1990, WB Saunders.

15 ❖ Cystic Fibrosis

PATHOPHYSIOLOGY

Cystic fibrosis is an inherited (autosomal-recessive trait) disorder affecting the exocrine glands (the bronchi, the small intestine, and the pancreatic and bile ducts). The mucus produced by these glands is viscous, causing obstruction of the small passageways of these organs. The effects of this biochemical defect on the involved organs are listed below.

1. Pancreas
   a. Degeneration and fibrosis of acini occur.
   b. Secretion of pancreatic enzymes is inhibited, causing impaired absorption of fats, proteins, and, to a limited degree, carbohydrates.
2. Small intestine — absence of pancreatic enzymes (trypsin, amylase, lipase) causes impaired absorption of fats and proteins, resulting in steatorrhea and azotorrhea.
3. Liver — biliary obstruction, fibrosis
4. Lungs
   a. Bronchial and bronchiolar obstruction from excessive pooling of secretions causes generalized hyperinflation and atelectasis.
   b. Pooled mucous secretions increase the susceptibility to bacterial infections. (*Pseudomonas aeruginosa* is the predominant organism found in sputum and lungs.)
   c. Altered oxygen and carbon dioxide exchange can cause varying degrees of hypoxia, hypercapnia, and acidosis.

   d. Fibrotic lung changes occur, and in severe cases, pulmonary hypertension and cor pulmonale can occur.
5. Skeletal
   a. Growth and onset of puberty are retarded.
   b. Retardation of skeletal maturation results in delayed bone aging and shortness of stature (38% to 42% of children with cystic fibrosis).
6. Reproductive
   a. Female—late menses, possible infertility because of thickness of cervical mucus
   b. Male—vas deferens often absent, sterile but not impotent

INCIDENCE

1. Cystic fibrosis affects 1 in 2000 white infants each year.
2. It affects 1 in 17,000 black infants each year.
3. It rarely affects infants of Asian descent.
4. Length and quality of life have greatly increased in recent years, but course of disease is ultimately terminal.
5. Odds are one in four (25%) that each subsequent pregnancy after birth of child with cystic fibrosis will result in child with cystic fibrosis.
6. Cystic fibrosis affects males and females equally.
7. Symptoms vary greatly, resulting in variable life span; many survive into adulthood; 95% survival to age 16, 50% to age 21.

CLINICAL MANIFESTATIONS

1. Presence of cyanosis
2. Wheezy respirations, moist crackles
3. Dry, nonproductive cough
4. Color of sputum—greenish tint during infection; yellow-grayish tint normally
5. Viscous sputum and increasing amount of sputum
6. Clubbed fingers and toes
7. Increased anteroposterior diameter of chest
8. Steatorrhea
9. Bulky, loose, foul-smelling stools
10. Distended abdomen
11. Thin extremities

12. Wasted buttocks
13. Failure to thrive (below norms for height and weight)
14. Meconium ileus (infants)
15. Degeneration and fibrosis of the exocrine organs
16. Shallow, pale skin color
17. Profuse sweating in warm temperature
18. Salty-tasting skin
19. Excessive loss of sodium and chloride

COMPLICATIONS

Gastrointestinal complications include cirrhosis, portal hypertension, esophageal varices, fecal impactions, hypersplenism, intussusception, cholelithiasis, pancreatitis, hemoptysis, and rectal prolapse.

Endocrine complications include diabetes mellitus and heat prostration.

Pulmonary complications include emphysema, pneumothorax, pulmonary pneumonia, and bronchiectasis.

LABORATORY/DIAGNOSTIC TESTS

1. Sweat test (to measure concentration of sodium and chloride in sweat; most definitive diagnostic test; not reliable for newborns less than 1 month old). Two positive sweat tests are diagnostic. Greater than 60 mEq/L, positive for CF.
2. Albumin in meconium (diagnostic for cystic fibrosis)
3. Urinalysis (to assess renal function)
4. Blood urea nitrogen (elevated)
5. Creatinine (elevated)
6. Serum glutamic-pyruvic transaminase (SGPT) and serum glutamic-oxaloacetic transaminase (SGOT) (to assess liver function)
7. Pulmonary function testing (used as diagnostic test to identify disease and its cause, to assess severity and degree of condition, and to determine therapy)

MEDICATIONS

1. Antibiotics—choice of medication depends on organisms involved, sensitivity to antibiotics, severity of infection, and patient response to therapy (see Appendix D, *Commonly Used Antibiotics*)

2. Pancreatic enzyme supplements — dose is determined by character of stool
3. Vitamins — fat-soluble A, K, D, and E
4. Hormone — testosterone; used to reverse protein loss associated with debilitating disease; restores and maintains positive nitrogen balance and reduces excretion of phosphorus, nitrogen, potassium, sodium, and chloride; 10 to 25 mg 2 to 3 times per week
5. Bronchodilators
   a. Acetylcysteine (Mucomyst) — used as adjuvant therapy to liquefy and loosen abnormal, viscid mucus; 1 to 10 ml of 20% solution through inhalation through oxygen mask or tracheostomy; 10% to 20% solution used for mist tent — dependent on amount needed for heavy mist
   b. Isoetharine (Bronkosol) — used as bronchodilator; facilitates expectoration of pulmonary secretions, increases vital capacity, and decreases airway resistance

NURSING ASSESSMENT

Refer to "Respiratory, GI, and Endocrine Assessment" in Appendix A.

NURSING DIAGNOSES

Ineffective airway clearance
Activity intolerance
Altered nutrition: less than body requirements
High risk for infection
Ineffective family coping: compromised
Altered growth and development
Impaired home maintenance management

NURSING INTERVENTIONS

1. Observe and monitor respiratory status and report any significant changes (respiratory rate, presence of intercostal retractions, presence of cyanosis, and color and amount of sputum).
2. Monitor effects of intermittent positive pressure breathing (IPPB) treatment (performed before postural drainage).

3. Administer and monitor effects of postural drainage and percussion.
4. Administer and monitor side effects and actions of medications.
   a. Antibiotics (to treat infection)
   b. Pancreatic enzymes (aid in digestion of protein, fat, and carbohydrates)
   c. Salt supplements (for salt depletion)
   d. Fat-soluble vitamins (needed because of impaired intestinal absorption of fat-soluble vitamins)
   e. Bronchodilators (cause bronchial tubes to dilate)
   f. Hormones (promote growth)
5. Teach and supervise breathing exercises (exhalation and inhalation).
6. Encourage physical activity as condition permits.
7. Obtain baseline information about dietary habits (food preferences, dislikes, eating attitudes, developmental abilities).
8. Monitor and record characteristics of stool (color, consistency, size, frequency).
9. Promote nutritional status.
   a. Administer high-protein, high-caloric, low-fat diet.
   b. Administer supplemental fat-soluble vitamins.
   c. Administer pancreatic enzymes before meals.
   d. Administer salt supplementation as needed.
   e. Assess need for supplemental protein formula.
10. Observe and report signs of complications (see "Complications").
11. Provide emotional support to patient and parents during hospitalization.
    a. Encourage verbalization of emotions (child and family).
    b. Perform age-appropriate teaching before procedures.
    c. Provide information about child's condition and hospitalization.
    d. Encourage use of social support network (e.g., neighborhood friends, relatives).
    e. Refer to social worker as needed.
    f. Provide age-appropriate toys and recreational activities.

    g. Elicit expression of fears concerning body mutilation, death, chronic disability.

Home Care

1. Instruct parents and child about techniques of home management.
   a. Dietary needs
   b. Postural drainage and percussion
   c. IPPB treatments
   d. Breathing exercises
   e. Administration of medications
   f. Avoid exposure to respiratory infections
   g. Management of constipation/diarrhea
2. Monitor family's compliance with home management.
   a. Monitor child's clinical course.
   b. Monitor frequency of hospital admissions.
   c. Assess family's level of knowledge.
3. Assist family in contacting support systems for financial, psychologic, and medical assistance (e.g., Cystic Fibrosis Foundation).
4. Genetic counseling

BIBLIOGRAPHY

Brissette S et al: Nursing care plan for adolescents and young adults with advanced cystic fibrosis, *Issues Compr Pediatr Nurs* 10(2):87, 1987.

Browing I, D'Alonzo G, Tobin M: Importance of respiratory rate as an indicator of respiratory dysfunction in patients with cystic fibrosis, *Chest: Cardiopulm J* 97(6):1317-1326, 1990.

Cappelli M, MacDonald N, McGrath P: Assessment of readiness to transfer to adult care for adolescents with cystic fibrosis, *Children's Health Care* 18(4):218-224, 1989.

Davidson A, Chandrase Karan K, Guida L, Holsclaw D: Enhancement of hypoxemia by atrial shunting in cystic fibrosis, *Chest: Cardiopulm J* 98(3):543-545, 1990.

Hartsell M: Chest physiotherapy and mechanical vibration, *J Pediatr Nurs* 2(2):135, 1987.

Henley L, Hill I: Global and specific disease-related information needs of cystic fibrosis patients and their families, *Pediatrics* 85(6):1015-1021, 1990.

Jacobs J: Cystic fibrosis as it affects the patient and his family, *Respir Ther* 52(60):116, 1977.

Landon C, Rosenfeld R: Short stature and pubertal delay in male adolescents with cystic fibrosis, *Am J Dis Child* 138:388, 1984.

Maccarato M, Cresevic D: Caring for adults who have cystic fibrosis, *American Journal of Nursing* 89(11):1462-1465, 1989.

McAnear S: Parental reaction to a chronically ill child, *Home Healthcare Nurse* 8(3):35-40, 1990.

McLeod S, McClowry S: Using temperament theory to individualize the psychosocial care of hospitalized children, *Children's Health Care* 19(2):79-55, 1990.

Nagy S, Ungerer J: Adaptation of mothers and fathers to children with cystic fibrosis: a comparison, *Children's Health Care* 19(3):147-154, 1990.

Passero M, Renoir B, Solomon J: Patient-reported compliance with cystic fibrosis therapy, *Clin Pediatr* 20(4):264, 1981.

Patterson J, McCubbin H, Warwick W: The impact of family functioning on health changes in children with cystic fibrosis, *Soc Sci Med* 31(2):159-164, 1990.

Reed S: Potential for alterations in family process: when a family has a child with cystic fibrosis, *Issues Comp Pediatr Nurs* 13(1):15-23, 1990.

Shwachman H, Khaw K, Kowalski S: The management of cystic fibrosis, *Clin Pediatr* 14(12):1115, 1975.

16 ❖ Cytomegalic Inclusion Disease

PATHOPHYSIOLOGY

Cytomegalic inclusion disease is the more severe expression of infection with the cytomegalovirus. A number of related strains of cytomegalovirus exist, and it is a member of the herpes family. It is also believed to play a role in acquired immunodeficiency syndrome, as well as Kaposi's sarcoma, but the relationship is inconclusive. The cytomegalovirus is probably transmitted through direct person-to-person contact with body fluids or tissues, including urine, blood, saliva, cervical secretions, semen, and breast milk. The period of incubation is unknown; the following are estimated incubation periods: after delivery—3 to 12 weeks; after transfusion—3 to 12 weeks; and after transplant—9 weeks. The urine often contains cytomegalovirus from months to years after infection. The virus can remain dormant in individuals and be reactivated. Currently, no immunizations exist to prevent its occurrence.

Three types of cytomegalovirus exist.

1. Congenital—acquired transplacentally in utero. In individuals with this type of cytomegalovirus, the most severe forms of cytomegalic inclusion disease occur in children. Approximately 40% of infants born to women experiencing a primary (first) cytomegalovirus illness during pregnancy will be infected, and only 5% to 10% of them will have signs of cytomega-

lic inclusion disease. Signs can appear at birth or up to 12 weeks after delivery.

2. Acute-acquired—acquired anytime during or after birth through adulthood. Symptoms resemble mononucleosis (malaise, fever, pharyngitis, splenomegaly, petechial rash, respiratory symptoms). Disease is not without sequelae, especially in young children, and can result from transfusions.

3. Generalized systemic disease—occurs in individuals who are immunosuppressed, especially if they have undergone organ transplantation. Symptoms include pneumonitis, hepatitis, and leukopenia, which can occasionally be fatal. Previous infection does not produce immunity and may result in reactivation of the virus.

INCIDENCE

1. Cytomegalovirus is the leading cause of congenital viral infections in North America.
2. The disease is apparent in 1% to 2% of live births; many more infants are symptomatic.
3. Sixty percent of the adult population is seropositive.
4. Lower rates occur in higher socioeconomic groups.
5. Twenty-five percent of affected infants die by 3 months of age; remaining 60% to 75% will have some form of intellectual impairment, and approximately 10% will be normal but will have minimal symptoms.

CLINICAL MANIFESTATIONS

In the newborn period, symptoms of cytomegaloviral infection are similar to other viral infections. Onset of congenital infection can occur immediately after birth or up to 12 weeks of age. There are no predictable indicators, but the following symptomatology is prevalent:

Petechiae and ecchymoses
Hepatosplenomegaly
Neonatal jaundice
Microcephaly
Intrauterine growth retardation
Prematurity

Other symptoms can occur in the newborn or older child.

Purpura
Intracerebral calcifications
Hearing loss
Chorioretinitis
Fever
Pneumonia
Tachypnea and dyspnea
Brain damage

Many individuals may be asymptomatic.

COMPLICATIONS

1. Variable hearing loss
2. Lower intelligence quotient (IQ)
3. Perceptual difficulties
4. Greater risk for microcephaly

LABORATORY/DIAGNOSTIC TESTS

1. Microscopic examination of urinary sediment, body fluids, tissues — reveals typical inclusion body in cells
2. Cytomegalovirus titer — diagnostic if results are >1:8
3. TORCH screen — used to assess presence of other viruses
4. Chest x-ray examination — used to reveal organ involvement
5. Computerized tomography scans — used to reveal organ
   involvement

MEDICATIONS

Only symptomatic relief is available at this time (e.g., fever
management, transfusions for anemia, respiratory support).
Some evidence exists that hyperimmunoglobulin can reduce the severity of an infection in immunocompromised
individuals.

NURSING ASSESSMENT

Refer to "Respiratory Assessment" and "Neuromuscular
Assessment" in Appendix A.

NURSING DIAGNOSES

High risk for infection
Altered nutrition: less than body requirements
Knowledge deficit

NURSING INTERVENTIONS

1. Institute and maintain isolation procedures to prevent contamination from blood and body fluids (urine is the most predictable source of spread, a fact that is especially significant when caring for any child in diapers).
   a. Private room is preferred; provide Isolette for infant.
   b. Laundry and diapers require special contamination disposal, using a covered, foot-operated receptacle. Keep receptacle a minimum of 3 feet from any other patient.
   c. Wear gown and gloves when in physical contact with nontoilet-trained child or with his or her secretions, blood, or body fluids.
   d. GOOD HAND WASHING IS ESSENTIAL for all staff *and* visitors.
   e. Decontaminate all respiratory equipment, blood drawing supplies, etc.
   f. Alert any pregnant personnel or visitors of risk.
2. Promote continuance of breastfeeding.
   a. Breastfeeding is contraindicated for infant with active infection.
   b. Use manual pump and freeze milk if feeding is temporarily discontinued.
   c. Test milk serologically if it is sent to milk bank; premature infants are at great risk if they are seronegative and receive milk from seropositive woman.
   d. Confer with infection control department.
3. Prevent spread of virus.
   a. Pregnant woman should avoid entering room of infant with cytomegalovirus.
   b. Immunosuppressed infants should be protected from unnecessary contact.
4. Provide emotional support to parents.
   a. Allow ventilation of family members' feelings (guilt, anger, grief).
   b. Support family by giving them attention.
   c. Reinforce information about asymptomatic aspects of this infection and about its widespread distribution to limit parents' guilt.
   d. Provide facts about the virus.

Home Care

1. Instruct parents about methods to prevent spread of infection.
   a. Advise parents of possibility that virus is secreted for more than a year.
   b. Pregnant friends should not perform child care (e.g., changing the child's diapers).
   c. Care should be taken to perform thorough hand washing after each diaper change and to dispose of diapers properly.
2. Instruct parents about long-term management of condition.
   a. Reinforce information about virus.
   b. If neurologic, cognitive, or developmental sequelae are evident, refer to community-based services.
   c. Emphasize importance of medical monitoring after acute episode.

Sequelae will necessitate further interventions beyond the scope of this section.

BIBLIOGRAPHY

Adler S: Molecular epidemiology of cytomegalovirus: viral transmission among children attending a day care center, their parents, and caretakers, *J Pediatr* 112(3):366, 1988.

American Academy of Pediatrics: *Report of the Committee on Infectious Diseases (The Red Book)*, Evanston, Ill, 1982, American Academy of Pediatrics.

Avery ME and Taeusch Jr HW: *Schaeffer's diseases of the newborn,* ed 5, Philadelphia, 1984, WB Saunders Co.

Friedman HM et al: Acquisition of cytomegalovirus infection among female employees at a pediatric hospital, *Pediatr Infect Dis* 3(3):233, 1984.

Haggerty L: TORCH: a literature review and implications for practice, *JOGN* 14(2):124, 1985.

Plotkin SA et al: The pathogenesis and prevention of human cytomegalovirus infection, *Pediatr Infect Dis* 3(1):67, 1984.

Pomeroy C et al: Cytomegalovirus: epidemiology and infection control, *Am J Infect Control* 15(3):107, 1987.

Urang S: Cytomegalovirus infection in pregnancy: case reports and literature review, *J Nurs Midwif Nurs* 13(1):44-53, 1990.

17 ❖ Diabetes Mellitus: Insulin-Dependent (Type I: IDDM)

PATHOPHYSIOLOGY

Insulin-dependent diabetes mellitus, or juvenile-onset diabetes (formerly known as juvenile onset diabetes mellitus) is caused by the negligible or complete lack of secretory capacity of the beta cells of the pancreas, resulting in insulin deficiency. Complete insulin deficiency necessitates the use of exogenous insulin to promote appropriate glucose use and to prevent complications related to elevated glucose levels, such as diabetic ketoacidosis and death. Insulin is necessary for the following physiologic functions: (1) to promote the use and storage of glucose in the liver, muscles, and adipose tissue for energy; (2) to inhibit and stimulate glycogenolysis or gluconeogenesis, depending on the body's requirements; and (3) to promote the use of fatty acids and ketones in cardiac and skeletal muscles. Insulin deficiency results in unrestricted glucose production without appropriate use, resulting in hyperglycemia and increased lipolysis and production of ketones, and, in turn, resulting in lipemia, ketonemia, and ketonuria. The insulin deficiency also heightens the effects of the counter-regulatory hormones—epinephrine, glucagon, cortisol, and growth hormone (refer to the box on p. 100 for the hormones' functions). Diagnosis of insulin-dependent diabetes mellitus is based on the patient's clinical history and initial symptoms. The cause is unknown, although the presence of human lymphocyte antigen (HLA) has been associated

Functions of Counterregulatory Hormones

Epinephrine

Inhibits uptake of glucose by muscle
Activates glycogenolysis and gluconeogenesis
Activates lipolysis, causing release of fatty acids and glycerol

Glucagon

Promotes production of glucose through glycogenolysis and gluconeogenesis

Cortisol

Limits glucose use by inhibiting muscle uptake
Increases glucose production by stimulating gluconeogenesis

Growth Hormones

Impede glucose uptake

---

with this disease. This presence suggests that the child may have a predisposition to a genetic defect in his or her immunologic response system, resulting in the destruction of pancreatic beta cells. Another relationship suggests that infection serves as a trigger (e.g., Coxsackie virus).

INCIDENCE

1. Fifteen percent of all diabetics have insulin-dependent diabetes mellitus.
2. Ninety-seven percent of newly diagnosed juvenile diabetics have insulin-dependent diabetes mellitus.
3. Mean age of onset is 11 years in females and 12.5 years in males.
4. The disease is more common in boys when diagnosed in preschool-age children.
5. The disease is more common in girls when diagnosed at 5 to 10 years of age.
6. Children are diagnosed more often in winter than in summer.

7. Diabetic ketoacidosis is a frequent cause of morbidity and sometimes of mortality.
8. Peak incidence age ranges: 5 to 7 years; puberty.

CLINICAL MANIFESTATIONS

Initial Effects

1. Polyuria
2. Polydipsia
3. Polyphagia
4. Yeast infections in girls
5. Recent weight loss (during a period of less than 3 weeks)
6. Fruity breath odor
7. Dehydration (usually 10%)
8. Diabetic ketoacidosis (see box on p. 102) — hyperglycemia, ketonemia, ketonuria, metabolic acidosis, Kussmaul respirations
9. Abdominal pain
10. Change in level of consciousness (due to progressive dehydration, acidosis, and hyperosmolality resulting in decreased cerebral oxygenation).

Long-Term Effects

1. Failure to grow at normal rate and delayed maturation
2. Neuropathy
3. Recurrent infection
4. Retinal and/or renal microvascular disease
5. Ischemic heart disease/arterial obstruction

COMPLICATIONS

1. Diabetic ketoacidosis
2. Coma
3. Hypokalemia and hyperkalemia
4. Hypocalcemia
5. Hypoglycemia
6. Osteopenia
7. Limited joint mobility (1%)
8. Microvascular changes resulting in retinopathy (maintaining a high degree of metabolic control is associated with delay and possible prevention of microvascular changes)

Signs of Diabetic Ketoacidosis

Kussmaul respirations (deep sighing respirations)

Hyperglycemia (serum glucose greater than 300 mg/dl)

Ketonuria (moderate to large amounts; positive ketostix)

Metabolic acidosis (pH <7.3; increased partial pressure of carbon dioxide [Pco_2]; decreased partial pressure of oxygen [Po_2]; sodium bicarbonate [$NaHCO_3$] <15 mEq/L)

Dehydration as a result of polyuria and polydipsia

Fruity breath odor

Electrolyte imbalance (falsely elevated potassium and sodium)

Potential for life-threatening cardiac arrhythmias (as a result of electrolyte imbalance)

Cerebral edema (caused by overzealous infusion of fluids)

Coma (caused by electrolyte imbalance and acidosis)

Death (mortality infrequent)

---

9. Myocardial infarction
10. Thromboemboli
11. Overwhelming infections

LABORATORY/DIAGNOSTIC TESTS

1. Initial serum blood glucose—300 mg/dl and higher
2. Serum ketones—greater than 3 mM/L
3. Serum pH—less than 7.3
4. Serum $NaHCO_3$—less than 15 mEq/L
5. Fasting blood glucose—venous plasma greater than or equal to 140 mg/dl; venous blood greater than or equal to 120 mg/dl; capillary blood greater than or equal to 120 mg/dl
6. Oral glucose tolerance—venous plasma greater than or equal to 200 mg/dl; venous blood greater than or equal

to 180 mg/dl; capillary blood greater than or equal to 200 mg/dl
7. Blood urea nitrogen (BUN), creatinine — increased because of interference of ketones in measurement
8. Serum calcium, magnesium, phosphate — decreased as a result of diuresis
9. Serum electrolytes (potassium [K^+] and sodium [Na^+]) — may be falsely elevated as a result of hyperosmolarity
10. White blood count — increased, with predominance of polymorphonuclear lymphocytes
11. Blood and urine cultures — increased in infections
12. Lead II electrocardiogram (ECG) — increased T wave with hyperkalemia
13. Immunoassay — to measure level of C-peptides after glucose challenge (to verify endogenous insulin secretion)
14. Twenty-four hour urine for glucose — considered more reliable parameter of urine glucose
15. Arterial blood gas values — to assess acidosis
16. Complete blood count

MEDICATION

Regular and NPH insulin is usually administered subcutaneously in highly individualized doses.

NURSING ASSESSMENT

1. Refer to Appendix A, *Nursing Assessments*.
2. Observe and document signs and symptoms of diabetic ketoacidosis.
3. Observe and document signs and symptoms of dehydration.

NURSING DIAGNOSES

Fluid volume deficit
High risk for injury
High risk for infection
Altered nutrition: less than body requirements
Knowledge deficit
Impaired home maintenance management

NURSING INTERVENTIONS

Diabetic Ketoacidosis

1. Monitor and observe child for change in status of diabetic ketoacidosis (see box on facing page).
2. Promote patient's hydration status.
   a. Monitor for dehydration.
      (1) Doughy or sticky skin turgor
      (2) Increased specific gravity
      (3) Depressed fontanels (in infants)
      (4) Dark circles under eyes
      (5) Vital signs (increased apical pulse, increased respiratory rate, decreased blood pressure)
   b. Monitor for fluid overload.
      (1) Signs of cerebral edema (decreased level of consciousness [LOC], fixed and dilated pupils)
      (2) Vital signs (increased apical pulse, increased respiratory rate, increased blood pressure)
   c. Record accurate input and output and specific gravity.
   d. Monitor administration of intravenous (IV) fluids.
      (1) Administer one half to two thirds of calculated fluid requirement during first 12 hours after admission; administer remaining amount during next 24 hours.
      (2) Administer IV fluids — initial dose — normal saline (NS) $\rightarrow$ 0.45 NS with K^+; 3 to 12 hours — 0.45 NS with K^+; 12 to 24 hours — 0.2 normal saline with 5% D_5W with K^+.
3. Monitor patient's glucose level hourly.
   a. Blood glucose should not fall below 250 mg/dl during first 12-hour treatment because too rapid a decline in osmolarity predisposes the patient to cerebral edema.
   b. Insulin can be administered by bolus or continuous infusion.
      (1) Bolus — initial dose of 2 U/kg regular insulin is followed by subcutaneous injections of 0.25 to 0.5 U/kg q6-8 hr until ketoacidosis has been treated.
      (2) Continuous infusion — priming dose of 0.1 U/kg is followed by 0.1 U/kg dose q1 hr. Regular insulin IV is administered separately from hydrating fluids. Decrease dose to 0.05 U/kg q1 hr when blood

glucose 300 mg/dl (dilution rate is 1 U/10 ml fluid). Follow with subcutaneous injections.
   c. Monitor urine for glucose and ketones with each voiding (dip stick).
4. Monitor for signs of complications.
   a. Acidosis
   b. Coma
   c. Hyperkalemia and hypokalemia
   d. Hypocalcemia
   e. Cerebral edema
   f. Hyponatremia

Recovery and Maintenance

1. Monitor and observe for signs of hypoglycemia and hyperglycemia.
2. Promote glucose control.
   a. Varying strengths of insulin are needed for the small doses required by small children and during periods of remission—with daily requirement of 25 U, less than 20 U; with daily requirement of 50 U, less than 30 U.
   b. Monitor urine and blood glucose TID to assess effectiveness of insulin.
   c. Adjust insulin requirements to food intake and exercise; with a total insulin dose of two thirds NPH and one third regular, administer two thirds of total dose ½ hour before breakfast and remaining one third dose ½ hour before dinner.
3. Promote adequate nutritional intake (see box on p. 106 for nutritional recommendations).
4. Monitor and establish appropriate relationship between insulin, dietary requirements, and exercise.
5. Provide emotional support to patient and family to promote psychosocial adaptation to diabetes.

Home Care

1. Instruct patient and parents about the management of diabetes.
   a. Insulin administration
   b. Dietary intake
   c. Urine testing

Diabetic Nutritional Requirements

Purpose of Dietary Plan

Provides the necessary intake of calories for energy requirements and appropriate distribution of nutrients (carbohydrates, fats, and proteins).

Energy Requirements

Carbohydrates	40% to 60% of total calories
Fats	25% to 40% of total calories
Proteins	15% to 30% of total calories

Rate of polyunsaturated to saturated fat should be at least 1:0. Total daily fat intake should be 420 g/day

Dietary Plans

Two exchange systems are used by diabetics: the American Diabetic Association (ADA) exchange group and the British Diabetic Association exchange system. The ADA exchange group has six exchange lists, which are for milk, fruit, vegetables, bread, meat, and fat. The exchange lists the equivalent amounts of calories and nutrients.

The British Diabetic Association exchange focuses on carbohydrate intake only. A liberal intake of protein is allowed and fats are less restricted.

General Information

1. Foods high in fiber retard carbohydrate absorption.
2. Foods have different glycemic responses (glycemic index).
3. Long delays between eating must be avoided.
4. Extra food must be consumed for increased activity (10 to 15 g of carbohydrate for every 30 to 45 minutes of activity).
5. Quantity of food needed between meals will vary according to increase or decrease in physical activity.

    d. Glucose monitoring
    e. Prevention of complications
    f. Care of hypoglycemic states
    g. Skin care
    h. Activity regimen
2. Initiate a home care referral to assess adherence and compliance to diabetic regimen.
3. Promote resumption of normal activities.
4. Promote ventilation by patient and parents of concerns and anxieties about diabetes as a chronic illness and its long-term management.

BIBLIOGRAPHY

Armstrong N: Coping with diabetes mellitus: a full time job, *Nurs Clin North Am* 22(3):559, 1987.

Bailie M: Heading off the complications of diabetes, *Contemp Pediatr* 6(1):87-102, 1989.

Chase HP: Monitoring glucose control and use of a diabetes control index in insulin-dependent diabetes mellitus, *Pediatr Ann* 12(9):643, 1983.

Clark L, Plotnick L: Insulin pumps in children with diabetes, *J Pediatr Health Care* 4:3-10, 1990.

Daneman D et al: Severe hypoglycemia in children with insulin-dependent diabetes mellitus: frequency and predisposing factors, *J Pediatr* 681-686, 1989.

Davis S et al: In-home bedside blood glucose control program; the importance of a quality control program, *J Pediatr Nurs* 4(5):353-356, 1989.

Drash A: The epidemiology of diabetes mellitus in children and adolescents, *Pediatr Ann* 12(9):629, 1983.

Frey M, Denyes M: Health and illness self care in adolescents with IDDM: a test of Orem's theory, *ANS* 12(1):67-75, 1989.

Gallo A: Family management style in juvenile diabetes: a case illustration, *J Pediatr Nurs* 5(1):23-32, 1990.

Jackson R: Growth and maturation of children with insulin-dependent diabetes mellitus, *Pediatr Clin North Am* 31(3):545, 1984.

Jenkins D: Lente carbohydrate: a newer approach to the dietary management of diabetes? *Diabetes Care* 5:634, 1982.

Lamborlane W, Press C: Insulin infusion pump treatment of type 1 diabetes, *Pediatr Clin North Am* 31(3):721, 1984.

Lebovitz H: Etiology and pathogenesis of diabetes mellitus, *Pediatr Clin North Am* 31(3):521, 1984.

Lipman T: What causes diabetes? *MCN* 13(1):40, 1988.

Lipman T et al: A developmental approach to diabetes in children: birth through preschool, *MCN* 14:255-259, 1989.

Lipman T et al: A developmental approach to diabetes in children: school age — adolescence, *MCN* 14:330-332, 1989.

Montana V: Glucose meters, *J Pediatr Nurs* 4(2):132-136, 1989.

Rosenbloom A: Skeletal and joint manifestations of childhood diabetes, *Pediatr Clin North Am* 31(3):569, 1984.

Skyler J: Dietary planning in insulin-dependent diabetes mellitus, *Pediatr Ann* 12(9):652, 1983.

Smith K et al: Issues of managing diabetes in children and adolescents: a multifamily group approach, *Child Health Care* 8:49-52, 1989.

Sperling M: Diabetic ketoacidosis, *Pediatr Clin North Am* 31(3):591, 1984.

18 ❖ Diarrhea

PATHOPHYSIOLOGY

Diarrhea refers to the loose consistency of stools rather than to the frequency of the stools. Chronic diarrhea is characterized by its severity and duration (greater than 2 weeks). The loss of fluids and electrolytes results in dehydration and acidosis. Furthermore, the constant movement of stools is irritating to the gastrointestinal tract, causing its inflammation and reducing its absorptive power. The undigested carbohydrates stimulate intestinal bacterial growth, resulting in increased peristalsis. In addition, the undigested carbohydrates ferment, resulting in the release of lactic and acetic acids, which cause further inflammation of the bowel and acidosis. The presence of carbohydrates in the gastrointestinal tract also causes greater amounts of fluids to be absorbed from the intestines, contributing to the watery stools. Chronic diarrhea occurs primarily in infants less than 3 months of age.

A variety of causative factors are associated with acute infectious and chronic diarrhea and include (1) infections caused by viral, bacterial, parasitic, and fungal agents (Table 1); (2) malabsorption syndromes; (3) immunoglobulin deficiencies (IgA and/or IgG deficiency); (4) inflammatory bowel disease; (5) endocrine and metabolic disorders; (6) GI food protein allergy; (7) carbohydrate intolerance; (8) dietetic candy and gum; (9) antibiotics; (10) malnutrition; and (11) postgastroenteritis syndrome. The most common causes of chronic diarrhea are postinfectious gastroenteritis syndrome, GI food protein allergy, and transient immunoglobulin deficiencies.

Diarrhea that resolves quickly is usually caused by dietary factors, whereas persistent diarrhea is associated with one of the previously mentioned causative factors. Prognosis is favorable with treatment. Death is rare, although in developing countries up to 15% of the children die from diarrhea and dehydration before their third birthday.

INCIDENCE

1. Five percent of pediatric office visits are for treatment of GI disorders.
2. Acute gastroenteritis is the second most common condition affecting children (the cold is first).
3. Fifteen percent to 45% of the specific causes of diarrhea are unknown.
4. Three to 5 billion cases of diarrhea occur worldwide.
5. Five to 10 million deaths from diarrhea occur in the countries of Asia, Africa, and Latin America annually.

CLINICAL MANIFESTATIONS

1. Electrolyte imbalance (especially Na^+ and K^+ loss)
2. Increased frequency and loose consistency of stools
3. Dehydration (poor skin turgor, dry mucous membranes, decreased weight, depressed fontanels, decreased urinary output, increased specific gravity)
4. Acidosis (Kussmaul respirations)
5. Anorexia
6. Generalized weakness
7. Malaise
8. Vomiting
9. Fever
10. Abdominal cramping due to increased peristalsis

COMPLICATIONS

1. Anemia (decreased absorption of iron and vitamin B_{12})
2. Decreased muscle tone (decreased protein intake)
3. Decreased subcutaneous tissue (decreased fat)
4. Skin hemorrhages (deficiency of vitamins C and K)
5. Cheilosis and small, red tongue (vitamin B deficiency)

6. Dry, scaly, flaking skin (fatty acid and vitamin A deficiency)
7. Enlarged liver and spleen (protein deficiency)
8. Peripheral edema (protein deficiency)
9. Delay in increase of height, weight, head size as indicated on growth curve, which is long-term effect of malabsorption

LABORATORY/DIAGNOSTIC TESTS

1. Hematest (to check for blood in stool because of excessive mucosal irritation)
2. Stools' culture and sensitivity, ova and parasites (to identify pathogen)
3. pH <6 (indicates disaccharide and monosaccharide malabsorption)
4. Reducing substances (plus result indicates lactose and glucose malabsorption)
5. Serum albumin and globulin (presence indicates protein malabsorption)
6. Sweat chloride (to rule out cystic fibrosis, positive results indicative of cystic fibrosis)
7. Serum folate (to assess small bowel absorption) — disease of small bowel results in decreased absorption of folate
8. Serum carotene and cholesterol (to assess bowel fat absorption) — decreased level indicates impaired absorption capacity
9. Serum radioallergosorbent (to determine presence of milk proteins)
10. Sigmoidoscopy (inspection of rectum and sigmoid colon)
11. Upper GI x-ray examination (uses contrast medium to visualize the esophagus, stomach, and duodenum for assessment of mucosal wall and GI tract motility)
12. Rectal biopsy (diagnostic for identification of specified bowel disease)
13. Urinalysis and culture (to detect urinary tract infection)

MEDICATIONS

Antibiotics are used to treat infections. The choice of antibiotic is dependent on culture and sensitivity results.

Table 1. Causative Factors Associated with Chronic Diarrhea

Pathogen	Epidemiologic features	Stool characteristics
Bacteria		
Escherichia coli		
Enterotoxigenic	Common cause of "summer" diarrhea in developing countries and of traveler's diarrhea	Profuse, watery, no pus or blood
Invasion	Not defined	Scanty; initially watery, later with pus and mucus; may become bloody
Enteropathogenic	Common cause of outbreaks of diarrhea in nurseries; usually occurs in summer	Profuse and watery
Campylobacter fetus *C. jejuni*	One of most common causes of bacterial diarrhea; peaks worldwide during warm season	Initially profuse and watery, foul smelling; later with pus, mucus, and blood
Yersinia enterocolitica	Most cases reported in Canada and Europe; occasional cases in USA; peak incidence in summer	Variable consistency; with pus and blood in one fourth of cases

Salmonella choleraesuis *S. paratyphi* *S. typhimurium* *S. agona*	Common cause of epidemics in nurseries	Watery, mucus, blood
Shigella dysenteriae *S. alkalescens* *S. flexneri* *S. sonnei*	Prevalent in developing countries and in Central America	Blood, mucus, pus
Viruses		
Rotavirus	Occurs during cooler months in temperate climates; accounts for 39% to 63% of hospitalizations	Watery
Norwalk	Occurs in epidemics; primarily affects school-age children and adolescents	Watery

Adapted from San Joaquin V, Marks M: New agents in diarrhea, *Pediatr Infec Dis* 1(1):53, 1982.

NURSING ASSESSMENT

Refer to "Gastrointestinal Assessment" in Appendix A.

NURSING DIAGNOSES

High risk for fluid volume deficit
Impaired skin integrity
Pain
Knowledge deficit

NURSING INTERVENTIONS

1. Promote and monitor child's fluid and electrolyte balance.
   a. Monitor intravenous (IV) fluids.
   b. Monitor intake and output (weigh diapers).
   c. Assess hydration status.
   d. Assess child's ability to rehydrate by mouth.
2. Prevent further GI irritability.
   a. Provide nothing by mouth initially to allow bowel rest.
   b. Assess child's ability to take nourishment by mouth (i.e., first provide clear liquid, then a soft diet, and then a regular diet).
   c. Avoid use of milk products.
   d. Consult with dietician about selection of foods.
3. Prevent skin irritation and breakdown.
   a. Lubricate dry, scaling skin to prevent cracking.
   b. Apply zinc oxide or lubricating ointment to rectum and perineum (acidic stools irritate skin).
   c. Change diapers frequently.
   d. Wash perineum with mild soap and water, and expose perineum to air.
4. Conserve child's expenditure of energy (lacks calories needed for metabolism).
   a. Maintain bed rest until status improves.
   b. Organize nursing activities to allow intermittent rest periods.
5. Enteric isolation for infectious gastroenteritis.
6. Provide for child's developmental needs during hospitalization.

   a. Provide age-appropriate toys (see Appendix B, *Growth and Development*).
   b. Incorporate home routine into hospitalization (e.g., feeding practices, bedtime ritual).
   c. Encourage ventilation of feelings through age-appropriate means.
7. Provide emotional support to family.
   a. Encourage ventilation of concerns.
   b. Refer to social service as needed.
   c. Provide for physical comforts (e.g., place to sleep, bathe).

Home Care

1. Instruct parents and child about personal and environmental hygiene.
   a. Safe drinking water
   b. Sanitary disposal of excreta
   c. Sanitary food preparation
   d. Toileting practices
2. Reinforce dietary information provided to parents about menu planning.

BIBLIOGRAPHY

Ament M, Barclay G: Chronic diarrhea, *Pediatr Ann* 11(1):124, 1982.

Bellet P: *The diagnostic approach to common symptoms and signs in infants, children and adolescents,* Philadelphia, 1989, Lea & Febiger.

Brown K et al: Effect of continual oral feeding on clinical and nutritional outcomes of acute diarrhea in children, *J Pediatr* 112(2):191, 1988.

Copeland F: Chronic diarrhea in infancy, *Am J Nurs* 77(3):461, 1977.

DeWitt T: Diarrhea. In Green M, Haggerty R, editors: *Ambulatory pediatrics,* Philadelphia, 1990, WB Saunders, pp 189-193.

Drumm B et al: *Campylobacter pylorides* — associated primary gastritis in children, *Pediatrics* 80:192-195, 1987.

Fleisher D, Ament M: Diarrhea, red diapers, and child abuse, *Clin Pediatr* 17(9):820, 1977.

Fontana M et al: Simple clinical score and laboratory-based method to predict bacterial etiology of acute diarrhea in childhood, *J Pediatr Infect Dis* 6(12):1088, 1987.

Gellis S, Kagan B: *Current pediatric therapy 13,* Philadelphia, 1990, WB Saunders.

Gryboski J: Chronic diarrhea. In Gluck L, editor: *Current problems in pediatrics,* St. Louis, 1979, Mosby–Year Book.

Merritt R et al: Treatment of protracted diarrhea of infancy, *Am J Dis Child* 138:770, 1984.

San Joaquin V, Marks M: New agents in diarrhea, *Pediatr Infect Dis* 1(1):53, 1982.

19 ❖ Disseminated Intravascular Coagulation

PATHOPHYSIOLOGY

Disseminated intravascular coagulation (DIC) is triggered by an illness such as sepsis, respiratory distress syndrome, shock, or malaria. DIC causes abnormal stimulation of the normal coagulation process, with ensuing development of widespread small thrombi in the microvasculature. DIC can be described in terms of the two processes that are activated. Initially, the injury to tissue caused by the primary disorder (e.g., infection or trauma) activates a mechanism that releases thrombin, which is necessary for blood clotting, into the circulation. Thrombin, in turn, activates the process that is necessary for the breakdown of fibrin and fibrinogen, resulting in fibrin/fibrinogen degradation products (FDP). FDP acts as an anticoagulant. DIC is characterized by the following three major symptoms: (1) generalized hemorrhage; (2) ischemia caused by thrombi, which results in organ ischemia (kidneys are particularly susceptible); and (3) anemia. Prognosis is dependent on the severity of the primary and secondary conditions.

CLINICAL MANIFESTATIONS

1. Spontaneous bleeding
2. Bruising
3. Pain

4. Hypoxia
5. Petechiae
6. Ecchymosis
7. Symptoms based on severity and extent of organic involvement
   a. Renal—hematuria
   b. Central nervous system—mental changes

COMPLICATIONS

1. Alteration in mental status
2. Coolness or cyanosis of extremity leading to gangrenous conditions

LABORATORY/DIAGNOSTIC TESTS

Refer to Table 2.
1. Clotting assays
2. Cellular tests
3. Fibrinolytic tests
4. Daily blood smears (to assess number of platelets and extent of microangiopathic hemolysis)
5. Hematocrit (Hct) q6-12 hr
6. Blood typing and cross match

MEDICATIONS

1. Heparin—used to decrease clot formation since it is an antagonist to thrombin. Heparin is discontinued as platelet count rises (used for specific types of DIC).
2. Whole blood or blood products—given to replace depleted clotting factor (risky—may cause increased clotting)

NURSING ASSESSMENT

1. Refer to "Hematologic Assessment" in Appendix A.
2. Assess bleeding sites.
3. Assess for signs of bleeding.

NURSING DIAGNOSES

High risk for injury
Altered tissue perfusion
High risk for impaired gas exchange
Pain

Table 2. Basic Tests for Disseminated Intravascular Coagulation

Test	Results
Clotting Assays	
Prothrombin time	Minimally to grossly prolonged
Activated partial thromboplastin time	Variable (short, normal, long)
Fibrinogen*	Usually depressed
Thrombin time*	Usually prolonged
Factor analyses	Variable (low, normal, elevated)
Cellular	
Platelet count*	Usually depressed
Red cell morphology	Often abnormal
Fibrinolytic	
Fibrinogen degradation products*	Usually present
Plasminogen	Usually depressed
Euglobulin lysis time	Variable (often long, sometimes short)
Serial thrombin time	Variable (often prolonged)
Paracoagulation	Often positive (low specificity)

Reprinted with permission from Daniel Deykin: The challenge of disseminated intravascular coagulation, *N Engl J Med* 283:12, 642, 1970.
*Rapid, usually diagnostic for DIC, but results may be due to liver disease.

NURSING INTERVENTIONS

1. Monitor child's clinical status; report any significant changes.
   a. Monitor for signs of hemorrhage—bleeding, dyspnea, lethargy, pallor, increased apical pulse, decreased blood pressure, headache, dizziness, muscle weakness, restlessness.

b. Test output (guaiac and stool, nasopharynx, urine) for bleeding.
2. Promote and monitor adequate oxygenation.
   a. Elevate head of bed.
   b. Monitor child's response to administration of oxygen.
   c. Monitor respiratory status (respiratory rate, signs of respiratory distress).
3. Provide comfort measures to alleviate or control pain (bone and joint).
   a. Immobilize joints.
   b. Apply hot or cold compresses.
   c. Use bed cradle.
   d. Administer medication.
4. Monitor child's therapeutic and untoward response to administration of blood products.
   a. Platelets—administer 1 u (10 to 50 mg)/5 to 10 kg; repeat q12-24 hr; used to decrease bleeding.
   b. Fresh frozen plasma—administer 10 to 15 ml/kg q12-24 hr; used to replace deficiencies of fibrinogen, prothrombin, factor II, factor VIII, and other deficient factors.
   c. Fresh whole blood and packed red blood cells—used to maintain Hct.
5. Monitor neonate's response to exchange transfusion (neonates cannot tolerate volume load of multiple infusions).
6. Monitor child's therapeutic and untoward response to administration of heparin; children with marked thrombosis (i.e., with a platelet count less than 20,000, fibrinogen level less than 75 mg/dl, prothrombin time [PT] greater than 25 seconds, and partial thromboplastin time [PTT] twice normal value) are managed with heparin.
   a. Loading dose—50 u/kg
   b. 10 to 20 u/kg q1 hr intravenous fast drip
   c. Intravenous push—50 to 75 u/kg q4 hr

BIBLIOGRAPHY

Esparaz B et al: Disseminated intravascular coagulation, *Crit Care Nurs Quart* 13(2):7-13, 1990.

Levin D, Morriss F, Moore G, editors: *A practical guide to pediatric intensive care*, St. Louis, 1984, Mosby–Year Book.

Mazer G: Disseminated intravascular coagulation, *Am J Nurs* 73(12):2067, 1973.

O'Brian B, Woods S: The paradox of DIC, *Am J Nurs* 78(11):1878, 1978.

20 ❖ Drowning and Near-Drowning

PATHOPHYSIOLOGY

Drowning causes death from hypoxia that results from submersion. Near-drowning refers to survival, at least temporarily, from the lethal effects of hypoxia. Drowning can be classified into four types: wet, dry, salt water, and fresh water. The factors affecting prognosis include the following: (1) length of time immersed; (2) temperature of immersion fluid; and (3) time until effective CPR provided. The extent of brain injury is strongly associated with cerebral hypoxia and metabolic acidemia.

Dry drowning (occurs in 10% of cases) results in airway obstruction after the aspiration of small amounts of fluids. It produces reflux closure of the glottis, as well as apnea.

Wet drowning (majority of cases) results in the initial aspiration of fluids, causing laryngospasm and vomiting. The resultant asphyxia causes the glottis to relax, allowing the lungs to be flooded with the immersion fluids.

Drowning results in aspirated fluids creating an inflammatory response in the alveoli, interfering with oxygen diffusion and disrupting ventilation. The sequence of physiologic reactions includes bronchospasm, which obstructs the airways, causing increased hypoxemia, and cerebral hypoxia, which results in severe metabolic acidosis and respiratory and cardiac failure. If hypertonic fluid is drawn into the alveoli, it causes hypovolemia, hemoconcentration, and increased serum electrolyte concentration.

Fresh-water drowning results in the aspirated fluid's being rapidly drawn out of the alveoli into the intravascular space. This shift of fluids causes hypervolemia, resulting in hemodilution and decreased serum electrolyte concentration.

INCIDENCE

1. Drowning is the second leading cause of death in children and young adults ages 1 to 25 years.
2. Drowning accounts for one third of the deaths in children less than 15 years old.
3. Between ages 5 and 13 years, 75% of the victims are boys.
4. Ratio of incidence of boys to girls less than 5 years old is 2:1.
5. Forty percent of the victims are less than 4 years old.
6. Highest incidence is among 10 to 19 year olds.
7. Drownings account for more than 6000 deaths per year.
8. More than 50% of victims under 10 years of age drown in pools.
9. Peak incidence occurs during summer months.
10. Younger children most often drown (1) in unprotected pools and ponds; (2) after falling through ice; and (3) in bathtubs after a fall.
11. Older children most often drown (1) while swimming; (2) during unsupervised water sports; (3) while boating; (4) after hyperventilating before diving; and (5) because of environmental hazards or associated alcohol ingestion.

CLINICAL MANIFESTATIONS

1. Respiratory rate—ranges from rapid, shallow breathing to apnea
2. Cyanosis
3. Pink, frothy sputum
4. Pulmonary edema
5. Tachycardia
6. Arrhythmias
7. Hypotension or hypertension
8. Headaches
9. Lethargy
10. Agitation

11. Disorientation
12. Twitching
13. Convulsions
14. Coma with irreversible brain injury
15. Decorticate or decerebrate posturing
16. Flaccidity
17. Hyperthermia (temperature above 42° C)
18. Metabolic or respiratory acidosis
19. Hyposthenuric diuresis (returns to normal renal function after several days)

COMPLICATIONS

1. Renal failure
2. Ventricular dysrhythmias
3. Aspiration pneumonia
4. Pulmonary interstitial fibrosis
5. Hypoxic encephalopathy
6. Pancreatic necrosis
7. Disseminated intravascular coagulation (DIC)
8. Secondary drowning

Secondary Drowning

Secondary drowning (edema in the lungs not due to the immediate drowning but to increased pulmonary capillary permeability) occurs in one out of five near-drowning cases. Increased intracranial pressure (ICP) and hypoxic brain cell injury may also develop. Secondary drowning symptoms may appear 24 to 72 hours after the near-drowning episode. The clinical manifestations include the following:

Coma
Increased pulmonary edema
Circulatory collapse
Hypoxemia
Respiratory acidosis
Development of hypercapnia

LABORATORY/DIAGNOSTIC TESTS

1. Chest x-ray examination — variable findings (from scattered parenchymal infiltrates to extensive pulmonary edema)

2. Electrocardiogram (ECG)
3. Computerized axial tomography (CAT) scan
4. ICP monitoring—maintain cerebral perfusion greater than 50 to 60 torr
5. Electroencephalogram (EEG)—to assess seizure activity and document brain death (seizure activity is decreased in fresh-water drowning and is increased in salt-water drowning)
6. Serum osmolarity—maintained at approximately 320 mOsm/L
7. Complete blood count (CBC), hematocrit (Hct), hemoglobin (Hgb)—decreased values caused by hemodilution (fresh-water drowning); increased values caused by hemoconcentration (salt-water drowning)
8. Serum electrolytes—decreased values caused by hemodilution except for an increase in serum potassium caused by hemolysis (fresh-water drowning); increased values caused by hemoconcentration (salt-water drowning)
9. Blood urea nitrogen (BUN)—increased in fresh-water drowning and decreased in salt-water drowning
10. Creatinine—increased in fresh-water drowning and decreased in salt-water drowning
11. Arterial blood gas values—to determine respiratory and metabolic acidosis
12. Chest x-ray examination—positive results are consistent with pulmonary edema and respiratory distress syndrome
13. Culture and sensitivity (C and S)—used to detect superimposed respiratory infection

MEDICATIONS

1. Pancuronium (Parulon)—for children more than 10 years of age; initial dose—0.04 to 1 mg/kg IV, then one fifth of initial dose q30-60 min
2. Furosemide (Lasix)—0.5 to 1 mg/kg/dose only if pulmonary edema or fluid retention present
3. Mannitol—1 to 2 g/kg IV over 30-60 min in 20% dextrose solution; 5 to 10 ml/kg IV over 30-60 min
4. Pentobarbital (Nembutal)—3 to 5 mg/kg intramuscularly (IM)

NURSING ASSESSMENT

Refer to "Respiratory Assessment" and "Neuromuscular Assessment" in Appendix A.

NURSING DIAGNOSES

Altered tissue perfusion
Ineffective airway clearance
Ineffective breathing patterns
Decreased cardiac output
Sensory/perceptual alterations
High risk for fluid volume excess
Altered nutrition: less than body requirements
High risk for injury
Altered growth and development
Guilt
Knowledge deficit

NURSING INTERVENTIONS

Emergency Care

Prompt action is essential since irreversible central nervous system (CNS) damage can occur within 3 to 7 minutes after immersion and within 1 minute after cardiopulmonary arrest. Cardiopulmonary resuscitation (CPR) should be instituted immediately.

Critical/Acute Care

1. Establish and maintain patency of airway.
   a. Suction as needed.
   b. Insert nasogastric (NG) tube (to prevent aspiration of vomitus).
2. Monitor and record child's response to oxygen therapy.
   a. Perform respiratory assessment (frequency is dependent on status).
   b. Monitor use of ventilator and respiratory equipment.
   c. Monitor CVP and arterial lines.
   d. Monitor use of intermittent positive pressure breathing (IPPB)/positive end-expiratory pressure (PEEP).
3. Monitor and record child's level of neurologic functioning.

    a. Perform neurologic assessment (frequency is dependent on status).

    b. Observe and report signs of ICP (lethargy, increased blood pressure, decreased respiratory rate, increased apical pulse, dilated pupils).

4. Monitor and maintain fluid balance.

    a. Record accurate input and output.

    b. Maintain patency and care for Foley catheter.

    c. Maintain fluid restriction with presence of cerebral edema (800 ml/m^2).

5. Monitor and maintain homeostatic temperature regulation (decreased oxygen requirements).

    a. Monitor temperature through flexible probe thermometers and telethermometers.

    b. Provide cooling mattress.

    c. Administer antipyretics.

6. Provide and maintain adequate nutritional intake.

    a. Assess child's capacity for route of nutritional intake (NG/po).

    b. Assess child's capacity to tolerate NG/po feedings (check for residuals and vomiting).

    c. Advance amount and type of nutritional intake.

7. Observe and report signs of complications (see "Complications").

8. Monitor child's response to physical therapy regimen.

9. Monitor child's therapeutic response to and any side effects from medications.

10. Provide age-appropriate quiet diversional activities and toys.

11. Provide emotional support to the child and family during child's hospitalization.

12. Provide family support in case of death.

    a. Provide emotional support during initial acute grief.

    b. Allow and encourage the parents' ventilation of feelings of guilt.

    c. Provide parents with names of community resources for long-term follow-up.

    d. Provide follow-up care with phone call or conference 1 to 2 months after death to assess and counsel the bereaved parents and family.

Preventive Care

Instruct parents about instituting the following preventive measures: CPR; water safety and swimming lessons for child; waterproof backyard (e.g., pool cover, fence enclosures); measures to raise awareness of environmental hazards; and appropriate supervision during use of pool.

Long-Term Care

1. Instruct parents about the proper administration of medication to enhance compliance.
   a. Correct dose, route, time
   b. Observation for side effects
2. Promote and maintain patency of airway.
   a. Suction to maintain patency of airway.
   b. Perform percussion and postural drainage as needed.
   c. Change position q2 hr.
   d. Raise head of bed to semi-Fowler's position to increase lung expansion.
   e. Provide or teach tracheostomy care if appropriate.
3. Provide for child's nutritional needs.
   a. Nasogastric (NG) tube
      (1) Check placement before feeding and q4 hr.
      (2) Check for residuals before feeding and q4 hr.
      (3) Monitor input and output.
      (4) Provide oral care q4 hr or every shift.
      (5) Monitor for problems (e.g., aspiration, abdominal distention).
   b. Gastrostomy tube
      (1) Raise head of bed to semi-Fowler's position and place patient on right side before feeding.
      (2) Check for reflux before feeding; feed residual again and subtract from amount of next feeding.
      (3) Provide oral care.
      (4) Monitor input and output.
4. Prevent and protect child from infection.
   a. Perform catheter care q24 hr.
   b. Change catheter every week.
   c. Provide pulmonary toilet.
   d. Prevent skin breakdown.
5. Provide skin care to prevent skin breakdown and infection.

a. Keep creases and folds of skin clean and dry.
b. Change position q2 hr.
c. Use sheepskin and/or waterbed.
d. Lubricate skin with lotion.
e. Change diapers frequently.
f. Use lubricating ointment in perineal area.

6. Prevent drying and ulceration of eyes.
   a. Lubricate eyes q2-4 hr.
   b. Tape eyes closed if necessary.

7. Provide environmental stimulation (child may hear even though unresponsive).
   a. Sing and talk to child as if he or she were awake.
   b. Use music box or favorite songs to provide musical stimulation.
   c. Provide different textures and shapes for child to touch.
   d. Massage and touch child during interactions.

8. Provide emotional support to parents (see "Critical/Acute Care," p. 127).

BIBLIOGRAPHY

Counseling to prevent household and environmental injuries, *Am Fam Physician* 42(1):135-142.

Florete O et al: Airway pressure release ventilation in a patient with acute pulmonary injury, *Chest: Cardiopulm J* 96(3):679-682, 1989.

Gonzalez-Rothi R: Near-drowning consensus and controversies in pulmonary and cerebral resuscitation, *Heart Lung* 16(5):474, 1987.

Hartsell M: New technology for safety and research . . . pool alert . . . wrist actigraph, *J Pediatr Nurs* 2(3):212, 1987.

Joy C: Pediatric cerebral resuscitation, *Critic Care Clin North Am* 1(1):181-187, 1989.

Martin L: Near-drowning and cold water immersion, *Ann Emerg Med* 13:263, 1984.

McKinley M: Near-drowning: a nursing challenge, *Critic Care Nurs* 9(10):52-54, 56, 58, 1989.

Nelson N, Beckel J: Near-drowning, *J Emerg Nurs* 16(2):119-123, 1990.

Sekar T et al: Survival after prolonged submersion in cold water without neurologic sequelae, *Arch Intern Med* 140:775, 1980.

Shea K, Folick M: Water sport injuries, *Orthoped Nurs* 8(6):11-17, 1989.

Shovein L et al: Near-drowning, *Am J Nurs* 89(5):680-686, 1989.

Sims J et al: Marine bacteria complicating sea water near-drowning and marine wounds: a hypothesis, *Ann Emerg Med* 12(4):212, 1983.

Stanford T: Near-drowning, *Emergency Medicine* 21(6):30, 32-33, 1989.

21 ❖ Epiglottitis

PATHOPHYSIOLOGY

Epiglottitis is an acute bacterial infection of the epiglottis and the surrounding areas (the aryepiglottic folds and the supraglottic area) that causes airway obstruction. The infection is caused by *Haemophilus influenzae* type B or, on rare occasions, streptococci or pneumococci. Onset is sudden and progresses rapidly, causing acute respiratory difficulty. This condition requires emergency medical measures because a fatal outcome can occur. The child is extubated when the epiglottis appears normal and the child is able to breathe around the tube (usually 48 to 72 hours after antibiotic treatment is started).

INCIDENCE

1. Boys, ages 2 to 7 years, most often are affected.
2. Incidence is highest in winter but can occur anytime.
3. Epiglottitis may be preceded by upper respiratory infection.

CLINICAL MANIFESTATIONS

1. Respiratory difficulty, which can progress to severe respiratory distress in a matter of minutes or hours (dyspnea)
2. Dysphagia
3. Drooling
4. Edematous, cherry-red epiglottis

5. Red and inflamed oral cavity
6. Breathing in tripod position
7. Complaining of intense sore throat
8. Sudden increase in temperature
9. Muffled voice
10. Pale, shallow color
11. Decreased breath sounds
12. Substernal or suprasternal and intercostal retractions
13. Bilateral cervical adenitis
14. Lethargy

COMPLICATIONS

1. Airway obstruction
2. Laryngospasm
3. Death

LABORATORY/DIAGNOSTIC TESTS

1. Arterial blood gas values (decreased pH, decreased partial pressure of oxygen [Po_2], increased partial pressure of carbon dioxide [Pco_2])
2. Lateral neck radiogram (to confirm diagnosis)
3. Throat culture (to rule out other bacterial infections)
4. Broad culture (to rule out other bacterial infections)
5. Direct laryngoscopy (performed in operating room to prevent complications; to confirm diagnosis)

MEDICATIONS

1. *Haemophilus influenzae* Type B (HIB) vaccination; vaccine schedule recommended by American Academy of Pediatrics — vaccinate beginning at 2 months in three-dose series with doses given at 2-month intervals
2. Antibiotics:
    a. Chloramphenicol (IV) 50 mg/kg/24 hr
    b. Ampicillin (IV) 200 mg/kg/24 hr
    c. Once antibiotic sensitivity results are obtained, the specific, effective antibiotic is continued and the others are discontinued

NURSING ASSESSMENT

Refer to "Respiratory Assessment" in Appendix A.

NURSING DIAGNOSES

High risk for suffocation
Ineffective airway clearance
Ineffective breathing pattern
Altered tissue perfusion
High risk for infection
High risk for fluid volume deficit
Anxiety
Altered family processes

NURSING INTERVENTIONS

1. Monitor respiratory status (including vital signs).
   a. Temperature, apical pulse, respiratory rate, blood pressure
   b. Presence of pulmonary congestion
   c. Presence of intercostal retractions
   d. Presence of circumoral cyanosis
   e. Use of accessory muscles
   f. Arterial blood gas values
2. Observe and report signs of increased respiratory distress or changes in respiratory status.
3. Maintain upright position (semi-Fowler's or high-Fowler's position) to facilitate breathing.
4. Prepare child preoperatively for airway insertion (endotracheal tube or a tracheostomy); prepare age-appropriate explanations before airway insertion.
5. Assist and support physician during emergency procedure.
   a. Ventilate through bag and mask if child becomes obstructed before reaches operating room.
   b. Observe and monitor respiratory status during airway insertion.
6. Maintain patency of airway.
   a. Apply mist collar to airway.
   b. Anticipate and assist in instituting emergency measures.
7. Provide tracheostomy care (if tracheostomy is inserted).
   a. Maintain patent airway.
   b. Monitor cardiopulmonary status through cardiac monitor.

   c. Use aseptic technique when suctioning.
   d. Clean tracheostomy site.
   e. Observe tracheostomy for incrustation.
8. Monitor action and side effects of prescribed medications.
   a. Chloramphenicol (for bone marrow depression; can cause aplastic anemia)
9. Assess hydration status: monitor input and output and specific gravity.
10. Provide for child's developmental needs during hospitalization.
    a. Provide age-appropriate toys (see Appendix B, *Growth and Development*).
    b. Incorporate home routines into hospital routine (e.g., feeding practices and bedtime rituals).
    c. Encourage ventilation of feelings through age-appropriate means.
11. Provide emotional support to family.
    a. Encourage ventilation of concerns.
    b. Refer to social service as needed.
    c. Provide for family's physical comforts (e.g., place to sleep, bathe).
12. Provide consistent nursing care to promote trust and to alleviate anxiety.

BIBLIOGRAPHY

Belkengren R et al: Pediatric management problems: diagnosis of epiglottitis, *Clin Pediatr* 13(4):257, 1987.

Forbes R: Acute epiglottitis: overcoming the challenge, *Can Oper Room Nurse J* 3(4):6, 1985.

Freid E: Acute epiglottitis, *Issues Compr Pediatr Nurs* 4:29, 1980.

Lepow M, Hethington S: Respiratory tract infections. In Green M, Haggerty R, eds: *Ambulatory pediatrics,* Philadelphia, 1990, WB Saunders.

Lewis J, Gartner J, Galvis A: A protocol for management of acute epiglottitis, *Clin Pediatr* 17(6):494, 1978.

Mauro R et al: Differentiation of epiglottitis and laryngotracheobronchitis in the child with stridor, *Am J Dis Child* 142:679-682, 1988.

Neff J: Epiglottitis, *J Emerg Nurs* 13(3):184, 1987.

Nemes J et al: Epiglottitis: ED nursing management, *J Emerg Nurs* 14(2):70, 1988.

Simkins R: Croup and epiglottitis, *Am J Nurs* 81(3):519, 1981.
Stokes D: The croup syndrome. In Gellis A, Kagan B: *Current pediatric therapy 13*, Philadelphia, 1990, WB Saunders, 111-112.
Wagener J: Respiratory emergencies: managing upper airway obstruction in children, *Consultant* 24(9):115, 1984.

22 ❖ Foreign Body Aspiration

PATHOPHYSIOLOGY

Foreign body aspiration refers to the lodgment of an object or substance in the airway. Eighty-seven percent of foreign body aspiration is caused by carelessness. This carelessness includes improper chewing of food, rapid eating, and laughing or running with food in the mouth.

The foreign body tends to lodge most often in the cricopharyngeal area because of the strong, propulsive pharyngeal muscles that move it to this location. Most objects aspirated by children are small enough to pass through the trachea and lodge in either of the main bronchi (most often the right main bronchus because the left main bronchus has a large angulation that impedes progression). Alveoli distal to the obstruction will collapse, resulting in atelectasis. Hyperinflation and pneumothorax occur as air passages enlarge during inspiration and decrease during expiration. Superior, basilar, and lateral lobes are most often affected.

The severity of symptoms depends on the size of the object and the degree of the obstruction. Generally, aspiration of a foreign body (e.g., a pin, coin, bone, button, marble, jelly bean, seed, small detachable part from a toy, popcorn, or pebble) follows a benign course. Aspiration of foreign bodies containing saturated fats (e.g., nuts) causes immediate irritation and inflammation of mucosal tissue. The longer a foreign body remains lodged in place, the less is the likelihood that it will move spontaneously because of the increasing edema, swelling, and inflammation. Prognosis is good even with presence of marked inflammation and dilated airways.

INCIDENCE

1. Forty percent of children who aspirate foreign bodies are not observed doing so by parents.
2. Children more than 5 years of age are less likely to be observed aspirating foreign bodies.
3. Foreign body aspiration accounts for more than 2000 deaths per year.
4. Age range most affected is children 6 months to 3 years old.
5. Eighty percent of affected children are under 4 years old.
6. Peanuts and nuts account for approximately 50% of inhaled foreign bodies.
7. Boys are affected twice as often as are girls.
8. Foreign body aspiration accounts for 500 deaths per year in children less than 5 years old.

CLINICAL MANIFESTATIONS

1. Suddenly wheezing when the child has not done so previously
2. Sudden violent coughing and hemoptysis
3. Gagging
4. Vomiting
5. Decreased breath sounds heard over affected side
6. Poor eating
7. Hypersalivation
8. Dysphagia
9. Fever
10. Acute respiratory infection that fails to resolve
11. Chronic coughing
12. Respiratory arrest
13. Leukocytosis
14. Purulent sputum

Symptoms Associated with Specific Site
Larynx (usually a medical emergency)

1. Hoarseness
2. Coughing

3. Aphonia
4. Hemoptysis
5. Wheezing
6. Dyspnea
7. Cyanosis
8. Apnea
9. Expiratory stridor

Trachea

1. Audible slaps
2. Palpable thuds
3. Asthmatic wheeze
4. Marked retractions

Bronchi

1. Coughing
2. Choking
3. Wheezing
4. Chest pain

These symptoms may not become apparent until several weeks after aspiration.

COMPLICATIONS

1. Laryngeal obstruction (object dislodged into larynx)
2. Asphyxia (a result of laryngeal obstruction)
3. Pneumothorax (results from increased coughing and anesthesia)
4. Retention of foreign body — likely to produce fatal complications or certain forms of morbidity
5. Subcutaneous emphysema (results from alveolar rupture)
6. Pneumonitis

LABORATORY/DIAGNOSTIC TESTS

1. Chest x-ray examination — anterior, posterior, lateral, and oblique (to evaluate foreign body's location; atelectasis, obstructive emphysema, and/or unilateral hyperextension are usual radiologic findings if foreign body is nonopaque)
2. Bronchoscopy — for direct visualization of foreign body
3. Force-expiration technique — demonstrates residual hyperinflation

4. Ventilation-perfusion scan—decreased ventilation and perfusion with obstructed lobe
5. Xerocardiography—for visualization of foreign body
6. Fluoroscopy—persistent inflation during all phases of breathing indicates obstruction; identifies location of foreign body
7. Barium swallow with simultaneous and delayed lateral films
8. Complete blood count—increased white blood count indicates acute respiratory infection
9. Arterial blood gas values—decreased pH, decreased partial pressure of oxygen (Po_2), and increased partial pressure of carbon dioxide (Pco_2) with acute respiratory distress

MEDICATIONS

1. Antibiotics—used to prevent and treat secondary infection; choice of antibiotic is dependent on culture and sensitivity.
2. Corticosteroids
   a. Hydrocortisone (Solu-Cortef)—four fifths of cortisone dose (1.5 to 5 mg/kg/24 hr) q12-24 hr intravenously (IV)
   b. Methylprednisolone (Solu-Medrol)—one sixth of cortisone dose (1.5 to 5 mg/kg/24 hr) q12-24 hr IV

NURSING ASSESSMENT

Refer to "Respiratory Assessment" in Appendix A.

NURSING DIAGNOSES

High risk for suffocation
Ineffective airway clearance
Ineffective breathing pattern
Altered tissue perfusion
Fluid volume deficit
Knowledge deficit
Anxiety

NURSING INTERVENTIONS

Emergency Measures

1. Perform Heimlich maneuver.
2. Use back-slap method (in infants).

3. Do NOT hang by feet (may move foreign body into vocal cords, causing complete obstruction).

Preoperative Care

1. Monitor and observe for changes in respiratory status.
2. Position to ensure adequate airway.
3. Provide nothing by mouth before surgery.
4. Perform postural drainage for 5 minutes every hour with close observation for respiratory effects (can cause foreign body to relodge in left bronchus, causing obstruction in left lung when right bronchus is edematous or occluded).
5. Monitor respiratory status after use of bronchodilators.
6. Prepare child emotionally for bronchoscopy or thoracotomy.

Postoperative Care

1. Monitor and observe for changes in respiratory status (edema of glottis or bronchus).
2. Monitor effects of administered medications.
   a. Corticosteroids for 24 to 48 hr postoperatively (to decrease swelling)
   b. Antibiotics (to treat infection)
3. Monitor hydration status.
   a. Monitor IV fluids.
   b. Introduce and increase fluids as condition improves.
   c. Assess for signs of dehydration.
   d. Record input and output and specific gravity.

Home Care

1. Instruct parents to observe for, and report immediately, signs of respiratory distress.
2. Provide list of resources for parents to call in case of emergency.
3. Instruct parents about use of Heimlich maneuver.
4. Instruct parents about environmental safety.
5. Make a referral or home visit to assess environmental safety before patient's discharge.

BIBLIOGRAPHY

Bailey P: Pediatric esophageal foreign body with minimal symptomatology, *Ann Emerg Med* 12:452, 1983.

Cotton E, Yasuda D: Foreign body aspiration, *Pediatr Clin North Am* 31(4):937, 1984.

Kendry E, Chernick V: *Disorders of the respiratory tract in children,* ed 4, Philadelphia, 1983, WB Saunders.

Phelan P, Landau L, Olinsky A: *Respiratory illness in children,* Oxford, 1982, Blackwell Scientific Publications, Ltd.

Pinney M: Foreign body aspiration, *Am J Nurs* 81(3):521, 1981.

Ryan C et al: Childhood deaths from toy balloons, *Am J Dis Child* 144(11):1221-1224, 1990.

Spala S: Pediatric management problems . . . foreign body aspiration, *Pediatr Nurs* 13(5):365, 1987.

Wolford R: Management of the pediatric airway, *Emerg Care Q* 3(3):52, 1987.

23 ❖ Fractures

PATHOPHYSIOLOGY

Fractures can have a variety of causes, including (1) a direct force applied to the bone; (2) a spontaneous fracture secondary to an underlying pathologic condition such as rickets; (3) abrupt, intense muscle contractions; and (4) an indirect force (e.g., being hit by a flying object) applied from a distance. There are a variety of fractures, which can be categorized using the Salter-Harris classification system (see box on facing page). The most common type seen in children less than 3 years of age is the greenstick fracture. It involves an incomplete break of the cortex, which results because the bone is softer and more pliable than bones in older children. Management varies according to the type of fracture. Management modalities include open reduction, traction, casting, and remodeling.

INCIDENCE

1. Greenstick fracture is the most common one in children less than 3 years of age.
2. Pelvic fracture constitutes a small portion of skeletal fractures in children; it ranks second in morbidity and mortality.
3. Most fractures occur to pedestrians.
4. Skull fracture ranks first in terms of morbidity and mortality.
5. Injuries to the growth plate occur in one third of skeletal traumas.

Salter-Harris Classifications

Type I

Fracture passes through growth plate without involvement of metaphysis or epiphysis

Occurs with mild traumatic injuries

Seen most often in distal fibula

Type II

Fracture extends through growth plate, involving metaphysis

Occurs as result of severe trauma such as car accident, fall from skateboard

Seen most often in distal radius and proximal humerus

Type III

Fracture extends through growth plate, involving epiphysis and joint

Occurs during moderately severe trauma

Seen most often in distal tibia

Type IV

Fracture involves metaphysis, extending through growth plate into epiphysis

Occurs as result of falls, skateboard and bicycle accidents

Seen most often in humerus

Can result in serious damage

Type V (Rare)

Growth plate is crushed

Compression fracture, resulting from falling or projectile impact

CLINICAL MANIFESTATIONS

1. Pain
2. Tenderness
3. Swelling

4. Impaired function
5. Limited motion
6. Ecchymosis surrounding site
7. Crepitus at site of fracture
8. Decreased neurovascular status distal to site of fracture

COMPLICATIONS

1. Deformity of limb
2. Limb-length discrepancy
3. Joint incongruity
4. Limitation of movement
5. Nerve injury resulting in numbness
6. Circulatory compromise
7. Volkmann's ischemic contracture
8. Gangrene
9. Compartment syndrome

LABORATORY/DIAGNOSTIC TESTS

1. X-ray examination of injury site
2. Complete blood count (CBC)

MEDICATIONS

Analgesics—dosage and type depend on child's level of pain intensity.

NURSING ASSESSMENT

Assess degree of trauma and position of limb.

NURSING DIAGNOSES

High risk for altered peripheral perfusion
High risk for injury
Impaired mobility
Impaired tissue integrity
High risk for infection
Pain
Self-care deficit
Diversional activity deficit
Knowledge deficit

NURSING INTERVENTIONS

Admission

1. Assess and document condition of injury.
    a. Amount of swelling
    b. Amount of pain
    c. Change in skin color
    d. Circulatory status of limb distal to injury (color, warmth, pulses)
    e. Neurologic status of limb distal to injury (tingling, numbness)
2. Apply splint or Jones dressing to affected limb to alleviate pain and prevent further injury (traction may be used).
    a. Apply to one side of affected limb.
    b. Immobilize fracture site and joints above and below it.
    c. Stabilize splints with bandages.
    d. Jones dressing—wrap extremity with two or three layers of cotton and cover with Ace bandage; repeat process three or four times.
3. Maintain nothing by mouth (NPO) until after treatment; child may have to be anesthetized.
4. Prepare child and family for selected treatment modality.

Later Treatment

1. Observe and report status of limb distal to fracture site.
    a. Neurovascular status
        (1) Upper limbs—radial and ulnar pulse
        (2) Lower limb—dorsalis pedis and posterior tibial pulses
        (3) Motor function and sensation
    b. Edema and swelling
    c. Skin color and warmth
2. Alleviate edema and swelling of trauma site and area distal to it.
    a. Elevate limb for 24 to 48 hours.
    b. Apply ice if necessary.

   c. Assess every hour immediately after treatment, then q4 hr for 48 hr.
3. Promote skin integrity.
   a. Apply alcohol to reddened areas.
   b. Petal cast edges to prevent skin irritation.
   c. Reposition q2 hr to alleviate increased pressure on bony prominences.
   d. Observe for reddened areas q4 hr.
4. Observe and report signs of infection.
   a. Elevated temperature
   b. Offensive odors
   c. Drainage
5. Observe for and record bleeding; note and outline amount.
6. Provide cast care (as indicated).
7. Maintain traction (as indicated).
8. Provide age-appropriate and diversional activities to alleviate and minimize effects of sensory deprivation and immobilization (refer to Appendix B, *Growth and Development*).
9. Promote adequate fluid and nutritional intake.
   a. Encourage fluid intake; maintenance fluids—0 to 10 kg: 100 ml/kg; 11 to 20 kg: 50 ml/kg; >20 kg: 20 ml/kg.
   b. Provide high-fiber and roughage diet to promote peristalsis.
   c. Provide well-balanced diet to promote healing.
10. Prevent complications of unaffected limb; provide daily exercises.

Home Care/Discharge

1. Assess child's and family's ability to keep follow-up appointments.
2. Instruct parents and child about signs and symptoms of potential complications to report.
3. Instruct parents about care of cast, use of crutches, etc.
4. Instruct parents to monitor and report signs of complications.
   a. Skin breakdown
   b. Signs of infection

c. Signs of bleeding
d. Contractures

BIBLIOGRAPHY

Conrad E, Rang M: Fractures and sprains, *Pediatr Clin North Am* 33(6):1523, 1986.

D'Ambrosia R, Zink W: Fracture of the elbow in children, *Pediatr Ann* 11(6):541, 1982.

Farrell J: Casts, your patients, and you, *Nurs 78* 4:65, Oct 1978.

Gross R: Ankle fractures in children, *Bull NY Acad Med* 63(8):739, 1987.

Ibrahim K: An overview of childhood fractures, *Pediatr Nurs* 12:57, Jan/Feb 1984.

Micheli L, Trepman E: Musculoskeletal trauma. In Gruen M, Haggerty R: *Ambulatory pediatrics,* Philadelphia, 1990, WB Saunders, pp 242-254.

Reichard S et al: Pelvic fractures in children: review of 120 patients with a new look at general management, *J Pediatr Surg* 15(6):727, 1980.

Salter R, Harris W: Injuries involving the epiphyseal plate, *J Bone & Joint Surg* 45A:587, 1963.

Stearns H: Radiology review, *Orthop Nurs* 5(3):46, 1986.

24 ❖ Gastroesophageal Reflux/ Fundoplication

PATHOPHYSIOLOGY

Gastroesophageal reflux refers to the presence of abnormal amounts of gastric contents in the esophagus, upper airways, and tracheobronchial area. The reflux of gastric contents can result in inflammation and stricture of tissue. Resultant effects include aspiration of the gastric contents, recurrent pneumonia, pulmonary disease, esophagitis, and esophageal stricture. Causative factors predisposing the infant or child to gastroesophageal reflux are (1) lower-esophageal sphincter pressure, (2) volume of reflux material in the esophagus, (3) rate of gastric secretion, and (4) ability of stomach to empty. Many children with gastroesophageal reflux improve spontaneously. A child may require surgery if he or she does not respond to medical management.

FUNDOPLICATION

Fundoplication, or Nissen's operation, is performed as a corrective measure for gastroesophageal reflux. The upper end of the stomach is wrapped around the lower portion of the esophagus, and the fundus is sutured in front of the esophagus, creating a circular acute-angle valve mechanism. The response to fundoplication results in complete relief of symptoms—the reflux is treated, vomiting ceases, and failure to thrive is resolved. The child retains feedings and regains weight.

INCIDENCE

1. Vomiting occurs in two thirds of children with gastro-esophageal reflux.
2. Failure to thrive occurs in 34% of these children.
3. Bleeding occurs in 28% of these children.
4. Pulmonary complications occur in 12% of these children.

CLINICAL MANIFESTATIONS

1. Chronic vomiting (most common)
2. Weight loss, failure to thrive
3. Hematemesis or melena due to esophageal bleeding

COMPLICATIONS

1. Aspiration pneumonia
2. Apnea and cyanosis
3. Esophagitis
4. Chest pain
5. Barrett esophagus
6. Esophageal carcinoma
7. Gastric fistula
8. Herniation

LABORATORY/DIAGNOSTIC TESTS

1. Esophageal sphincter pressure (<6 mm Hg is diagnostic)
2. Lower pH in esophagus (direct measure of reflux)
3. Radionuclide gastroesophagraphy (noninvasive test for gastroesophageal reflux)
4. Barium esophagram (often fails to detect intermittent reflux)
5. Acid reflux test (detects acid regurgitation)
6. Endoscopy (detects presence of gross and microscopic esophagitis)
7. Biopsy (assesses severity of esophagitis)

MEDICATIONS

Use antacids between feeding to treat esophagitis.

NURSING ASSESSMENT

1. Refer to "Gastrointestinal Assessment" in Appendix A.
2. Assess for "gas-bloat syndrome."

3. Assess for presence of vomiting and lack of weight gain.
4. See "Postoperative Care" for assessment after fundoplication.

NURSING DIAGNOSES

Fluid volume deficit
High risk for activity intolerance
Altered nutrition: less than body requirements
Knowledge deficit
Ineffective coping
High risk for impaired home maintenance management

NURSING INTERVENTIONS

Conservative Management/Preoperative Care

1. Promote adequate nutritional and fluid intake.
    a. Maintain head of bed in 60-degree position for 30 to 40 minutes after feeding.
    b. Raise head of bed with 6-inch blocks.
    c. Provide small, frequent feedings every 2 to 3 hours.
    d. Thicken formula with cereal.
    e. Provide last meal of day several hours before bedtime.
    f. Avoid serving fat or chocolate.
    g. Monitor daily weights.
    h. If does not respond to feedings by mouth, do the following:
        (1) Monitor continuous nasogastric (NG) feedings.
        (2) Monitor hyperalimentation infusion.
2. Observe, monitor, and report signs of respiratory distress; assess for changes in respiratory status.
3. Prepare parents preoperatively for child's surgery.
    a. Provide information about preoperative routine and surgery (fundoplication; see p. 148).
    b. Encourage participation during induction of anesthesia and recovery (if applicable).

Postoperative Care

1. Assess and monitor child's status postoperatively.
    a. Monitor vital signs q2 hr (for 24 hours), then q4 hr.
    b. Monitor for signs of bleeding—decreased blood pressure, increased apical pulse, frank blood.

   c. Monitor input and output; assess hydration status.
   d. Monitor surgical site for intactness.
   e. Observe for postoperative complications.
      (1) Inability to vomit when necessary
      (2) Inability to burp when necessary
      (3) Gas-bloat syndrome
      (4) Inability to eliminate excessive swallowed air (produces postprandial distress)
      (5) Repeat herniation
      (6) Diarrhea
      (7) Leaking suture in esophagus or stomach (rare but potentially fatal)
2. Prevent abdominal distention and gas-bloat syndrome.
   a. Maintain patency of NG tube (irrigate with normal saline q4 hr).
   b. Check position of NG tube (aspirate contents and auscultate for bowel sounds).
   c. Remove NG tube if vomiting occurs.
   d. Check patency of NG tube used for intermittent suctioning.
3. Monitor for signs and symptoms of gas-bloat syndrome.
   a. Severe distention
   b. Tachycardia
   c. Dyspnea
4. Monitor for signs and symptoms of postoperative hemorrhage.
   a. Decreased blood pressure and increased apical pulse
   b. Gross blood in NG drainage
   c. Coffee-ground NG drainage expected for first 24 hours
5. Assist parents in expression of feelings—may express anger, guilt, frustration because they feel inadequate or responsible.
6. Provide developmentally appropriate stimulation activities (see Appendix A, *Growth and Development*).
7. Provide consistent one-to-one nursing care as a means of establishing a secure environment for the infant.

Home Care/Discharge Plans

1. Instruct parents about signs and symptoms of gas-bloat syndrome.

2. Instruct parents to report any vomiting or presence of frank blood.
3. Provide name of resource to contact for medical or nursing problems.
4. Instruct parents about feeding techniques (review information about nutritional and fluid intake in "Preoperative Care").

BIBLIOGRAPHY

Berquist W: Gastroesophageal reflux in children: a clinical review, *Pediatr Ann* 11(1):135, 1982.

Berquist W: Diagnosis and treatment of gastroesophageal reflux. In Moss A, ed.: *Pediatrics update reviews for physicians,* New York, 1984, Elsevier/North Holland Biomedical Press.

Bowen A: The vomiting infant: recent advances and unsettled issues in imaging, *Radiol Clin North Am* 26(2):377, 1988.

Holder T, Ashcraft K: *Pediatric surgery,* Philadelphia, 1980, WB Saunders Co.

Lynn M: Use of infant seats for gastroesophageal reflux, *J Pediatr Nurs* 1(2):127, 1986.

Peterson M: Esophageal pH monitoring, *J Pediatr Nurs* 1(5):354, 1986.

Skinner D, Belsey R: Surgical management of esophageal reflux and hiatus hernia, *J Thorac Cardiovasc Surg* 53:33, 1967.

Sondheimer J: Gastroesophageal reflex: update on pathogenesis and diagnosis, *Pediatr Clin North Am* 35:103, 1988.

Weissbluth M: Gastroesophageal reflux: a review, *Clin Pediatr* 20(1):7, 1981.

25 ❖ Gastrostomy

PATHOPHYSIOLOGY

A gastrostomy provides a direct route for nutrition, although, with the use of total parenteral nutrition (TPN), gastrostomies are not performed as frequently as in the past. Gastrostomy is indicated in the following circumstances: (1) gastric decompression; (2) for infants with esophageal atresia and tracheoesophageal fistula; (3) for infants with intestinal obstructions; (4) for infants with poor tolerance to nasogastric (NG) feedings; and (5) for infants with swallowing and respiratory difficulties. The anterior surface of the stomach is used for the gastrostomy site. A procedure using the Malecot catheter is most frequently performed. Other procedures use the Pezzer, Foley balloon, or Robinson catheters. After the surgery the infant should begin to regain nutritional status and gain weight because the gastrostomy provides a direct route for feedings. Five to 7 days are required for the gastrostomy and the abdominal wall to establish a good seal.

INCIDENCE

Perioperative morbidity for gastrostomy is 2.5% to 16%.

CLINICAL MANIFESTATIONS

1. Swallowing difficulties
2. Respiratory difficulties

COMPLICATIONS

1. Perforation of posterior gastric wall
2. Leakage of gastric contents causing extensive loss

153

of fluid and electrolytes and erosion of skin
3. Bleeding around tube or stoma
4. Vomiting related to blockage or irritability of pylorus by tube
5. Diarrhea from tube migration into duodenum or jejunum
6. Intussusception
7. Peritonitis, sepsis

LABORATORY/DIAGNOSTIC TESTS

1. Complete blood count — routine preoperative workup
2. Hematocrit
3. Platelet count — to assess platelet function
4. Urinalysis — routine preoperative workup

MEDICATION

An analgesic such as acetaminophen (Tylenol) may be used for mild pain.

NURSING ASSESSMENT

1. Refer to "Gastrointestinal Assessment" in Appendix A.
2. Assess gastrostomy site, output, and patency of tube.

NURSING DIAGNOSES

Altered nutrition: less than body requirements
Fluid volume deficit
High risk for impaired skin integrity
Activity intolerance
Pain
High risk for impaired home maintenance management

NURSING INTERVENTIONS

1. Monitor for patency of gastrostomy to provide sufficient nutritional intake.
   a. Record all intake and drainage.
   b. Attach drainage bag to gastrostomy; hang below level of insertion site to promote decompression.
   c. Check for residuals before each feeding; subtract them from next feeding.
   d. Feed slowly; too rapid infusion of formula can cause vomiting, respiratory distress, and bradycardia.
   e. Prevent air from entering stomach; seal and close end after feeding; fill tubing with formula.

    f. Offer pacifier for infant to suck during feedings as means of stimulating sucking activity.
2. Monitor and prevent complications postoperatively.
    a. Erosion of skin surrounding stoma
    b. Dislodged gastrostomy (surgically replaced within 5 to 7 days postoperatively; placement is verified through use of meglumine diatrizoate [a contrast medium])
    c. Peritonitis or sepsis
    d. Bleeding
    e. Perforation
3. Provide skin care to maintain integrity and prevent erosion of skin.
    a. Keep skin clean and dry.
    b. Apply lubricant to area surrounding stoma.
    c. Tape tubing to abdomen to prevent undue strain and possible dislodgment.
4. Provide comfort measures to alleviate or minimize postoperative pain.
    a. Prevent abdominal distention (monitor feedings).
    b. Provide position of comfort.
    c. Hold, cuddle, and rock as needed.
    d. Monitor infant's response to pain medication.

Home Care/Discharge Planning

Instruct parents about care of gastrostomy
1. Feeding
2. Complications
3. Replacing dislodged tube
4. Evaluating outcome of feedings in terms of weight gain and growth, hydration status, and general appearance

BIBLIOGRAPHY

Bagnell P: Evaluation and examination of the gastrointestinal tract in children, *Curr Opin Pediatr* 1:339, 1989.

Holder T, Ashcroft K: *Pediatric surgery*, Philadelphia, 1980, WB Saunders.

Huth M et al: The gastrostomy feeding button, *Pediatr Nurs* 13(4):241, 1987.

Latchao L: Preoperative and postoperative care of patients undergoing gastrointestinal surgery. In Gellis S, Kagan B: *Current pediatric therapy 13*, Philadelphia, 1990, WB Saunders.

Welch K: *Complications of pediatric surgery: prevention and management*, Philadelphia, 1982, WB Saunders.

26 ❖ Glomerulonephritis

PATHOPHYSIOLOGY

Glomerulonephritis is a term used for a collection of disorders that involve the renal glomeruli (the renal glomeruli are responsible for filtering body fluids and wastes). There are two types of this disease: acute and chronic, with chronic being the progressive form. Acute glomerulonephritis is the most common form of nephritis in children. It is an inflammation of the glomeruli that usually follows a streptococcal infection. It is considered an immune complex disease. The glomerular injury is induced by antigen-antibody complexes trapped in the glomerular filter. The glomeruli become edematous and are infiltrated with polymorphonuclear leukocytes, which occlude the capillary lumen. This condition results in decreased plasma filtration, causing excessive accumulation of water and retention of sodium. The resultant plasma and interstitial fluid volumes lead to circulatory congestion and edema. Hypertension is associated with glomerulonephritis.

INCIDENCE

1. Glomerulonephritis is most common in school-age children.
2. It rarely occurs in children less than 2 years of age or more than 13 years of age.
3. Peak incidence is from ages 5 to 6 years.
4. Incidence in boys is twice that of girls.

It is difficult to estimate incidence because there are many unreported asymptomatic cases.

CLINICAL MANIFESTATIONS

1. Sixty percent to 80% of children with acute glomerulo-nephritis have a history of a preceding upper respiratory infection or otitis media (typically, the child has been in good health before the infection).
2. Nephritis tends to have an average latent period of approximately 10 days, with onset of symptoms 10 days after the initial infection.
3. Initial signs are puffiness of the face, periorbital edema, anorexia, and dark urine.
4. Edema tends to be more prominent in the face in the morning; then it spreads to the abdomen and the extremities during the day (moderate edema may not be recognized by someone who is unfamiliar with the child).
5. Urinary output is severely decreased.
6. Urine is cloudy, smoky, or described as the color of tea or cola.
7. The child is pale, irritable, and lethargic.
8. Younger children may appear ill but seldom express specific complaints.
9. Older children may complain of headaches, abdominal discomfort, vomiting, and dysuria.
10. Mild-to-moderate hypertension is present.

COMPLICATIONS

Once acute glomerulonephritis progresses to the chronic stage, the following complications may be seen.

1. Deteriorating renal function (generally reflected by clinical manifestations and laboratory findings)
2. Frequently, development of nephrotic syndrome
3. Hypertension
4. Edema
5. Discolored urine
6. Hematuria
7. Proteinuria
8. Anemia and osteodystrophy (manifestations of progressive disease)

9. Hypertensive encephalopathy (characterized by head-ache, vomiting, irritability, convulsions, and coma)—can result from the chronic hypertension
10. Cardiac failure, possibly a result of an increase in blood volume secondary to retention of sodium and wa-ter—associated with pulmonary congestion
11. Severe renal failure (characterized by oliguria and anuria)—a final complication

LABORATORY/DIAGNOSTIC TESTS

No diagnostic tests are specifically indicated for the diagno-sis of glomerulonephritis.
1. Examination of urine—proteinuria (one to four plus), hematuria; presence of casts, red blood cells, and white blood cells; decreased creatine clearance rates
2. Blood results—elevated blood urea nitrogen, serum cre-atinine, and uric acid; electrolyte alterations (metabolic acidosis, decreased sodium and calcium; increased potas-sium, phosphorus, serum albumin, and cholesterol); mild anemia and leukocytosis; elevated antibody titers (antistreptolysin, antihyaluronidase, or anti-DNAase B) and erythrocyte sedimentation rate
3. Renal biopsy—may be indicated in rare cases; if it is performed, possible findings are an increased number of cells in each glomerulus and subepithelial "humps" con-taining immunoglobulin and complement

MEDICATIONS

Acute glomerulonephritis has no specific treatment; thus therapy is targeted at the symptoms. Marked hypertension may be treated with diuretics and/or antihypertensives. Ap-propriate antibiotics are used for acute infections. Some medicinal approaches for chronic glomerulonephritis have included glucocorticoids and immunosuppressive agents.

NURSING ASSESSMENT

Refer to "Renal Assessment" in Appendix A.

NURSING DIAGNOSES

Fluid volume excess
Altered nutrition: less than body requirements

High risk for infection
Pain
Diversional activity deficit

NURSING INTERVENTIONS

1. Maintain bed rest, and keep the child comfortable until diuresis occurs; after diuresis, encourage quiet activity.
2. Closely monitor vital signs (especially blood pressure).
3. When hypertension is present, limit sodium intake, and administer ordered medications.
4. Monitor urine for protein and occult blood.
5. Promote adequate nutritional intake—encourage high carbohydrate meals, serve preferred foods, and try small, frequent feedings.
6. Limit potassium intake if hyperkalemia occurs.
7. Perform daily weights, and record accurate intake and output.
8. Assess edema and fluid status daily.
9. Monitor for complications—significant changes in vital signs, change in appearance or volume of urine, excessive weight gain, visual disturbances, motor disturbances, seizure activity, severe pain, or any behavioral changes.

Home Care/Long-Term Care

1. Provide the family with education about the child's illness and treatment plan.
2. Instruct about any medications the child will take at home.
3. Instruct parents and child to monitor blood pressure and to obtain urinalyses for several months; follow-up appointments should be arranged.
4. Instruct parents to contact the physician if there is any change in the child's condition such as signs of infection, alteration in eating habits, abdominal pain, headaches, change in appearance or amount of urine, or lethargy.
5. Explain any dietary restrictions to the parents.

BIBLIOGRAPHY

Bergstein J: Hematuria in the young, *Emerg Med* 18(17):20, 1986.
Vernies R, Chavers B: Glomerular permeability: new concepts, *Pediatr Ann* 17:590, 1988.

Weachter EH, Phillips J, Holaday B: *Nursing care of children,* ed 10, Philadelphia, 1985, JB Lippincott.

Whaley LF, Wong DL: Essentials of pediatric nursing, ed 3, St. Louis, 1989, Mosby–Year Book.

Wieczorek RR, Natapoff JN: A conceptual approach to the nursing of children: health care from birth through adolescence, Philadelphia, 1981, JB Lippincott.

27 ❖ Hemolytic-Uremic Syndrome

PATHOPHYSIOLOGY

Hemolytic-uremic syndrome is an intravascular coagulation condition that primarily affects the kidney. It consists of the following symptomatology: (1) renal failure; (2) hemolytic anemia with fragmented red blood cells (RBCs) and platelets; and (3) thrombocytopenia. The exact cause is unknown, although findings suggest the majority of cases of idiopathic hemolytic-uremic syndrome are associated with the enteric pathogens *Escherichia coli* or *Shigella dysenteriae*. The clinical manifestations and features result from changes in the capillary endothelium caused by the etiologic agent. The endothelial changes result in the following pathologic responses: (1) mechanical trauma to erythrocytes and platelets, shortening their life span and resulting in anemia and thrombocytopenia; and (2) decreased renal blood flow and glomerular filtration rate, resulting in cortical necrosis, which leads to renal failure and acquired hemolytic anemia in infants and children. The severity of the condition varies. The length of the oliguria phase correlates with the ultimate prognosis for recovery. In addition, the prognosis is related to the efficiency and promptness of treatment.

INCIDENCE

1. No figures on overall incidence are available.
2. A seasonal variation exists, with an increased prevalence during spring and fall.
3. The incidence of hypertension as a long-term complication varies from 10% to 50%.

161

4. Hemolytic-uremic syndrome affects males and females equally.
5. It is uncommon for a sibling to be affected.
6. Mortality is 10% to 25%.

CLINICAL MANIFESTATIONS

Prodromal Period

1. Hemolytic-uremic syndrome usually follows gastroenteritis or viral illness.
2. Prodromal illness in older children resembles upper respiratory illness.
3. Prodromal symptoms may last a week, whereas other symptoms may recur in children who appear to have recovered; severity varies (see box on p. 163 for four types of clinical manifestations).

Acute Phase

1. Oliguric, amber urine
2. Renal failure (metabolic disturbance or acidosis; hypocalcemia or hyperkalemia)
3. Oligoanuric for more than 1 week, then diuresis
4. Abdominal pain (caused by splenic enlargement or gastrointestinal [GI] involvement)
5. Edema
6. Hypertension
7. Mild icterus
8. Pallor
9. Systemic bleeding manifestations—purpura, petechiae
10. Irritability, lethargy
11. Anemia associated with uremia
12. Anorexia
13. Seizures
14. Moderate-to-severe respiratory distress caused by congestive heart failure (CHF) and circulatory overload

COMPLICATIONS

1. Neurologic—mortality rate in children with neurologic symptoms (seizures, coma) is 90%, compared to overall mortality rate of 45%.
2. Disseminated intravascular coagulation (DIC)—primarily affects vasculature of kidney, nervous system, and GI tract.

Clinical Manifestations

Mild

No anemia
Oliguria*
Hypertension*
Convulsions*

Severe

Anuric for more than 24 hours

Deteriorating Renal Function

Progressively oliguric
Azotemia
Complete renal failure — may not occur
Severe hypertension
Cardiac failure

Recurrent Hemolytic-Uremic Syndrome

First occurrence — mild
Recurrent occurrence — mild to severe

*Child may manifest one or more symptoms but not all three.

LABORATORY/DIAGNOSTIC TESTS

1. Renal scan (to assess renal perfusion)
2. Renal biopsy (to assess renal involvement)
3. Serum protein (increased)
4. Complete blood count (CBC) (decreased Hgb; increased white blood count [WBC]; significant reticulocytosis; reticulocyte count >2%)
5. Platelet count (<140,000; remains low for 7 to 14 days)
6. Serum albumin decreased
7. Arterial blood gas values (decreased pH; acidosis with acute renal failure)
8. Electrolytes consistent with renal failure (hyponatremia, hyperkalemia)
9. Hyperuricemia, hypocalcemia, hyperphosphatemia
10. Urinalysis (gross hematuria, proteinuria, casts)
11. Blood urea nitrogen (BUN), creatinine (increased; reflects severity of renal failure)

MEDICATIONS

Drugs such as corticosteroids, anticoagulants, or antiplatelet agents have not been found effective.

NURSING ASSESSMENT

Refer to "Renal Assessment" in Appendix A. Assess for signs and symptoms of hypervolemia and circulatory overload.

NURSING DIAGNOSES

Fluid volume excess
High risk for injury
Decreased cardiac output
High risk for infection
Impaired tissue integrity
Knowledge deficit
Anxiety

NURSING INTERVENTIONS

1. Monitor and maintain fluid and electrolyte balance.
    a. Monitor types of fluids and administration rate to avoid fluid overload and cerebral edema.
    b. Record accurate input and output.
    c. Record daily weights (BID during acute phase).
    d. Monitor blood pressure and pulse pressure to assess hydration.
    e. Replace fluids from urinary loss with isotonic solution (normal saline or lactated Ringer's).
    f. Assess hydration status q4-6 hr during acute phase.
    g. For hypovolemic shock, replace fluids.
    h. Perform arterial pressure and central venous pressure (CVP) monitoring.
2. Monitor and observe for signs of electrolyte imbalance.
    a. Hyperkalemia—muscular instability; electrocardiogram (ECG) changes—peaked T waves, wide QRS complex, prolonged PR interval; cardiac arrhythmias
    b. Hypocalcemia—coma, convulsions
    c. Hyponatremia—seizures
    d. Hypoglycemia—seizures
3. Transfuse with blood products as indicated
    a. Washed PRBCs for low hemoglobin; transfuse slowly; do not raise Hgb greater than 7 to 8 g

b. Platelets — prn for bleeding
4. Observe and report signs and symptoms of impending complications.
   a. Shock
   b. Infection
   c. Disseminated intravascular coagulation (DIC)
   d. Heart failure
   e. Potassium intoxication
   f. Overhydration
   g. Seizures
   h. Neurologic disturbance — lethargy, coma, hyperactivity
   i. Pulmonary edema
   j. Hypertension
5. Monitor for nutritional status; NG feedings or hyperalimentation may be needed.
6. Prepare child and family for peritoneal dialysis or hemodialysis if indicated; indications include the following
   a. Anuria for 24 to 48 hr
   b. Central nervous system (CNS) disturbance
   c. Congestive heart failure (CHF)
   d. Bleeding (GI and cutaneous)
   e. BUN >150 mg/100 ml
   f. Uncontrollable hyperkalemia
   g. Hyponatremia <130 mEq/L
   h. Change in neurologic status — lethargy to coma or hyperactivity
   i. Hyperphosphatemia >8 mg/100 ml
   j. Uncontrollable acidosis
   k. Hypocalcemia <8 mg/100 ml
7. Encourage child and parents to ventilate feelings of concern regarding child's condition. The child's response will be affected by the following
   a. Developmental needs
   b. Presence of primary caretakers
   c. Extent of immobilization
   d. Nutritional needs
   e. General malaise
8. Provide information about procedures before they are performed, and reinforce data provided to parents.

BIBLIOGRAPHY

Callahan D et al: Recurrent oliguria in a "well controlled" child, *Hosp Pract* 30(9A):36, 1986.

Hagg R, Buchanan G: Hemolytic-uremic syndrome. In Levin D, Morris F, Moore G: *A practical guide to pediatric intensive care*, St. Louis, 1984, Mosby–Year Book.

Kaplan B, Thompson P, Chadarevian J: The hemolytic-uremic syndrome, *Pediatr Clin North Am* 23:761, 1976.

Kavi J, Wise R: Causes of hemolytic-uremic syndrome, *Brit Med J* 298:65, 1989.

Musgrave J et al: The hemolytic-uremic syndrome, *Clin Pediatr* 17(B):218, 1978.

Rezzoni G et al: Plasma infusion for hemolytic uremic syndrome in children: results of a multi-center controlled trial, *J Pediatr* 112(2):284, 1988.

Stiegler R: Management of hemolytic-uremic syndrome, *J Pediatr* 112:1014, 1988.

28 ❖ Hemophilia

PATHOPHYSIOLOGY

Hemophilia refers to a group of blood coagulation disorders that are secondary to the deficiency of factor VIII (hemophilia A) or factor IX (hemophilia B or Christmas disease). It is an inherited disorder that is transmitted by an X-linked recessive gene from the maternal side. Factor VIII and factor IX are plasma proteins that are necessary components of blood coagulation; they are needed for the formation of fibrin clots at the site of vascular injury. Severe hemophilia results when plasma concentrations of factors VIII and IX are less than 1%. Moderate hemophilia is associated with plasma concentrations between 1% and 5%. The clinical manifestations depend on the child's age and the severity of the deficiency of factors VIII and IX. Severe hemophilia is characterized by recurrent hemorrhages, occurring either spontaneously or after relatively minor trauma. The most common sites of hemorrhage are within the joints of the knees, elbows, ankles, shoulders, and hips. The muscles most often affected are the forearm flexor, the gastrocnemius, and the iliopsoas. Because of improvements in treatment, almost all hemophiliacs are expected to live a normal life span.

INCIDENCE

1. Incidence is 1 in 10,000 male births.
2. Twenty-five thousand males are severely affected.

3. The family history of two thirds of the patients reveals an X-linked recessive form of inheritance.
4. Noncompliance rates range from 4% to 92%, with an average of 35%.
5. Central nervous system (CNS) bleeding occurs in 3% of children.
6. Spontaneous bleeding and posttraumatic intracranial bleeding are associated with a 34% mortality rate and 50% long-term morbidity.
7. Ten percent of patients with hemophilia A and hemophilia B develop IgG antibodies that inhibit the activity of factors VIII and IX.

CLINICAL MANIFESTATIONS
Infancy (for Diagnosis)
1. Prolonged bleeding after circumcision
2. Subcutaneous ecchymoses over bony prominences (at 3 to 4 months of age)
3. Large hematomas after infections
4. Bleeding from oral mucosa
5. Soft-tissue hemorrhages

Bleeding Episodes (Throughout Life Span)

1. Initial symptom — pain
2. After pain — swelling, warmth, and decreased mobility

Long-Term Sequelae

Prolonged bleeding into the muscle causes nerve compression and muscle fibrosis.

COMPLICATIONS
1. Progressive, crippling arthropathy
2. Muscular contracture
3. Paralysis
4. Intracranial bleeding
5. Hypertension
6. Renal impairment
7. Splenomegaly
8. Hepatitis
9. Acquired immunodeficiency syndrome (AIDS) from exposure to blood products

10. Antibodies formed as antagonist to factors VIII and IX
11. Allergic transfusion reaction to blood products
12. Hemolytic anemia
13. Thrombosis and/or thromboembolism

LABORATORY/DIAGNOSTIC TESTS

1. Screening tests for blood coagulation
   a. Platelet count
   b. Prothrombin time (normal)
   c. Partial thromboplastin time (increased; measures adequacy of intrinsic coagulation cascade)
   d. Bleeding time (normal; assesses formation of platelet plugs in capillaries)
   e. Functional assays of factors VIII and IX (confirm diagnosis)
   f. Thrombin clotting time
2. Liver biopsy (sometimes) used to obtain tissue for pathologic examination and culture
3. Liver function tests (sometimes) used to detect presence of liver disease (e.g., serum glutamic-pyruvic transaminase [SGPT], serum glutamic-oxaloacetic transaminase [SGOT], alkaline phosphatase, bilirubin)

MEDICATIONS

See Table 3.

NURSING ASSESSMENT

1. Refer to "Neuromuscular Assessment" in Appendix A.
2. Assess site of involvement for extent of bleeding and extent of sensory, nerve, and motor impairment.

NURSING DIAGNOSES

High risk for fluid volume deficit
Pain
High risk for injury
Knowledge deficit
Diversional activity deficit
Impaired home maintenance management
High risk for infection
High risk for impaired physical mobility

Table 3. Plasma Products Used to Treat Patients with Hemophilia

Product	Major contents	Clinical indications	Unit volume per bag or vial
Fresh frozen plasma	All coagulation factors*	Unknown type of hemophilia; mild hemophilia A or B with history of few prior transfusions; von Willebrand's disease	200-300 ml
Cryoprecipitate	Factor VIII† Fibrinogen	Hemophilia A; von Willebrand's disease	10-30 ml
Factor VIII concentrate§	Factor VIII	Hemophilia A	10-30 ml
Factor IX (prothrombin complex) concentrate	Factor IX Factors II, VII, X Contaminating procoagulants	Hemophilia B; hemophilia A with inhibitor	20-30 ml

From Buchanan GR: Hemophilia, *Pediatr Clin North Am* 27(2):314, 1980.
*Factors V and VII may be diminished if stored for more than 2 to 3 months.
†Factor IX is not present.
‡Tremendous variations from bag to bag.

Table 3. Plasma Products Used to Treat Patients with
Hemophilia — cont'd

Average number of factor VIII or IX per bag or vial	Storage conditions	Advantages	Disadvantages
100-200 units	Below −20° C for several years	Low risk of hepatitis Readily available	Transfusion reactions Volume overload Inconvenient Impossible to raise factor level more than 15% to 20%
75-100 units‡	Below −20° C for 6 to 12 months	Moderate hepatitis risk Less expensive than concentrates	Bags contain widely variable amounts of factor VIII Inconvenient to use
250-1200 units (recorded on label)	4° C for 2 years; room temperature for variable periods	Convenient Ability to infuse known numbers of units	Hepatitis Hemolytic anemia Expensive
400-600 units (recorded on label)	4° C for 2 years; room temperature for variable periods	Convenient Ability to infuse known number of units	Hepatitis Venous thrombosis Expensive

§Products currently available in the United States include Profilate (Abbott Pharmaceuticals), Factorate (Armour Pharmaceutical Co.), Koãte (Cutter Biological), Hemofil (Hyland Therapeutics Division), and Humafac (Parke-Davis).

‖Products currently available in the United States include Konŷne (Cutter Biological) and Proplex (Hyland Therapeutics).

NURSING INTERVENTIONS

Acute Episodes

1. Monitor child's or adolescent's response to administration of plasma products (Table 3).
2. Monitor child's response to administration of pain medication and to measures to relieve pain.
   a. Acetaminophen
   b. Narcotic analgesics
   c. Application of ice to affected joint
   d. Immobilization of affected limb
   e. Bed cradle
3. Monitor child or adolescent for further bleeding episodes; observe for signs and symptoms of bleeding.
4. Protect child or adolescent from further injury.
   a. Pad child's or infant's crib.
   b. Apply pressure after venipunctures.
   c. Apply fibrin or gelatin foam to bleeding sites.
5. Instruct and monitor child regarding dental care.
   a. Use of soft-bristle toothbrush
   b. Good nutritional intake
   c. Avoidance of excessive amounts of sweets
   d. Chewing of sugarless gum
   e. Need for regular dental visits
   f. Use of factor replacement before dental work
6. Instruct child about monitoring self for bleeding episodes — an intuitive feeling or "knowing" that bleeding is occurring.
7. Encourage quiet age-appropriate play or diversional activities (see Appendix A, *Growth and Development*).
8. Provide age-appropriate explanations before treatments and procedures.
9. Provide emotional support to family.
   a. Encourage ventilation of concerns (e.g., guilt, fear).
   b. Refer to social service as needed.
   c. Provide for physical comforts (e.g., place to sleep or bathe).
   d. Encourage use of preexisting support systems.

Home Care/Discharge

1. Instruct child and parents about administering replacement for deficient factor.

2. Instruct child and parents about signs and symptoms of bleeding episodes.
3. Problem solve and plan life-style activities to support (sedentary) living and to prevent further injuries.
4. Discuss with parents and child methods to make life-style more normal and to avoid being labeled "handicapped."
5. Encourage parents and child to express feelings about the disease and the limitations it imposes on activities.
6. Link family to appropriate community-based resources.

BIBLIOGRAPHY

Buchanan G: Hemophilia, *Pediatr Clin North Am* 27(2):309, 1980.

Dykstra D: Pediatric rehabilitation: joint and connective tissue diseases part 5, *Arch Phys Med Rehabil* (Supplement) 70(5-5): Study Guide Issue: 5179, 1989.

Huckstadt A: Hemophilia: the person, family and nurse, *Rehab Nurs* 11(3):25, 1986.

Greer R, Ballard J: Musculoskeletal bleeding in hemophilia, *Pediatr Ann* 11(6):521, 1982.

Markova I: Self and other awareness of the risk of HIV/AIDS for behavioral change, *Soc Sci Med* 31(1):73, 1990.

Sergis-Deavenport E, Darni J: Behavioral techniques in teaching hemophilia factor replacement procedures to families, *Pediatr Nurs* 10:416, Nov/Dec 1982.

Steed D et al: Surgery on the hemophiliac patient. Special considerations, *J Assoc Oper Room Nurses* 45(6):1412, 1987.

Varni J, Wako G, Katz E: A cognitive behavioral approach to pain associated with pediatric chronic diseases, *J Pain Sympt Manag* 4(4):238, 1989.

Wilson P, Wasserman K: Psychological responses to the threat of HIV exposure among people with bleeding disorders, *Health Soc Work* 14(3):176, 1989.

29 ❖ Hepatitis

PATHOPHYSIOLOGY

Hepatitis, a liver disease that is typically self-limiting and uncomplicated, is caused by a viral agent. Hepatitis viruses can be classified into four types: hepatitis A (HAV); hepatitis B (HBV); non-A, non-B (NANB); and hepatitis D (HDV, formerly called *delta* hepatitis). The most common form in children is hepatitis A.

Hepatitis A

Hepatitis A is the most highly contagious form of hepatitis. It is transmitted primarily through the fecal-oral route. It can also be transmitted by unsanitary food handlers, contaminated food supplies, and shellfish from sewage-contaminated waters. It is rarely transmitted through transfusions. Epidemics of hepatitis A have been reported in institutions housing or caring for large numbers of children such as day-care centers, schools, and homes for the mentally retarded. The incubation period is approximately 1 month. Jaundice appears 4 to 6 weeks after exposure. The child is contagious up to 1 week after the onset of jaundice. Hepatitis A manifests a wide spectrum of symptoms; it rarely (10% of cases) leads to chronic hepatitis. Children may have minimal symptoms or be asymptomatic. The child is rarely hospitalized; if hospitalization is necessary it is because of a decrease in the child's clotting factors, his or her inability to retain oral fluids, and fulminating hepatic failure.

Hepatitis B, Non-A, Non-B Hepatitis, and Hepatitis C (Parenterally Transmitted Non-A, Non-B Hepatitis)

These forms of hepatitis are uncommon in children. The virus is transmitted through blood or blood derivatives and body secretions (semen, saliva, breast milk, urine). Hepatitis B occurs most commonly in the following populations of children: (1) infants whose mothers are chronic carriers of the viral antigen HB_sAg; (2) children receiving frequent transfusions or hemodialysis. The incubation period is 2 to 6 months. Children with non-A, non-B hepatitis are asymptomatic, although a few fulminating cases have been reported. In the United States more than 90% of the cases of NANB hepatitis are associated with transfusions of blood or blood products. Approximately 70% to 90% of parenterally transmitted NANB cases are caused by the hepatitis C virus (HCV). Fecal transmission is presumed to be another route of infection. The distinguishing feature of non-A, non-B hepatitis is the fluctuating enzyme levels during the acute and chronic phases of illness.

Hepatitis D

This virus can only cause infection and clinical manifestations in association with HBV infection. The virus acts as a parasite of HBV. Coinfection with HDV increases the severity of the HBV infection, creating a more fulminating course and enhancing the potential for chronic liver disease.

INCIDENCE

1. Hepatitis A is the most common type of hepatitis.
2. Approximately 30,000 cases of hepatitis A are reported each year; they represent a small proportion of actual cases.
3. Ten percent of children with hepatitis B or non-A, non-B hepatitis develop chronic hepatitis.
4. Approximately 90% of children and infants with hepatitis do not exhibit jaundice.
5. Day-care centers figure prominently in the epidemiology of hepatitis A; they account for 13% of cases in Phoenix and 40% of cases in New Orleans (the risk increases in centers accepting children less than 2 years old).

6. Tropical and developing nations have a higher incidence than industrialized and temperate-zone nations.
7. Highest incidence in the United States is in southwestern, western, and Rocky Mountain states.
8. About 50 individuals die from hepatitis annually.
9. Non-A, non-B hepatitis is responsible for 90% to 95% of posttransfusion hepatitis.
10. Approximately 200,000 persons, mainly young adults, acquire hepatitis B annually.
11. Incidence of hepatitis D is difficult to measure because it occurs concurrently with hepatitis B and may not be readily diagnosed.

CLINICAL MANIFESTATIONS

Hepatitis A

1. Acute febrile illness
2. Jaundice (develops as fever drops)
3. Anorexia
4. Nausea
5. Malaise
6. Dark urine (precedes jaundice)
7. Children under three — often asymptomatic
8. Hepatomegaly
9. Splenomegaly

Hepatitis B; Non-A, Non-B Hepatitis; Hepatitis C; and Hepatitis D

1. Insidious onset
2. Jaundice
3. Anorexia
4. Malaise
5. Nausea
6. Papular acrodermatitis (Gianotti-Crosti syndrome)
7. Prodromal symptoms — arthralgia, arthritis, erythematous maculopapular rash
8. Polyarteritis nodosa
9. Glomerulonephritis
10. Hepatitis D intensifies the symptoms of hepatitis B and increases the possibility of a chronic condition
11. Hepatitis C is characterized by mild asymptomatic infection with insidious onset of jaundice and malaise

COMPLICATIONS

Hepatitis A

1. Progresses to fulminating disease (rare)
2. Encephalopathy
3. Aplastic anemia

Hepatitis B, Non-A, Non-B Hepatitis, and Hepatitis C

1. Hepatocellular cancer
2. Liver failure
3. Aplastic anemia
4. Cirrhosis
5. Fulminating hepatitis
6. Hepatic failure (75% mortality rate)
7. Massive hepatic necrosis
8. Carrier state (persistent viral infection without symptoms)
9. Fifty percent of patients with hepatitis C can develop chronic liver disease.

LABORATORY/DIAGNOSTIC TESTS

1. SGOT increased
2. SGPT increased
3. Bilirubin—elevated
4. IgM antibodies (hepatitis A virus antibody and anti-HAV-IgM)—diagnostic for hepatitis A
5. IgM antibodies (hepatitis B core antigen; antiHB$_c$-IgM)
6. IgG antibodies (hepatitis A virus antibody and anti-HAV)—indicates susceptibility or past exposure to hepatitis A.
7. Hb$_s$Ag titers—diagnostic for hepatitis B; if persists more than 6 months, indicates acute chronic hepatitis B
8. AntiHb$_c$Ag titers—diagnostic for chronic hepatitis
9. AntiHb$_s$—presence indicates recovery and immunity to hepatitis B
10. AntiHb$_e$—presence indicates low titers of hepatitis B and insufficient disease transmission
11. Aspartate aminotransferase (AST)—increase indicates acute hepatitis
12. Alanine aminotransferase (ALT)—increased in acute hepatitis
13. AntiHDV (in certain situations)

MEDICATIONS

1. Immune globulin (Ig) — used for prophylaxis before and after exposure to hepatitis A (administered within 2 weeks of exposure)
2. HBIG — given as prophylaxis after exposure — unvaccinated: 0.06 ml/kg IM, STAT; initiate HB vaccine series. Vaccinated: 0.06 ml/kg plus booster doses of vaccine. Perinatal: 0.5 ml IM within 12 hours of birth.
3. Hepatitis B vaccine — used to prevent occurrence of hepatitis B. Heptavax-B (MSD — 20 μg of Hb_sAg protein/ml) — perinatal: 0.5 ml (10 μg) IM within 12 hours of birth; repeat at 1 and 6 months. Children younger than 10 years old: three doses of 0.5 ml (10 μg) IM (anterolateral thigh/deltoid); first two doses are given 1 month apart, a booster is given 6 months after the first dose. Children older than 10 years old: three doses of 1 ml (20 μg) into the deltoid muscle. NOTE: Children undergoing long-term hemodialysis and children with Down syndrome should be routinely vaccinated because of increased risk for acquisition of hepatitis B infection.

NURSING ASSESSMENT

1. Refer to "Gastrointestinal Assessment" in Appendix A.
2. Assess for areas of jaundice — skin and sclera.

NURSING DIAGNOSIS

Fluid volume deficit
Altered nutrition: less than body requirements
High risk for infection
Pain
Impaired home maintenance management
Knowledge deficit

NURSING INTERVENTIONS

1. Provide and maintain adequate fluid and food intake.
   a. Monitor for signs of dehydration.
   b. Monitor and record input and output.
   c. Provide small, frequent meals; may need antiemetics.
   d. Offer child's favorite foods.
2. Prevent secondary infections.
   a. Avoid contact with infectious sources.

    b. Use and encourage appropriate hand washing technique.

    c. Monitor for signs of infection.

    d. Provide for additional rest periods.

3. Prevent or control spread of hepatitis.

    a. Refer to institutional procedures for isolation techniques.

    b. Inoculate those people exposed to hepatitis during the incubation period.

      (1) Immune globulin (Ig)

      (2) HBIG vaccine

    c. Vaccinate those individuals at high risk with hepatitis B vaccine.

4. Monitor for bleeding.

    a. Monitor coagulation studies.

    b. Vitamin K, IM may be ordered.

5. Monitor child closely for progression into fulminating hepatitis.

    a. Behavioral changes.

    b. Lethargy.

    c. Coma.

Home Care/Discharge Instructions

1. Ensure that all family members and others exposed to child receive inoculation of Ig or HBIG.

2. Instruct parents and child about signs and symptoms of hepatitis so they can observe for them in those individuals exposed to child.

3. Provide instruction to parents about sanitary measures to institute in home.

4. Refer to public health nurse or community nurse for assessment of use of preventive measures for hepatitis.

BIBLIOGRAPHY

American Academy of Pediatrics: Report of the Committee of Infectious Diseases, Elk Grove Village, Ill, 1991, AAP.

Balistreri W: Viral hepatitis, *Pediatr Clin North Am* 35(3):637, 1988.

Belkengren R, Supala S: Pediatric management problems: hepatitis A, *Pediatr Nurs* 15(6):638, 1989.

Brady M: Preventing the perinatal spread of hepatitis B, *J Pediatr Health Care* 3(1):49, 1989.

Chilton L: Viral hepatitis in school-aged children, *Pediatr Rev* 4(4):105, 1982.

Gershon A: Immunization practices in children, *Hosp Pract* 25(9):91, 1990.

Harris J, Fischer R, Parks B: Pediatric drug information, *Pediatr Nurs* 10(3):228, May/June 1984.

Hicks R, Cullen J, Jackson W, Burry V: Work-related risk factors for hepatitis B virus infection in personnel of a children's hospital, *Clinic Pediatr* 28(6):245, 1989.

Lanphear B: Hepatitis B immunoprophylaxis: developing a cost-effective program in the hospital setting, *Infect Contr Hosp Epidemiol* 11(1):47, 1989.

NANB test hailed, but HBU nearing a "national tragedy," *Hosp Infect Contr* 16(6):73, 1989.

Position Paper: human immunodeficiency virus and hepatitis B virus, *J Intraven Nurs* 12(6):344, 1989.

Poss J: Hepatitis B virus infection in Southeast Asian children, *J Pediatr Health Care* 3(6):311, 1989.

Poss J: Hepatitis D virus infection, *Nurs Pract: Am J Prim Health Care* 14(8):12, 1989.

Powers R: Taking care of bite wounds, *Emerg Med* 22(13):131, 1990.

Rosenblum C: A multifocal outbreak of hepatitis A traced to commercially distributed lettuce, *Am J Publ Health* 80(9):1075, 1990.

Shoop N: Prepare for the 1990s; update: tuberculosis, hepatitis and acquired immunodeficiency syndrome, part 1, *Gastroenterol Nurs* 12(3):200, 1990.

Stehlin D: Hepatitis B: available vaccine safe, but underused, *Emerg Med Serv* 19(7):70, 1990.

Thomas D: Neonatal nosocomial infections, *Critic Care Nurs Quart* 11(4):83, 1989.

Treem W, Etienne N, Hyams J: Pediatric liver transportation: choosing and caring for the transplant candidate, part 1, *Gastroenterol Nurs* 12(4):261, 1990.

Triolo P, Montgomery L: Occupational health hazards: implications for perinatal and neonatal nurses, *J Perinat Neonat Nurs* 3(4):34, 1990.

Van-de-Linden J: Hepatitis B: the disease, the risk, the answer, *J Post Anesth Nurs* 4(6):416, 1989.

Weber D, Rutula W: Hepatitis B immunization update, *Infect Contr Hosp Epidemiol* 10(12):541, 1989.

West K: Viral hepatitis: non A, non B and delta hepatitis: hepatitis C and D, *Emerg Med Serv* 19(3):37, 1990.

West K, Yuras R: Screening costs in a hepatitis B vaccine program, *J Emerg Med Serv* 15(8):40, 1990.

Wolfe M: Vaccines for foreign travel, *Pediatr Clin North Am* 37(3):757, 1990.

30 ❖ Hernia (Inguinal)/Hernia Repair

PATHOPHYSIOLOGY

Inguinal hernia refers to the prolapse of a portion of the intestine into the inguinal ring above the scrotal sac, caused by a congenital weakness or failure of closure. An incarcerated hernia occurs when the prolapsed intestine causes constriction of the blood supply to the scrotal sac. The infant then develops pain and symptoms of intestinal obstruction (abdominal distention, no flatus, no stool, vomiting). A communicating hydrocele is always associated with hernia. The child is initially seen with an intermittent lump or bulge in the groin, scrotum, or labia. It becomes prominent with intraabdominal pressure such as that resulting from crying or straining. A 2- to 4-cm transverse incision is made in the area overlying the right inguinal canal. Herniorrhaphy is usually performed on an outpatient basis.

INCIDENCE

1. Herniorrhaphy is the most frequently performed surgery in children.
2. One percent to 3% of children have a hernia.
3. The incidence is greater in premature infants (3% to 4.8%).
4. The prevalence is greatest during infancy (more than 50%).

5. The remaining 50% occur in children 1 to 5 years of age.
6. Prevalence is greatest in males as compared with females (6:1).

CLINICAL MANIFESTATIONS

If hernia is incarcerated:
1. Continuous crying
2. Vomiting
3. Abdominal distention
4. Bloody stools

COMPLICATIONS

1. Recurrence of hernia
2. Incarcerated hernia
3. Atrophy of gonad

LABORATORY/DIAGNOSTIC TESTS

1. Complete blood count (CBC) — routine preoperative testing
2. Urinalysis — routine preoperative testing

MEDICATIONS

Analgesic — acetaminophen (Tylenol) is administered postoperatively because surgical pain is minimal. The dosage is as follows:
1. <1 year — 60 mg by mouth (po)
2. 1 to 3 years — 60 to 120 mg po
3. 3 to 6 years — 120 mg, not to exceed 480 mg/day
4. 6 to 12 years — 150 to 325 mg, not to exceed 1.2 g/day; administered po as needed q4-6 hr

NURSING ASSESSMENT

1. Refer to "Gastrointestinal Assessment" in Appendix A.
2. Assess for presence of lump in area of groin, scrotum, or labia.

NURSING DIAGNOSES

Impaired tissue integrity
High risk for injury
Altered nutrition: less than body requirements

Fluid volume deficit
Activity intolerance
Pain
Ineffective individual coping
Knowledge deficit

NURSING INTERVENTIONS

Preoperative

1. Assess child's clinical status before surgery.
   a. No signs of infection
   b. Hemoglobin (Hgb) > 10 g
2. Prepare child physically for surgery; obtain routine laboratory tests (CBC, urinalysis).
3. Provide explanations to parents about surgical preparation as means of alleviating anxiety.
4. Provide age-appropriate explanations to child before surgery.

Postoperative

1. Monitor child's clinical status.
   a. Vital signs as often as q2 hr for first 24 hr, then q4 hr
   b. Patency of dressing
   c. Signs and symptoms of infection
   d. Temperature, drainage from site, redness, inflammation
2. Monitor for signs and symptoms of complications.
   a. Recurrence of hernia
3. Promote nutritional and fluid intake.
   a. Record input and output.
   b. Advance diet as tolerated.
   c. Monitor for signs of dehydration.
4. Promote and maintain respiratory function.
   a. Turn, cough, and deep breathe.
   b. Perform postural drainage and percussion.
   c. Change position q2 hr.
   d. Keep head of bed in semi-Fowler's position.
5. Alleviate child's pain as needed.
   a. Maintain position of comfort.
   b. Use recreational and diversional activities and toys.
   c. Administer analgesics.

6. Provide emotional support to child.
   a. Provide age-appropriate diversional and recreational activities (see Appendix B, *Growth and Development*).
   b. Encourage parental participation in care.
   c. Incorporate child's routines (e.g., bedtime routine) into care.
7. Provide and reinforce information given to parents about child's condition.

Home Care

1. Instruct parents about care of dressing (if present).
   a. Keep incision covered with plastic-coated dressing.
   b. Bathe with incision covered by a dressing.
   c. Protect incision from fecal and urinary contamination.
2. Instruct parents about short- and long-term management.
   a. Do not restrict activities.
   b. Administer acetaminophen (Tylenol) for pain as needed.
   c. Monitor for complications.

BIBLIOGRAPHY

Ashby D: Susan's first pregnancy and first surgery, *J Post Anesth Nurs* 4(6):406, 1990.

Ashby D: The pediatric patient . . . a left inguinal hernia, *J Post Anesth Nurs* 4(2):116, 1989.

Fonkalsrud E, DeLorimier A, Clatworthy H: Femoral and direct inguinal hernias in infants and children, *JAMA* 192:597, 1965.

Halder T, Ashcraft K: *Pediatric surgery*, Philadelphia, 1980, WB Saunders.

Kingsley A, Lichtenstein I, Sieber W: Common hernias in primary care, *Patient Care* 24(7):98, 1990.

Welch K: *Complications of pediatric surgery: prevention and management*, Philadelphia, 1982, WB Saunders.

31 ❖ Hirschsprung's Disease/Surgical Repair

PATHOPHYSIOLOGY

Hirschsprung's disease, or congenital megacolon, refers to the absence of ganglion cells in the rectum or the rectosigmoid portion of the colon. This absence results in the lack of peristalsis and the total absence of spontaneous bowel evacuation. Also, the rectal sphincter fails to relax, preventing the normal passage of stool. Intestinal contents are propelled to an aganglionic segment, causing fecal material to accumulate there and to dilate the bowel proximal to this area. It is speculated that Hirschsprung's disease is caused by both genetic and environmental factors. The environmental factors include nutritional deficiencies, irradiation, rubella and other viruses, and medications (thalidomide). Hirschsprung's disease may manifest at any age, although it is most commonly observed in neonates. A colostomy is performed initially; then corrective surgery is performed when the child is 6 to 9 months old or when he or she is two to three times his or her birth weight.

INCIDENCE

1. Hirschsprung's disease occurs once in 20,000 live births.
2. It affects 700 neonates per year in the United States.
3. Ninety-five percent of affected infants are white.

4. Eighty percent of affected infants are males.
5. Incidence increases in siblings and offspring of affected children.
6. Among affected infants, 3.5% to 10% are premature or have low birth weight.
7. Among affected infants, 5% to 9% are diagnosed with Down syndrome.
8. This disease accounts for 25% of neonatal obstructions.
9. Among affected infants, 2.5% to 3.6% have associated urinary tract conditions.

CLINICAL MANIFESTATIONS

Neonatal Period

1. Failure to pass meconium within 48 hours of birth
2. Bile-stained vomitus
3. Reluctant to ingest fluids
4. Abdominal distention

Preschool and School-Age Periods

1. Constipation
2. Recurrent diarrhea
3. Ribbonlike, foul-smelling stool
4. Abdominal distention

COMPLICATIONS (PRIMARILY IN NEONATAL PERIOD)

1. Respiratory distress
2. Enterocolitis

LABORATORY/DIAGNOSTIC TESTS

1. Abdominal x-ray films (supine, erect, prone, lateral decubitus)—diagnostic
2. Barium enema—diagnostic
3. Rectal biopsy—to detect absence of ganglion cells
4. Anorectal manometry—records reflux response of internal and external rectal sphincter

MEDICATIONS

An analgesic, acetaminophen (Tylenol), is administered for mild to moderate pain. For children less than 1 year of age, the dosage is 60 mg by mouth (po).

NURSING ASSESSMENT

Refer to "Gastrointestinal Assessment" in Appendix A.

NURSING DIAGNOSES

High risk for infection
High risk for injury
Fluid volume deficit
Impaired tissue integrity
Knowledge deficit
Impaired home maintenance management
Ineffective family coping: compromised

SURGICAL MANAGEMENT

Surgical treatment of Hirschsprung's disease is a two-stage process. Initially, a double-barrel or loop colostomy is performed so that the dilated and hypertrophied portion of the bowel can regain normal tone and size (takes approximately 3 to 4 months). When the infant is between 6 and 12 months of age (or when the infant weighs 18 to 20 pounds), one of three procedures is performed as a means of resectioning the aganglionic bowel and of anastomosing the ganglion-containing bowel to the rectum within 1 cm of the anus. The Duhamel procedure is generally performed on infants less than 1 year old. It consists of pulling down the normal colon and anastomosing it behind the aganglionic bowel, creating a double wall composed of both the aganglionic sheath and the posterior section of the normal pulled-through colon. In the Swenson procedure, the aganglionic portion of colon is resected. An end-to-end anastomosis of the ganglionic colon to the dilated anal canal is performed. A sphincterotomy is performed posteriorly. The Soave procedure is performed on older children and is the most frequently used procedure for treating Hirschsprung's disease. The muscular wall of the rectal segment is left intact. The normally innervated colon is pulled through to the anus where an anastomosis between the normal colon and the remaining rectosigmoid muscular tissue is performed.

Response to Surgery

The response to surgery results in the amelioration of symptoms (see "Pathophysiology"). Peristaltic activity throughout the colon is established.

NURSING INTERVENTIONS

Preoperative Care

1. Assess and monitor clinical status preoperatively.
   a. Monitor vital signs q2 hr as needed.
   b. Monitor intake and output.
   c. Observe for signs of bowel perforation.
      (1) Vomiting
      (2) Increased tenderness
      (3) Abdominal distention
      (4) Irritability
      (5) Respiratory distress (dyspnea)
   d. Observe for enterocolitis.
   e. Measure abdominal girth q4 hr (to assess for abdominal distention).
2. Prepare infant and family emotionally for surgery.
   a. Provide explanations before all procedures.
   b. Reinforce information given about surgery.
   c. Encourage expression of concern about temporary colostomy.
   d. Use age-appropriate means for explaining body image changes and eliciting concerns from child.
3. Monitor infant's reactions to presurgical preparations.
   a. Enemas until clear (to sterilize bowel preoperatively)
   b. Intravenous (IV) tube insertion
   c. Foley catheter insertion
   d. Preoperative medication
   e. Diagnostic testing
   f. Decompression of stomach and bowel (nasogastric [NG] or rectal tube)
   g. Nothing by mouth for 12 hours before surgery
4. Promote nutritional status before surgery.
   a. Offer diet high in calories, protein, and residue.
   b. Use alternative route of intake if cannot take oral fluids.
   c. Assess intake and output accurately q8 hr.
   d. Weigh every day.

Postoperative Care

1. Assess and monitor child's postoperative status.
   a. Auscultate for return of bowel sounds.
   b. Monitor vital signs q2 hr until stable, then q4 hr.
   c. Monitor for abdominal distention (to maintain patency of NG tube).
2. Monitor child's hydration status.
   a. Observe for signs of dehydration or fluid overload.
   b. Measure and record NG drainage.
   c. Measure and record colostomy drainage.
   d. Measure and record Foley catheter drainage.
   e. Monitor IV infusion (amount, rate, infiltration).
   f. Observe for electrolyte imbalances (hyponatremia or hypokalemia).
3. Observe and report signs of complications.
   a. Intestinal obstruction caused by adhesions, volvulus, or intussusception
   b. Leakage from anastomosis (especially with Swenson's procedure)
   c. Sepsis
   d. Fistula
   e. Enterocolitis (especially with Swenson and Duhamel procedures)
   f. Frequency of stooling (with Swenson and Soave procedures, pulled-through colonic segment acts as propelling conduit)
   g. Constipation (Swenson)
   h. Bleeding (Duhamel)
   i. Recurrence of symptoms (Soave)
4. Promote return of peristalsis.
   a. Maintain patency of NG tube.
   b. Check frequency of suction machine.
   c. Irrigate with normal saline solution q4 hr and as needed.
5. Promote and maintain fluid and electrolyte balance.
   a. Record intake per route (IV, NG, oral).
   b. Record output per route (urine, stool, emesis, stoma).
   c. Consult with physician about disparities.
6. Alleviate or minimize pain and discomfort.
   a. Maintain patency of NG tube.

b. Maintain position of comfort.
c. Monitor child's response to administration of medications.
7. Prevent infection.
   a. Provide Foley catheter care every shift.
   b. Change dressing as needed (perianal and colostomy).
   c. Monitor incision site.
   d. Refer to institutional procedure manual for care related to specific procedure.
   e. Change diaper frequently; diaper to avoid fecal contamination.
8. Perform interventions specific to procedure; refer to institutional procedures manual.
9. Provide emotional support to child and family.
   a. Actively listen to concerns regarding colostomy and surgical correction.
   b. Listen to expression of parental guilt in feeling responsible for condition.
   c. Listen to expression of feelings of inadequacies in long-term care of colostomy.
   d. Listen to expression of parents' fears of death and mutilation aroused by surgery.

Home Care

1. Provide instructions to parents and child about colostomy care.
   a. Skin preparation
   b. Use of colostomy equipment
   c. Stomal complications (bleeding, failure to pass stool, increased diarrhea, prolapse, ribbonlike stools)
   d. Care and cleaning of colostomy equipment
   e. Irrigation of colostomy (refer to Chapter 39 for further information)
2. Provide and reinforce instructions about dietary management.
   a. Low-residue diet
   b. Unlimited fluid intake
   c. Signs of electrolyte imbalance or dehydration
3. Instruct parents to monitor for signs and symptoms of the following long-term complications.
   a. Stenosis

  b. Soiling
  c. Inadequate emptying
4. Encourage parents' ventilation of concerns related to colostomy.
  a. Appearance
  b. Odor
  c. Discrepancy between this child and "ideal" child
5. Refer to specific institutional procedures for information distributed to parents about home care.

BIBLIOGRAPHY

Ehrenpreis T: *Hirschsprung's disease,* St Louis, 1970, Mosby–Year Book.

Hanani M et al: Nerve mediated responses to drugs and electrical stimulation in aganglionic muscle segments in Hirschsprung's disease, *J Pediatr Surg* 21(10):848, 1986.

Martin L: Hirschsprung's disease. In Hardy J, ed: *Rhoads textbook of surgery: principles and practice,* Philadelphia, 1977, JB Lippincott.

Soave F: Hirschsprung's disease: a new surgical technique, *Arch Dis Child* 30:116, 1964.

Vane D et al: Hirschsprung's disease: current management, Perinatol Neonatol 11(6):26, 1987.

32 ❖ Hodgkin's Disease

PATHOPHYSIOLOGY

Hodgkin's disease is a malignancy of the lymphatic system. The cause of the disease is unknown. It is characterized by a proliferation of Reed-Sternberg cells, eosinophils, histiocytes, and lymphocytes. Extension occurs to adjacent and distant lymphoid areas; the disease spreads serially through the lymphatic system. Extralymphatic sites include the spleen, liver, bone marrow, and lungs. Hodgkin's disease can be diagnosed according to four histologic types. They are: (1) lymphocytic predominant (with best prognosis); (2) lymphocytic depletion (rapidly progressive); (3) mixed cell (moderately progressive); and (4) nodular sclerosis (long-term survival). Hodgkin's disease has the highest incidence of secondary malignancies.

Prognosis and treatment are based on the Hodgkin's disease staging system (Table 4).

INCIDENCE

1. Evident in late childhood or adolescence
2. Rare before 5 years of age
3. More common in females
4. Accounts for 6.5% of childhood cancers
5. Ninety percent survival rate for stages I and II
6. Seventy-five percent survival rate for stages III and IV

Table 4. Hodgkin's Disease Staging System — Ann Arbor Staging of Hodgkin's Disease

Stage	Description
I	Involvement of a single lymph node region or a single extralymphatic organ or site
II	Involvement of two or more lymph node regions on the same side of the diaphragm or localized involvement of an extralymphatic organ or site and one or more lymph node regions on the same side of the diaphragm
III	Involvement of lymph node regions or extralymphatic organs or sites or spleen on both sides of the diaphragm
IV	Diffuse involvement of one or more extralymphatic organs or tissues with or without associated lymph node involvement
Subdivision	A — no defined symptoms B — symptoms include unexplained recent weight loss or fever or night sweats

CLINICAL MANIFESTATIONS

1. Fatigue
2. Anorexia
3. Swollen lymph nodes
4. Fever
5. Weight loss
6. Night sweats
7. Involvement of liver, spleen, lungs, central nervous system, bones, and mediastinum
8. Secondary malignancy; e.g., acute nonlymphocytic leukemia (ANLL)
9. Hypothyroidism
10. Gonadal dysfunction
11. Infertility
12. Skeletal growth retardation
13. Long-term asplenia

LABORATORY/DIAGNOSTIC TESTS

1. Complete blood count (CBC) — diagnostic
2. Bone scan — to assess for bone involvement
3. Intravenous pyelogram (IVP) — to assess for renal involvement
4. Bone marrow biopsy — to assess for marrow involvement
5. Renal and liver function tests — to assess for renal and liver involvement
6. Exploratory laparotomy — used for staging purposes
7. Lymphangiogram — to assess extent of lymph node involvement
8. Tissue biopsy (Reed-Sternberg cells are diagnostic)

MEDICATIONS

1. Antibiotics are administered prophylactically if splenectomy is performed.
2. MOPP, a combination chemotherapeutic regimen, is used for 6 months:
   a. Mechlorethamine (nitrogen mustard) — interferes with DNA replication and RNA protein synthesis; has potent myelosuppressive and weak immunosuppressive action
   b. Vincristine (Oncovin) — an antineoplastic agent that inhibits cell division by arresting mitosis at metaphase
   c. Procarbazine (Matulane) — antineoplastic agent that inhibits cell division; suppresses mitosis at interphase and causes chromatin derangement; used as an adjunct medication in treatment of Hodgkin's disease; dosage is highly individualized
   d. Prednisone — a corticosteroid used for its antiinflammatory effects; inhibits phagocytosis and suppresses other clinical symptoms of inflammation; dosage is highly individualized
3. COPP, also a combination chemotherapeutic regimen, is used for 6 to 18 months of chemotherapy (cyclophosphamide is substituted for vincristine). Cyclophosphamide (Cytoxan) is an antineoplastic agent used to block the synthesis of DNA, RNA, and protein. It has pronounced immunosuppressive effects and is used as an adjunct with other chemotherapeutic agents for the treatment of Hodgkin's disease.

SURGICAL TREATMENT: STAGING PROCEDURES

Staging refers to the exact determination of the extent of the disease at the time of diagnosis. Two major types of staging systems are currently used in pediatric practice: (1) the tumor nodes metastasis (TNM) method of classification, based on the anatomic factors present; and (2) the stage grouping, which uses both anatomic and biologic variables. Staging can be achieved through three methods:

1. Clinical diagnostic staging, which is noninvasive and relies on physical examination and diagnostic studies
2. Surgical evaluation staging, which uses biopsy results
3. Postoperative (pathologic) treatment staging, which relies on the holistic examination of cancer tissue after its surgical removal

NURSING ASSESSMENT

Refer to "Respiratory Assessment" and "Gastrointestinal Assessment" in Appendix A.

NURSING DIAGNOSES

High risk for infection
High risk for injury
Impaired skin integrity
Constipation
Diversional activity deficit
Altered nutrition: less than body requirements
Knowledge deficit
Pain
Anxiety

NURSING INTERVENTIONS

Preoperative Care

1. Monitor child's clinical status.
    a. Vital signs
    b. Swollen lymph nodes
    c. Fever
2. Prepare child with age-appropriate explanations.
3. Provide and reinforce information given to parents about child's condition, upcoming surgery, and hospitalization.

4. Assist and support child in the collection of laboratory specimens.
   a. Routine preoperative laboratory tests — CBC, urinalysis, chest x-ray examination, bleeding times
   b. Bone marrow aspiration (BMA)
   c. Computed tomography (CT) scans

Postoperative Care

1. Monitor signs and symptoms of infection (immunosuppressive drugs increase susceptibility to infection).
2. Monitor gastrointestinal (GI) functioning.
   a. Presence of bowel sounds
   b. Abdominal distention
   c. Tolerance for food and fluid intake
   d. Stooling
3. Promote fluid and electrolyte balance.
   a. Monitor infusion of intravenous (IV) fluids.
   b. Monitor input and output (i.e., nasogastric [NG] output, urine, IV infusion).
   c. Observe for signs and symptoms of dehydration or fluid overload.
   d. Observe for signs and symptoms of alkalosis (caused by GI drainage).
   e. Observe for signs and symptoms of electrolyte imbalances (hypokalemia, hypochloremia).
4. Promote GI functioning.
   a. Maintain patency of NG tube.
   b. Irrigate NG tube with 15 ml normal saline q4 hr and as needed.
   c. Check functioning of intermittent suctioning.
5. Monitor side effects of radiotherapy and chemotherapy.
6. Monitor side effects of the following.
   a. Prophylactic antibiotics (penicillin) if splenectomy performed
   b. MOPP used for 6 months (mechlorethamine, vincristine, procarbazine, and prednisone)
   c. COPP used for 6 to 18 months (cyclophosphamide, vincristine, procarbazine, and prednisone)
7. Promote respiratory functioning.
   a. Elevate head of bed to semi-Fowler's position.

    b. Turn, cough, and deep breathe.
    c. Perform chest physiotherapy.
8. Provide child or adolescent the opportunity to ventilate feelings about disease, prognosis, and threats to body image.
    a. Use age-appropriate methods to encourage expression (see Appendix B, *Growth and Development*).
    b. Refer to child support group.
    c. Refer to social worker, child psychologist, or psychiatrist as needed.
9. Provide emotional support to parents.
    a. Refer to parents' support group.
    b. Refer to mental health specialist.
    c. Use active listening.
    d. Encourage ventilation of feelings.
    e. Provide for physical comforts (e.g., sleeping arrangements and hygienic needs).
    f. Encourage use of preexisting support systems.

Home Care

1. Instruct parents about the following aspects of medical management.
    a. Therapeutic response to medications
    b. Untoward reactions to medications
    c. Compliance with appointments for clinic visits
2. Provide information to parents about the following.
    a. School resources
    b. Financial resources
3. Provide emotional support and referral to support groups for parents, siblings, and affected child.

BIBLIOGRAPHY

Brecher M: Diagnosis and treatment of childhood malignancies, *Hosp Med* 22(1):83, 1986.

Fraser M, Tucker M: Second malignancies following cancer therapy, *Sem Oncol Nurs* 5(1):43, 1989.

Hdzik C: Late effects of chemotherapy: implications for patient management and rehabilitation, *Nurs Clin North Am* 25(2):423, 1990.

Hockenberry M, Coody J, Bennett B: Childhood cancers: incidence, etiology, diagnosis and treatment, *Pediatr Nurs* 16(3):239, 1990.

Kaplan H: *Hodgkin's disease,* Cambridge, Mass, 1980, Harvard University Press.

Lachner M, Redmon J: *Hodgkin's disease: the consequences of survival,* Philadelphia, 1990, Lea & Febiger.

Nirenberg A et al: Malignancies in adolescents, *Sem Oncol Nurs* 2(2):75, 1986.

Pilch Y: *Surgical oncology,* New York, 1984, McGraw-Hill.

Sullivan M: Hodgkin's disease in children, *Hematol Oncol Clin North Am* 4(1):603, 1987.

33 ❖ Hydrocephalus/ Surgical Repair

PATHOPHYSIOLOGY

Hydrocephalus results from (1) overproduction of cerebrospinal fluid (CSF) (rare), (2) obstruction of CSF flow, and/or (3) interference with absorption of CSF. Several causative factors account for hydrocephalus, including tumors, vascular malformations, abscesses, intraventricular cysts, intraventricular hemorrhage, meningitis, aqueductal stenosis, and cerebral trauma. There are two types of hydrocephalus. *Noncommunicating hydrocephalus* is a result of obstruction within the ventricular system (also called "obstructive"). *Communicating hydrocephalus* refers to blockage distal to the outlets of the fourth ventricle (CSF "communicates" with the subarachnoid space).

INCIDENCE

1. Hydrocephalus is the most common cause for an enlarging head circumference in children.
2. Seventy percent of the children with untreated hydrocephalus have a 5-year survival rate, and 75% of these children have an intelligence quotient (IQ) greater than 75.

CLINICAL MANIFESTATIONS

Signs and symptoms are the results of increased intracranial pressure (ICP).

1. Vital signs (decreased apical pulse, decreased respiratory rate, increased blood pressure)
2. Vomiting
3. Increased head circumference
4. Irritability
5. Lethargy
6. Decreased activity level
7. Change in cry (pitch)
8. Seizure activity

Infants

1. Progressive head enlargement
2. Prominence of frontal portions of the skull
3. Bulging, tense fontanels
4. Distention of superficial scalp veins
5. Symmetrically increased transillumination over the skull
6. Down-turned eyes ("sunset eyes")

Older Children

1. Headache, nausea, and vomiting
2. Anorexia
3. Ataxia
4. Lower-extremity spasticity
5. Deterioration in child's school performance or cognitive ability

COMPLICATIONS

1. Increased ICP
2. Infection
3. Obstructed shunt
4. Delays in cognitive, psychosocial, and physical development
5. Decreased intelligence quotient (IQ)

LABORATORY/DIAGNOSTIC TESTS

1. Lumbar puncture—hazardous in noncommunicating hydrocephalus because of brain and ventricular displacement
2. Computed tomography (CT) scan—most useful method of diagnosis
3. Direct puncture into ventricle through anterior fontanel—to monitor CSF pressure

MEDICATIONS

1. Anticonvulsant—phenobarbital; used for treating seizures (generalized tonic-clonic and partial simple); limits
   seizure activity by increasing the threshold for motor
   cortex stimuli; dosage—2 mg/kg/24 hr q8 hr by mouth
   (po) as needed
2. Antibiotics—choice of antibiotic is dependent on results
   of culture and sensitivity (if infection is present)

SURGICAL TREATMENT: SHUNT INSERTION

A shunt is inserted into the right ventricle as a surgical
treatment for hydrocephalus. The shunt removes the excessive cerebrospinal fluid (CSF) and decreases intracranial
pressure (ICP). The proximal end is inserted in the lateral
ventricle; the distal end is extended to the peritoneal cavity
or right atrium as a means of draining excessive fluid into
another body cavity. The ventricular peritoneal shunt is
used most frequently because the atrioventricular (AV)
shunt requires repeated revisions because of growth and
the risk of bacterial endocarditis.

CLINICAL MANIFESTATIONS

The symptoms of increased ICP are relieved. After surgery,
the child is more alert, and vomiting, anorexia, and bulging
of the fontanel are decreased.

COMPLICATIONS

1. Shunt malfunction
2. Shunt infection
3. Meningitis
4. Progressive mental deterioration

NURSING ASSESSMENT

1. Refer to "Neuromuscular Assessment" in Appendix A.
2. Assess ICP.

NURSING DIAGNOSES

Altered tissue perfusion, cerebral
Impaired physical mobility
Sensory-perceptual alteration
High risk for infection
High risk for injury

Altered growth and development
Altered family processes
Knowledge deficit

NURSING INTERVENTIONS

Preoperative Care

1. Monitor vital signs; report deviations to prevent further deterioration in condition.
   a. Temperature, apical pulse, respiratory rate, blood pressure
   b. Neurologic assessment
2. Prepare child and parents for surgical procedure.
   a. Provide age-appropriate explanations.
   b. Provide and reinforce information given to parents about child's condition and treatment.
3. Prepare or provide information about upcoming procedures.
   a. Complete blood count (CBC)
   b. Urinalysis
   c. CT scan
4. Place child in position of comfort; raise head of bed to 30 degrees (to decrease congestion and increase drainage).
5. Monitor for signs of ICP.
   a. Increased respiratory rate, decreased apical pulse, increased blood pressure
   b. Decreased level of consciousness (LOC)
   c. Seizure activity
   d. Vomiting

Postoperative Care

1. Monitor child's vital signs and neurologic status; report signs of ICP (size, fullness, tension of anterior fontanel), LOC, anorexia, vomiting, convulsions, seizures, sluggishness.
2. Monitor and report signs of infection.
   a. Shunt infection (irritability, decreased LOC, vomiting)
   b. Site infection (fever, tenderness, inflammation, nausea, and vomiting)
3. Monitor and maintain functioning of shunt.

    a. Check shunt for fullness.
    b. Elevate head of bed 30 degrees (to increase drainage and decrease venous congestion).
    c. Position on left side (nonoperative side).
    d. Maintain bed rest for 24 to 72 hours.
4. Monitor dressing for drainage and intactness.
    a. Check for drainage and outline of the drainage on the dressing.
    b. Notify physician of excessive drainage.
5. Promote nutritional and fluid intake.
    a. Monitor intake and output.
    b. Assess bowel sounds before feeding.

Home Care/Discharge Planning

1. Instruct parents to monitor and report signs of the following.
    a. Shunt malfunction
    b. Shunt infection
2. Provide parents with assistance in contacting community resources.
    a. Follow-up by public health nurse
    b. Selection of preschool and recreational programs
3. Assess cognitive, linguistic, adaptive, and social behaviors to determine development; use developmental history to assess early milestones, and refer to appropriate specialists as needed.

BIBLIOGRAPHY

Chuang S: Parental and neonatal hydrocephalus; clinical presentation and radiologic studies part 2, *Perinatol Neonatol* 10(6):10, 1986.

Conway B: *Carini and Owens' neurological and neurosurgical nursing*, ed 7, St. Louis, 1978, Mosby–Year Book.

Jackson P: Peritoneal shunting for hydrocephalus, *Crit Care Update* 10(4):33, 1983.

Jackson P: Primary care needs of children with hydrocephalus, *J Pediatr Health Care* 4(2):54, 1990.

Nickel R et al: Developmental prognosis for infants with benign enlargement of the subarachnoid spaces, *Dev Med Child Neurol* 24(2):181, 1987.

Pleasants D: Managing hydrocephalus with a ventricular shunt, *AORN J* 35(5):885, 1982.

Scheinblum S, Hammond M: The treatment of children with shunt infections: extraventricular drainage system care, *Pediatr Nurs* 16(2):139, 1990.

Scott R: *Hydrocephalus: concepts in neurosurgery* (vol 3), Baltimore, 1990, Williams & Wilkins.

Shaw N: Common surgical problems in the newborn, *J Perinat Neonat Nurs* 3(3):50, 1990.

Thompson J, Thompson H: Applying the decision-making model: case studies, *Neonat Network: J Neonat Nurs* 9(4):57, 1990.

34 ❖ Hypertension

PATHOPHYSIOLOGY

Hypertension in the pediatric patient is described as blood pressures that are persistently between the 90th and 95th percentile. The box on p. 206 identifies guidelines (based on age and sex) for suspect blood pressure values. A variety of mechanisms are associated with hypertension. The renin-angiotensin-aldosterone system maintains fluid volume and vascular tone through the production of angiotensin II (a vasoconstrictor) and the stimulation of aldosterone production (for sodium retention). The sympathetic nervous system affects peripheral vascular resistance, cardiac output, and renin release, influencing the regulation of blood pressure.

Hypertension is classified as primary or secondary. Primary hypertension can be attributed to no identifiable cause, whereas secondary hypertension is attributable to a structural abnormality or to an underlying disease (renal, cardiovascular, endocrine, central nervous system [CNS], and collagen). A variety of factors have been identified as contributing to hypertension, including diet (high in calories, saturated fats, and sodium), contraceptives, positive family history, obesity, and minimal physical exercise. Children generally manifest no overt symptoms. If symptomatic, the disease may be quite severe. Prognosis is variable, depending on the age of onset and response to treatment. Problems evident in adults may have originated during the first or second decade of life. The earlier the onset, the more severe the disease will be.

Approximate Guidelines for Suspect Blood Pressures

Blood Pressure Values
Supine position — lowest of three readings

	Boys and Girls		
Age in Years	3-5	6-9	1-14
Blood pressure mm Hg	>110/70	>120/75	>130/80

Seated position — average of second and third readings

	Girls	Boys		
Age in years	14-18	14	15	16-18
Blood pressure mm Hg	>125/80	>130/75	>130/80	>135/85

From Gilles S and Kagan B: *Current Pediatric Therapy* 13, Philadelphia, 1990, WB Saunders, p. 148.

INCIDENCE

1. There is an increased incidence among children in a lower socioeconomic status.
2. There is an increased incidence among black adolescents.
3. Age has no direct relationship to blood pressure.
4. Incidence rates vary from 0.6% to 20.5% (depends on methodology used).
5. Noncompliance with treatment occurs among more than 50% of the children; compliance improves when child is dependent on parent.
6. Males are affected more often than females.
7. Forty-five percent to 100% of cases of hypertension in individuals 2 to 18 years of age are attributed to primary hypertension.
8. Twenty-five percent of children with primary hypertension have positive family history.
9. One percent to 2% of children and 11% to 12% of adolescents are affected.

CLINICAL MANIFESTATIONS

1. Blurred vision; symptoms of ICP
2. Severe headaches

3. Marked irritability
4. Nosebleeds
5. Dizziness
6. Fatigue
7. Nervousness
8. Anorexia, failure to thrive (FTT), weight loss
9. Focal or generalized seizures
10. Severe back and/or abdominal pain
11. Papilledema
12. Retinal hemorrhage or exudate
13. Left-ventricular hypertrophy
14. Altered renal function

COMPLICATIONS

1. Ischemic (coronary) heart disease
2. Side effects associated with use of antihypertensives (e.g., postexercise syncope, depression, and dizziness)

LABORATORY/DIAGNOSTIC TESTS

1. Urinalysis, urine culture — to assess for renal cause
2. Serum electrolytes — to assess for renal and metabolic status
3. Complete blood count (CBC) — to assess for infection, fluid overload
4. Creatinine, blood urea nitrogen (BUN) — to assess for renal function
5. Serum cholesterol — greater than 250 mg/100 ml
6. Serum triglyceride level — increased
7. Lipoprotein electrophoresis — elevated
8. Electrocardiogram (ECG) — left-ventricular hypertrophy
9. Chest x-ray film — left-ventricular hypertrophy
10. Rapid-sequence intravenous pyelogram — to assess activation of renin-angiotensin system
11. Plasma renin activity — to assess activation of renin-angiotensin system
12. Excretory venography — to detect renal and renovascular abnormalities
13. Arteriography — to detect renal and renovascular abnormalities
14. Radionuclide studies — to detect renal and renovascular abnormalities

MEDICATIONS

This list is not inclusive; a variety of medications can be used, depending on severity of symptoms.

1. Diuretics (initial pharmacologic treatment)
   a. Chlorothiazide (Diuril) — produces diuresis by reducing sodium reabsorption and increasing potassium excretion in the distal convoluted tubules; antihypertensive mechanism is unclear; acts by reducing cardiac output, thereby decreasing peripheral vascular resistance; used to reduce blood pressure or treat essential hypertension
      (1) Initial dose — 10 mg/kg/day by mouth (po); gradually increased over 2 weeks to maintenance dose
      (2) Maintenance dose — 20 mg/kg/day po
   b. Hydrochlorothiazide (HydroDiuril) — similar to chlorothiazide in action; used in managing hypertension
      (1) Initial dose — 1 mg/kg/day po
      (2) Maintenance dose — 1 to 2 mg/kg/day po
2. Beta blockers
   a. Methyldopa (Aldomet) — reduces concentration of serotonin and dopamine, which is a precursor of norepinephrine; used to treat sustained moderate to severe hypertension (particularly if caused by renal dysfunction)
      (1) Initial dose — 10 mg/kg/day po (increased over 1 week to maintenance dose)
      (2) Maintenance dose — 40 mg/kg/day po; 20 mg up to 65 mg/kg/24 hr q6 hr intravenously (IV)
   b. Propranolol (Inderal) — lowers blood pressure by decreasing cardiac output, suppressing renin activity, and blocking sympathetic pathways; used with a thiazide or another antihypertensive in the treatment of essential hypertension; dosage — 20-40 mg TID/QID po. Dosages have been established for *adults* only.
3. Vasodilator
   a. Hydralazine (Apresoline) — reduces blood pressure by direct relaxation of vascular smooth muscles, with greater effect on arterioles than on veins (increases

renal and cerebral blood flow as a result); used as an adjunct with other antihypertensives

(1) Initial dose — 1 mg/kg/day po (increased over 1 week to maintenance dose)
(2) Maintenance dose — 5 mg/kg/day po; 1.7 to 3.5 mg/kg/day q4-6 hr po

NURSING ASSESSMENT

Refer to "Renal Assessment" in Appendix A.

NURSING DIAGNOSES

Altered tissue perfusion
Decreased cardiac output
Pain
Knowledge deficit

NURSING INTERVENTIONS

1. Monitor and assess child's clinical status for changes.
   a. Blood pressure (see Appendix E)
   b. Neurologic status
   c. Presence of bleeding
   d. Blurred vision
   e. Renal function
2. Monitor and observe child's therapeutic and untoward response to administered medications.
3. Monitor and encourage child's nutritional intake.
   a. Administer diet restricted in sodium, fats, and calories.
   b. Reinforce dietary information and management plan provided by dietician.

Home Care

Instruct child and family about management of hypertension.

1. Explanation of hypertension
2. Medications
3. Dietary restrictions and weight control
4. Use of oral contraceptives
5. Salt intake
6. Exercise
7. Smoking

BIBLIOGRAPHY

Adeyanju M et al: A 3 year study of obesity and its relationship to high blood pressure in adolescents, *J School Health* 57(3):109, 1987.

Carman M: Cardiovascular screening programs: implications for school nurses, *Pediatr Nurs* 16(5):509, 1990.

DeCastro F et al: Hypertension in adolescents, *Pediatr Nurs* 5:30, July/Aug 1975.

Harris J: High blood pressure in children and adolescents, *Health Educ* 18(3):31, 1987.

Kaplan N: *Clinical hypertension*, ed 5, Baltimore, 1990, Williams & Wilkins.

Kelsall J, Watson A: Should school nurses measure blood pressure? *Publ Health* 104(3):191, 1990.

O'Brien P, Elixson E: The child following the Fontan procedure: nursing strategies, *ANCN Clinic Issues Critic Care Nurs* 1(1):46, 1990.

Rauh W: Hypertension in childhood and adolescence, *Pediatr Ann* 10(9):59, 1981.

Vogel M: Hypertension in children, *Pediatr Nurs* 5:37, Nov/Dec 1977.

Wilson D, Killon D: Urinary tract infections in the pediatric patient, *Nurse Pract: Am J Prim Health Care* 14(7):38, 1989.

Winer H: Hypertensive crisis, *Critic Care Nurs Quart* 13(3):23, 1990.

35 ❖ Hypertrophic Pyloric Stenosis

PATHOPHYSIOLOGY

Hypertrophic pyloric stenosis is one of the more frequently occurring conditions of infancy that cause malnutrition. Hypertrophy and hyperplasia of the circular muscle of the pylorus cause obstruction at the pyloric sphincter. The circular muscle thickens as much as four times normal, and the pylorus increases in length, with narrowing of the lumen as a result. In addition, the stomach dilates in size, and hypertrophy of the antrum occurs. The cause is unknown, although several factors have been identified as causative agents, including gastrointestinal (GI) hormones, environmental postnatal factors, muscle enzymes, autonomic neurons, and genetic predisposition. Diagnosis is based on history, initially seen symptoms, and confirmatory x-ray findings.

INCIDENCE

1. Occurs in 2.6 of 1000 live births
2. Mortality—less than 1%
3. Rare in blacks and Chinese
4. Gender ratio of males to females—4:1
5. Seasonal peak prevalence of hypertrophic pyloric stenosis—spring (April to June) and fall (September to November)
6. Increased incidence in breastfed infants
7. Increased incidence associated with younger maternal age

8. Increased incidence associated with ovarian dysgenesis and X/XX mosaicism

CLINICAL MANIFESTATIONS

1. Projectile vomiting emerging from mouth and nares
2. Feeds hungrily; eager to be fed after vomiting
3. Does not vomit after each feeding; retained feeding vomited with current feeding
4. Vomitus contains milk and mucus, blood (20% of cases), and no bile
5. May be constipated (stool q48 hr)
6. Increased frequency and decreased size of stool
7. Paleness
8. Signs of dehydration (decreased tears, poor skin turgor, dark circles under eyes, sunken fontanel)
9. Failure to gain weight
10. Loss of fat pads
11. Pain behaviors—arching back, stretching, screaming
12. Visible right-to-left gastric waves
13. Palpable olive-size pyloric tumor during feeding

COMPLICATIONS

1. Jaundice (8% of cases) caused by deficiency of hepatic glucuronide transferase
2. Metabolic alkalosis
3. Severe dehydration

Long-Term Effects (Adulthood)

1. Dyspeptic symptoms—heartburn, feeling of fullness in stomach
2. Ulcer
3. Diarrhea, ranging from periodic to constant
4. No correlation between severity of pyloric stenosis and presence of later GI disturbances

LABORATORY/DIAGNOSTIC TESTS

1. Complete blood count (CBC) (anemia)
2. Serum electrolytes (hypochloremia, hypokalemia)
3. Serum glucose and Dextrostix (hypoglycemia)
4. Blood urea nitrogen (BUN) (increased; indicative of dehydration)

5. Arterial blood gas values (metabolic alkalosis)
6. Upper GI x-ray examination (diagnostic; delayed gastric emptying)
7. Ultrasound: diagnostic
8. Hematest of vomitus

MEDICATIONS

Anticholinergics (e.g., scopolamine and atropine) are the principal medications used for treating hypertrophic pyloric stenosis.

NURSING ASSESSMENT

Refer to "Gastrointestinal Assessment" in Appendix A.

NURSING DIAGNOSES

Fluid volume deficit
Altered nutrition: less than body requirements
Pain
High risk for infection
Impaired tissue integrity
Knowledge deficit

NURSING INTERVENTIONS

1. Promote and maintain fluid and electrolyte balance.
    a. Monitor replacement of intravenous (IV) fluids 12 to 24 hours after hospital admittance; replacement fluids include the following:
        (1) 0.25 normal saline with potassium (K^+) replacement
        (2) 0.5 normal saline with K^+ replacement
    b. Monitor urinary output.
    c. Assess clinical status for treatment of dehydration.
    d. Feed again, if ordered, immediately after child vomits.
    e. Perform gastric lavage with normal saline through nasogastric (NG) tube until clear (preoperative preparation).
2. Observe and monitor child's response to electrolyte imbalance.
    a. Monitor for clinical signs of hypokalemia and report as indicated.
    b. Monitor and report symptoms of compensatory re-

sponse to metabolic alkalosis (decreased pulmonary ventilation, hypercapnia [usually of minimal significance]).

3. Prepare parents preoperatively for child's upcoming surgery.
    a. Provide information about preoperative and postoperative care and surgery itself (Fredet-Ramstedt operation).
    b. Encourage ventilation of concerns; gather information from medical and support personnel to assist in coping with stressful event.

Postoperative Care

1. Promote and maintain fluid and electrolyte balance.
    a. Monitor IV infusions until oral fluids are tolerated.
       (1) Maintenance dose—D_5W or 0.2 normal saline solution with K^+
       (2) Replacement dose of K^+ is not started until urinary status is ascertained
    b. Monitor child's response to feedings by mouth.
    c. Assess for signs of hydration (urinary output, serum electrolytes, and blood gases within normal limits).
2. Monitor child's response to oral intake.
    a. Initiate fluids by mouth 3 to 4 hours postoperatively; assess response.
    b. Provide small, frequent feedings (15 to 20 ml per feeding) as tolerated.
    c. Begin with D_5W; increase to full-strength formula as tolerated (progression of fluids—D_5W, one-fourth, one-half, three-fourths, full-strength formula).
    d. Feed with infant in upright position.
    e. Monitor blood sugars with Dextrostix.
    f. Observe for signs of vomiting and hematemesis (may delay feedings by mouth 48 hours).
    g. Monitor for weight gain.
3. Provide pain relief measures as indicated.
    a. Observe for signs of pain—crying, irritability, stretching, arching back, increased motor activity.
    b. Monitor child's response and untoward reactions to medications.
4. Monitor and maintain integrity of incisional site.

   a. Observe for signs of infection — redness, drainage, inflammation, warm to touch.
   b. Cleanse with normal saline solution or hydrogen peroxide as needed.
   c. Change dressing as needed.
5. Provide psychosocial support.
   a. Provide age-appropriate stimulation.
   b. Promote parent to infant or child bonding.
   c. Encourage parents to ventilate concerns.

Home Care

1. Instruct parents to observe child's response to feedings and untoward symptoms.
   a. Persistent vomiting
   b. Signs of infection
2. Instruct parents about care of incisional site.
3. Provide follow-up support and management for parents.
   a. Name and phone number of primary physician
   b. Phone number of clinic
   c. Name and phone number of clinical nurse specialist and primary nurse

BIBLIOGRAPHY

Bowen A: The vomiting infant: recent advances and unsettling issues in imaging, *Radiol Clin North Am* 26(2):377, 1988.

Breaux C et al: Changing patterns in the diagnosis of hypertrophic pyloric stenosis, *Pediatrics* 81(2):213, 1988.

Breaux C et al: The significance of alkalosis and hypochloremia in hypertrophic pyloric stenosis, *J Pediatr Surg* 24:1250, 1989.

Jedd M et al: Factors associated with infantile hypertrophic pyloric stenosis, *Am J Dis Child* 142:334, 1988.

Rollins M et al: Pyloric stenosis: congenital or acquired, *Arch Dis Child* 64:138, 1989.

Solowiejczk O, Holtzman M, Michowitz M: Congenital hypertrophic pyloric stenosis: a long-term follow-up of 41 cases, *Am Surg* 46(10):737, 1980.

Spenner D: When the baby's sick and the mother's concerns are ignored, *Am J Nurs* 80(12):2221, 1980.

Spicer R: Infantile hypertrophic pyloric stenosis: a review, *Br J Surg* 69:128, 1982.

36 ❖ Hypothyroidism

PATHOPHYSIOLOGY

Hypothyroidism is one of the most common childhood endocrine disorders. It results from inadequate thyroid hormone production as a result of congenital or acquired causes (see box on facing page). The thyroid hormone performs the following functions: (1) regulates body metabolism by increasing oxygen consumption; (2) enhances protein synthesis, affecting tissue growth and differentiation; (3) plays a role in temperature regulation, cardiovascular functioning, gastrointestinal (GI) motility, and neurologic reflexes; and (4) affects the growth and development of the skeletal and central nervous systems.

One third of the cases are initially seen in infancy; the remaining two thirds are seen in childhood. Only 5% of cases are suspected clinically before diagnosis.

Thyroid dysgenesis accounts for 80% of the known causes of hypothyroidism. Inborn errors of thyroid hormone synthesis account for 10% to 15% of the diagnosed cases. Development of the symptoms of hypothyroidism and its prognosis depend on the following factors: (1) type of defect; (2) age of onset and duration; and (3) severity of hormonal deficiency. Effects are devastating if not treated.

INCIDENCE

1. Occurrence — 1 in 7000 births
2. Male to female ratio — 1:2

Causes of Hypothyroidism

Congenital

Thyroid dysgenesis (aplasia, hypoplasia, ectopia)
Maternal ingestion of medications
Goitrogens
Propylthiouracil
Methimazole
Iodides
Radioactive iodine
Autoimmune thyroiditis
Hypopituitarism
Inadequate hormonal secretion
Inadequate hormonal use
Impaired hormonal synthesis

Acquired

Chronic lymphocytic thyroiditis
Thyroidectomy
Hypopituitarism
Prolonged administration of thyroid (transient)

CLINICAL MANIFESTATIONS
Infants
1. Majority appear normal at birth; signs and symptoms absent
2. Decreased GI peristalsis, causing decreased stooling or constipation
3. Decreased appetite, resulting in poor feeding
4. Lethargy
5. Increased periods of sleeping
6. Prolonged jaundice
7. Classical facial appearance — edematous, wide fontanels and sutures, flattened nasal bridge with pseudohypertelorism, large protruding tongue
8. Hoarse cry
9. Protuberant abdomen with umbilical hernia
10. Cold, mottled skin

Children

1. Short, stocky frame
2. Proportionally longer upper torso
3. Dull facial expression
4. Obese
5. Sexual precocity — premature breast development, testicular enlargement
6. Elevated serum hormonal levels — increased thyroid-stimulating hormone (TSH); increased follicle-stimulating hormone (FSH); increased luteinizing hormone (LH); increased serum prolactin
7. Galactorrhea
8. Premature menstrual spotting
9. Delayed bone age

COMPLICATIONS (IF UNTREATED)

1. Retarded skeletal growth
2. Delayed dental eruption
3. Mental retardation
4. Retarded somatic growth
5. Ataxia
6. Muscular hypotonia
7. Strabismus

LABORATORY/DIAGNOSTIC TESTS

1. Radioimmunoassays — T_3 (decreased), thyroxine (T_4) (decreased), thyroxine-binding globulin (TBG), TSH (decreased); to measure thyroid hormones
2. Skeletal x-ray examination — to assess bone age
3. Antithyroglobulin antibody titer
4. Antimicrosomal titer
5. Serum cholesterol — normal in infants; increases to 275 to 600 mg/100 ml
6. Serum glucose — low
7. Plasma carotene level — increased; abnormality in conversion of carotene to vitamin A
8. Protein-bound iodine (PBI) — normal for first 2 months of life; then increased
9. Creatine phosphokinase (CPK) — increased
10. Electrocardiogram (ECG) — flat or inverted T waves and prolonged PR

11. Electroencephalogram (EEG)—slow alpha rhythm
12. Electromyogram (EMG)—slow nerve conduction

NEWBORN SCREENING

1. TSH assay
2. Technetium-99m pertechnetate—to determine whether thyroid gland is present and its size, shape, location

MEDICATIONS

Synthetic levothyroxine is used to treat hypothyroidism.
1. First year—5 to 6 μg/kg
2. Second year—4 μg/kg
3. Late childhood and adolescence—3 to 4 μg/kg

NURSING ASSESSMENT

Refer to "Endocrine Assessment" in Appendix A.

NURSING DIAGNOSES

Impaired physical mobility
Sensory-perceptual alterations
Constipation
Fatigue
Knowledge deficit

NURSING INTERVENTIONS

1. Provide emotional support to parents during phase of diagnosis.
   a. Encourage ventilation of feelings of guilt and/or fear.
   b. Reinforce information provided about diagnosis.
   c. Clarify misconceptions parents may have about etiology, manifestations, prognosis.
2. Monitor infant's or child's response to administration of thyroid replacement.
   a. Monitor therapeutic responses—linear growth, activity level, sleep, eating, and elimination pattern.
   b. Monitor untoward effects of overdosage—irritability, nervousness, sweating, diarrhea, tremors, tachycardia, wide pulse pressure, and craniosynostosis.
   c. Schedule follow-up appointments to monitor serum levels.
      (1) First year—every 3 months

(2) Second year—every 6 months
(3) Third year through adulthood—every year

Home Care

1. Instruct parents about the administration of thyroid replacement.
   a. Dosage *must* be given every day.
   b. If dose is missed, two doses must be given.
   c. Demonstrate methods of crushing and administering with food.
   d. Describe untoward effects.
   e. Explain action and therapeutic outcomes (may have unrealistic expectations).
   f. Explain necessity for long-term continuous monitoring of hormonal levels.
2. Assist, support, and counsel parents to seek genetic counseling (recurrence in subsequent children is dependent on cause).

BIBLIOGRAPHY

Allen D et al: Screening programs for congenital hypothyroidism. How can they be improved? *Am J Dis Child* 142(2):232, 1988.

Coody D: Congenital hypothyroidism, *Pediatr Nurs* 12(6):342, 1984.

Iodine-containing antiseptics, *Nurses Drug Alert* 14(2):12, 1990.

Isley W: Thyroid disorders, *Critic Care Nurs Quart* 13(3):39, 1990.

La Franchi S: Hypothyroidism, *Pediatr Clin North Am* 26(1):33, 1979.

Muir A et al: Thyroid scanning ultrasound and serum thyroglobulin in determining the origin of congenital hypothyroidism, *Am J Dis Child* 142(2):214, 1988.

Newborn screening fact sheets, *Pediatrics* 83(3):449, 1990.

Schneider R, Tenore A: *Hypothyroidism and the infant,* Evanston, Ill, 1981, Arthur Retlan and Assoc.

Shiminski-Maher T, Rosenberg M: Late effects associated with treatment of craniopharyngiomas in childhood, *J Neurosci Nurs* 22(4):220, 1990.

Smith J: Pregnancy complicated by thyroid disease, *J Nurs Midwif* 35(3):143, 1990.

Yeomans A: Assessment and management of hypothyroidism, *Nurse Pract: Am J Prim Health Care* 15(11):11, 1990.

37 ❖ Idiopathic Thrombocytopenic Purpura

PATHOPHYSIOLOGY

Idiopathic thrombocytopenic purpura (ITP) refers to an acquired syndrome in which there is a reduction in the number of circulating platelets in the presence of normal marrow. The exact cause of this condition is unknown, although it is speculated to be caused by viral agents that damage platelets. Generally, ITP is preceded by a vaguely defined febrile illness 2 to 3 weeks before onset of symptoms. Clinical manifestations vary considerably. ITP can be classified into three types: acute, chronic, and recurrent (see box on p. 222). Children are initially seen with the following symptoms: (1) fever, (2) bleeding, (3) purpura with thrombocytopenia, and (4) anemia. Prognosis is favorable, especially in children with the acute form.

INCIDENCE

1. The peak periods of occurrence are 2 to 6 years of age.
2. ITP affects males and females equally.
3. It occurs more commonly in whites.
4. Eighty percent of ITP in children is the acute type.
5. Seasonal prevalence — this illness occurs more frequently in winter and spring.
6. Fifty percent to 85% of the children have a viral illness before ITP.

Types of ITP

Acute

Child is initially seen with thrombocytopenia.

Platelet count returns to normal within 6 months of diagnosis (spontaneous remission).

Subsequent relapses are not seen.

Chronic

Thrombocytopenia persists more than 6 months after diagnosis.

Onset is insidious.

Platelet count remains below normal throughout disease.

This form is seen primarily in adults.

Recurrent

Individual is initially seen with thrombocytopenia.

He or she has repeated relapses.

Platelet count returns to normal between relapses.

---

7. Ten percent to 25% of the children develop the chronic form of ITP.

CLINICAL MANIFESTATIONS

1. Prodromal period—fatigue, fever, and abdominal pain
2. Spontaneous appearance on skin of petechiae and ecchymoses
3. Easily bruised
4. Epistaxis (initially seen symptom in one third of children)
5. Hematuria (infrequent)
6. Bleeding from oral cavity (infrequent)
7. Melena (infrequent)

COMPLICATIONS

1. Transfusion reaction
2. Relapse

LABORATORY/DIAGNOSTIC TESTS

1. Platelet count (decreased to less than 20,000 when child admitted to hospital)
2. Complete blood count (CBC) (anemia results from inability of red blood cells [RBCs] to use iron)
3. Bone marrow aspiration (increased megakaryocytes)
4. White blood count (WBC) (mild to moderate leukocytosis; mild eosinophilia)
5. Platelet antibody test: The following tests are done with questionable diagnosis:
    a. Tissue biopsy of skin and gingiva (diagnostic)
    b. Antinuclear antibody test (to rule out systemic lupus erythematosus [SLE])
    c. Slitlamp examinations (screen for uveitis)
    d. Renal biopsy (to diagnose renal involvement)
    e. Chest x-ray examination and pulmonary function test (diagnostic for pulmonary manifestations—effusion, interstitial pulmonary fibrosis)

MEDICATIONS/TREATMENTS

1. Antibiotics (sulfa drugs and penicillin)—selection of antibiotic is dependent on culture and sensitivity (not used often).
2. Prednisone (a corticosteroid)—used for antiinflammatory effects (a glucocorticoid); inhibits phagocytosis and suppresses inflammatory reaction; used to suppress inflammatory and immune responses in rheumatic disorders.
3. Immunosuppressive agents:
    a. Vincristine (Oncovin)—immunosuppressive used in difficult cases.
    b. Cyclophosphamide (Cytoxan)—immunosuppressive used in difficult cases.
4. Iron—treats anemia. Dosage—6 mg/kg/24 hr po of elemental iron; 7 mg/0.6 ml po of ferrous sulfate drops.
5. Gamma globulins—intravenous gamma globulin (IVGG): high dose given to elevate platelet count.
6. Splenectomy: may be performed if ITP lasts more than 1 year. Done in children more than 5 years old.

NURSING ASSESSMENT

1. Refer to "Hematologic Assessment" in Appendix A.
2. Determine location of purpuric areas.
3. Determine sites of bleeding.

NURSING DIAGNOSES

High risk for injury
Impaired tissue integrity
Altered tissue perfusion
Fluid volume deficit
Diversional activity deficit
Knowledge deficit

NURSING INTERVENTIONS

1. Monitor child's clinical status.
   a. Vital signs as often as q2 hr during acute phase
   b. Bleeding sites
   c. Level of activity
   d. Purpuric area
   e. Areas susceptible to bruising
2. Monitor and prevent infection.
   a. Screen contacts with child.
   b. Institute clean techniques when in contact with child.
   c. Monitor for signs of infection (pulmonary, systemic, localized).
   d. Administer medications.
3. Monitor child's response to blood products transfusions (whole blood, packed cells, platelets).
4. Monitor child's therapeutic and untoward response to administration of medications.
   a. Antibiotics
   b. Antipyretics
   c. Iron preparations
   d. Immunosuppressives
5. Promote rest and conservation of the child's energy.
   a. Maintain complete bed rest during acute stages.
   b. Assess child's response to activity as means of assessing tolerance and progression.
6. Provide diversional and age-appropriate activities for child during periods of limited activities (see Appendix B, *Growth and Development*).

7. Provide age-appropriate explanations before procedures and treatments.
8. Provide preoperative instruction to child and parents to prepare for surgery (if splenectomy indicated).

Home Care/Discharge Instructions

1. Provide parents and child with instructions about administration of medications.
   a. Time and route of administration
   b. Monitoring for untoward effects
2. Instruct parents and child to monitor for signs and symptoms of relapse.
3. Instruct parents to monitor child's tolerance for activities.
   a. Look for signs of fatigue—lower activity level, longer periods of sleep, flat affect, irritability, cries easily, low tolerance for frustration.
   b. Provide intermittent rest periods.

BIBLIOGRAPHY

Burstein Y, Berns L: Immune thrombocytopenic purpura, *Pediatr Ann* 11(3):323, 1982.

Byrnes J: Thrombotic thrombocytopenic purpura: an epidemiologic study, *J Pediatr* 83:31, 1980.

Reynolds M: Role of immune globulin in the treatment of idiopathic thrombocytopenic purpura, *J Pediatr Health Care* 3(2):109, 1989.

Tammi A, Touric U: Idiopathic thrombocytopenic purpura: an epidemiologic study, *J Pediatr* 83:31, 1973.

Thomas G, O'Brien R: Idiopathic thrombocytopenic purpura in children, *Nurs Pract: Am J Prim Health Care* 12(4):24, 1987.

Thomas G et al: Idiopathic thrombocytopenic purpura in children, *Nurs Pract* 12(4):24, 1987.

Tucker J, Iyer R: Idiopathic thrombocytopenic purpura in children, *Semin Thromb Hemost* 3:175, 1977.

38 ❖ Imperforate Anus

PATHOPHYSIOLOGY

A variety of anorectal malformations are classified collectively as imperforate anus, or anal atresia. They are listed in the box on the facing page. Depending on the level of anorectal anomaly, definitive surgery is delayed until the child is 12 to 18 months old. This delay allows the pelvis to enlarge and the musculature to develop and enables the child to gain weight and attain satisfactory nutritional status. A temporary transverse colostomy, which remains until definitive surgery can be performed, is performed within a few days of birth. Infants are diagnosed shortly after birth when meconium is not passed and taking a rectal temperature is attempted unsuccessfully. The appearance of the defect varies, depending on its severity. A less involved imperforate anus appears as a deep anal dimple and exhibits strong muscular reaction to pin prick, indicating innervation of that area. More severe involvement is initially seen as a flat perineum with no dimple and poor muscular response to pin prick, a result of defective perineal innervation and muscle formation. A highly involved defect includes other anomalies as well (Table 5). The infant may initially be seen with poorly developed labia, undescended testicles, and ambiguous genitalia. Outcomes are favorable after definitive surgery is performed.

Types of Imperforate Anus

Anal Stenosis

Gastrointestinal tract is normal in terms of both structure and function. It narrows at the distal end within 1 cm of the anus. Treatment is uncomplicated and simple. The anus is dilated at frequent intervals until it passes stool normally.

Imperforate Anal Membrane

The gastrointestinal tract is normal in terms of both structure and function. The anus is intact. The epithelial membrane covering the anus is incised. The anus is dilated at frequent intervals until normal passage of stool occurs.

Anal Agenesis

This type of imperforate anus is primarily found in males; however, anal agenesis with fistula most frequently occurs in females. The fistula opens into the vulva or the perineal region. The gastrointestinal tract is normal in structure and function. The bowel ends 0.5 to 2 cm above the anus. An incision is made over the external sphincter. The blind end of the intestine is anastomosed to the external sphincter. The anal orifice is dilated for 1 to 2 months following surgery.

Rectal Agenesis

This is the most common type of imperforate anus. The end of the intestine is more than 2 cm from the anus. Rectal agenesis is frequently accompanied by a fistula.

Rectal Atresia

The anus is normal in structure. The intestine ends in a blind pouch. Because of the normal appearance of the anus, it is mistaken as normal.

Table 5. Associated Anomalies of Imperforate Anus.

Type	Incidence*(%)
Esophageal atresia	13
Intestinal atresia	4
Intestinal malrotation	4
Cardiovascular defects	7
Skeletal deformities (spina bifida, agenesis of sacrum)	6
Genitourinary anomalies (renal agenesis, hypospadias, epispadias)	40

*Approximate percentage.

PATIENT RESPONSE TO SURGERY

In most instances, correction of the imperforate anus requires a two-stage surgical approach. For mild to moderate defects, the prognosis is favorable. The defect can be repaired, and normal peristalsis and continence can be obtained. More serious defects are usually associated with other anomalies, compounding the surgical outcomes.

CLINICAL MANIFESTATIONS

1. Meconium not passed within first 24 hours after birth
2. Inability to take patient's rectal temperature
3. Varying clinical appearance according to severity of defect (see "Pathophysiology")

COMPLICATIONS

1. Hyperchloremic acidosis
2. Continuing urinary tract infection
3. Urethral damage (result of surgical procedure)
4. Extravasation of urine into pelvis

Long-Term Complications

1. Eversion of anal mucosa
2. Stenosis (result of contraction of scar from anastomosis)
3. Impactions and constipation (result of sigmoid dilation)
4. Problems/delays associated with toilet training

5. Incontinence (result of anal stenosis or impaction)
6. Prolapse of anorectal mucosa (results in persistent seepage and incontinence)
7. Recurrent fistulas (result of tension in surgical site and infection)

NURSING ASSESSMENT

1. Refer to "Gastrointestinal Assessment" in Appendix A.

NURSING DIAGNOSES

Fluid volume deficit
Altered nutrition: less than body requirements
Impaired tissue integrity
High risk for infection
High risk for injury
Pain
Impaired home maintenance management

NURSING INTERVENTIONS

Preoperative Care

1. Prepare parents emotionally for surgery.
    a. Provide understandable explanations in lay terms.
    b. Encourage ventilation of feelings (guilt, anger, anxiety).
    c. Encourage parents to room-in and participate in child's care as means of promoting security and decreased anxiety.
2. Monitor child's condition before surgery.
    a. Measure abdominal girth (assess for abdominal distention).
    b. Monitor vital signs q4 hr.
    c. Monitor for bowel complications (perforation and enterocolitis).
    d. Monitor fluid and electrolyte balance (input and output, nasogastric [NG] drainage).
3. Prepare infant for surgery.
    a. Monitor infant's response to evacuation of bowel.
    b. Using NG tube, decompress stomach.
    c. Using catheter, decompress bladder.
    d. Provide only clear liquids 24 to 48 hours before surgery.

    e. Monitor child's response to antibiotics (e.g., neomy-
       cin) used to sterilize bowel.
4. Prepare infant for procedures and surgeries.
    a. Intravenous pyelogram (IVP) (to assess associated
       urologic anomalies)
    b. Voiding cystourethrogram (diagnostic, confirmatory
       for urologic abnormality)
    c. Electrocardiogram (ECG)
    d. Chest x-ray examination
    e. Serum electrolytes
    f. Abdominal x-ray examination
    g. Complete blood count (CBC)
    h. Type and crossmatch blood

Postoperative Care

1. Monitor child's response to surgery.
    a. Vital signs
    b. Intake and output—report discrepancies
    c. Surgical site—bleeding, intactness, signs of infection
2. Monitor for signs and symptoms of complications.
    a. Urinary tract infection
    b. Hyperchloremic acidosis
    c. Decreased urinary output
    d. Constipation
    e. Obstruction
    f. Bleeding
3. Promote and maintain fluid and electrolyte balance.
    a. Record intake per route (intravenous [IV], NG, oral).
    b. Record output per route (urine and stool, NG drain-
       age, emesis, Penrose drain).
    c. Assess hydration status (signs of dehydration, electro-
       lyte imbalance).
4. Provide dressing care; maintain integrity of surgical site
   (depends on type of surgery).
    a. Monitor dilation of anus.
    b. Monitor endorectal pullthrough (incision made over
       anal dimple and colon directly through to muscle
       cuff).
    c. Keep anus clean and dry.
    d. Apply zinc oxide for skin lesions and irritation sur-
       rounding surgical site.

  e. Elevate surgical site off mattress; position on pillow for elevation or use Bryant's traction.
5. Promote adequate nutritional intake.
   a. Monitor bowel sounds; begin fluids when bowel sounds are heard.
   b. Advance to full diet as tolerated.
6. Protect child from infection.
   a. Provide Foley catheter care every shift.
   b. Change dressing and note drainage.
   c. Monitor incisional site for drainage, redness, inflammation.
   d. Clean anal area frequently to prevent fecal contamination.
   e. Perform pulmonary toilet q2-4 hr.
   f. Change position q2 hr.
   g. Monitor for signs of systemic infection or local abscess.
7. Promote functioning and maintain integrity of colostomy.
8. Promote comfort and minimize pain.
   a. Provide sitz bath (initiate 1 week after surgery).
   b. Apply zinc oxide to excoriated and irritated areas of skin.
   c. Provide position of comfort.
   d. Use distractions (play activities).
   e. Monitor child's response to medication.

Home Care/Discharge Instructions

1. Encourage parents to ventilate concerns about outcomes of surgery.
2. Refer to specific institutional procedures for information distributed to parents about home care.
3. Instruct parents about follow-up techniques to promote optimal surgical outcomes.
   a. Colostomy care
   b. Dilation of anus
   c. Sitz bath

BIBLIOGRAPHY

Bellet P: *The diagnostic approach to common symptoms and signs in infants, children and adolescents,* Philadelphia, 1989, Lea & Febiger.

Golladay E et al: Pyloric stenosis—a timed perspective, *Arch Surg* 122(7):825, 1987.

Kieswelter W, Hoon A: Imperforate anus: an analysis of mortalities during a 25 year period, *Prog Pediatr Surg* 13:211, 1979.

Seashore J: Disorders of the anus and rectum. In Gellis S, Kagan B: *Current pediatric therapy 13,* Philadelphia, 1990, WB Saunders, pp. 225-227.

Ukabiala O et al: The extract of muscle hypertrophy in infantile hypertrophic pyloric stenosis does not depend on age and duration of symptoms, *J Pediatr Surg* 22(3):200, 1987.

Weiner E, Kiesewelter W: Urologic abnormalities associated with imperforate anus, *J Pediatr Surg* 81:151, 1973.

Welsh S et al: Imperforate anus: diagnosis and surgical treatment, *J Assoc Oper Room Nurses* 42(5):492, 1985.

39 ❖ Inflammatory Bowel Disease

PATHOPHYSIOLOGY

Inflammatory bowel disease refers to two gastrointestinal conditions: ulcerative colitis and Crohn's disease. Differentiating ulcerative colitis from Crohn's disease may be difficult; in 10% of the cases, a differential diagnosis is not made. The causes of both diseases are unknown. No association has been found between the incidence of inflammatory bowel disease and environmental factors, viral agents, and immunologic disorders. An association between ankylosing spondylitis and the histocompatibility of HLA-B27 and inflammatory bowel disease is a possibility. Ulcerative colitis and Crohn's disease have similar initial signs, including diarrhea, rectal bleeding, abdominal pain, fever, malaise, anorexia, weight loss, and anemia. Children may initially be seen with vague symptoms such as growth failure, anorexia, fever, and joint pains with or without gastrointestinal symptoms. Both conditions are characterized by remissions and exacerbations. Extracolonic manifestations such as joint problems, skin rashes, and eye irritation can occur. Although the peak incidence of inflammatory bowel disease occurs between 15 and 25 years of age, 15% of all cases occur at age 15 years and younger. Prognosis is dependent on the following factors: (1) an early and rapid onset; (2) poor response to medical treatment; and (3) severe extensive involvement.

Ulcerative colitis refers to a recurrent inflammatory and ulcerative disease affecting primarily the large intestine. Lesions are continuous and involve the superficial mucosa, causing vascular congestion, capillary dilation, edema, hemorrhage, and ulceration. Muscular hypertrophy and deposition of fibrous tissue and fat result, giving the bowel a "lead pipe" appearance because of narrowing of the bowel itself.

Crohn's disease refers to an inflammatory and ulcerative disease affecting any portion of the intestines. The disease affects the deep walls of the bowel. The lesions are discontinuous, resulting in a "skipping" effect, with the diseased portions of the bowel separated by normal tissue. Fissures, fistulas, and thickened intestinal walls result. Granulomas occur in approximately 50% of cases.

INCIDENCE

1. Annual incidence of ulcerative colitis and Crohn's disease is 4 to 10 cases per 100,000 children.
2. Ulcerative colitis represents over half of the 20,000 to 25,000 newly diagnosed cases of inflammatory bowel disease each year.
3. Peak incidence is at 15 to 20 years of age.
4. Geographic locale — inflammatory bowel disease is most common in the United States, England, and Scandinavia.
5. Whites are affected more than blacks.
6. There is a high preponderance among American Jews.
7. Familial incidence is 29% with ulcerative colitis.
8. Familial incidence is 35% with Crohn's disease.
9. No association is found with socioeconomic status or psychologic, dietary, and urban-rural factors.

CLINICAL MANIFESTATIONS
Ulcerative Colitis

1. Major symptom — frequent, bloody stools (number of stools varies from 4 to 24)
2. Pain relief after defecation
3. Rectal bleeding
4. Anorexia, pallor, and fatigue
5. Fever

6. Tachycardia
7. Peritoneal irritation
8. Electrolyte imbalance
9. Ten- to 20-pound weight loss over 2 months
10. Anemia
11. Extraintestinal symptoms—skin rashes, arthritis
12. Flatulence
13. Severe pain
14. Growth retardation

Crohn's Disease

1. Diarrhea
2. Cramping abdominal pain aggravated by eating
3. Pain in the right lower quadrant of abdomen
4. Growth retardation
5. Weight loss
6. Abscess formation
7. Spiking fever
8. Leukocytosis
9. Perianal disease—fistula and fissures
10. Nutritional deficiencies—malnutrition, electrolyte imbalances
11. Amenorrhea, delay in sexual maturation
12. Cachexia
13. Finger clubbing
14. Arthritis

COMPLICATIONS

Ulcerative Colitis

1. Predisposed to cancer—20% risk is associated with each decade after the first 10 years
2. Toxic megacolon
3. Hemorrhage
4. Sepsis

Crohn's Disease

1. Perforation
2. Toxic megacolon
3. Hemorrhage
4. Liver abscess and liver disease
5. Ureteral obstruction

Retroperitonitis
Erythema nodosum

LABORATORY/DIAGNOSTIC TESTS

1. Complete blood count (CBC) (anemia)
2. White blood count (WBC) (increased with inflammation)
3. Sedimentation rate (increased with inflammation)
4. Hematocrit (decreased because of blood loss)
5. Serum electrolytes (decreased potassium)
6. Serum protein (decreased proteins)
7. Stool culture (for presence of infectious organisms)
8. Hematest of stool (for presence of blood in stool)
9. D-Xylulose absorption blood and urine test (to measure intestinal absorption when there are fatty stools)
10. Lactose tolerance test
11. Sigmoidoscopy (to evaluate mucosa, rectum, sigmoid colon directly)
12. Colonoscopy (to evaluate colon directly)
13. Upper gastrointestinal x-ray series with small bowel follow through (differential diagnosis)
14. Barium enema (differential diagnoses)
15. Biopsy (to determine type of inflammatory bowel disease; tissue specimens are taken from several sites)
16. Bone studies

MEDICATIONS

1. Antidiarrheal preparations—used to control diarrhea
   a. Diphenoxylate hydrochloride with atropine sulfate (Lomotil)
      (1) Dosage at 2 to 5 years—6 mg/24 hr TID by mouth (po)
      (2) Dosage at 5 to 8 years—8 mg/24 hr TID po
      (3) Dosage at 8 to 12 years—10 mg/24 hr 5 doses/day po
   b. Paregoric—0.25 to 0.5 ml/kg/dose po
   c. Propantheline bromide (Pro-Banthine)—1.5 mg/kg/24 hr po in 4 doses after meals and at bedtime
2. Antiinflammatory—used to control or suppress inflammatory process

a. Sulfasalazine (Azulfidine) — has both antibacterial and antiinflammatory action
b. Azathioprine (Imuran) — immunosuppressive therapy (2 mg/kg/24 hr); may prolong remissions
   (1) Initial dose — 37.5 to 150 mg/kg/24 hr, q4-8 hr po
   (2) Maintenance dose — 40 mg/kg/24 hr QID
c. Hydrocortisone (Solu-Cortef) — short-acting corticosteroid; has antiinflammatory effects by inhibiting phagocytosis and suppressing other clinical manifestations of inflammation; used in the treatment of ulcerative colitis and Crohn's disease
   (1) Divided doses — 20 to 240 mg qd intravenously (IV) or po
d. Methylprednisolone sodium succinate (Solu-Medrol) — used as an antiinflammatory agent in the treatment of both acute and chronic inflammatory diseases; used in the treatment of ulcerative colitis and Crohn's disease; dosage is highly individualized — 10 to 500 mg IV q6 hr; 10 to 40 mg IV q6 hr
e. Prednisone — has same action as hydrocortisone; dosages are highly individualized; initial dose — 2 mg/kg/24 hr, then reduced to lowest effective dose

3. Analgesics and narcotics for pain control
4. Iron supplements

SURGICAL TREATMENT

Ileostomy

This surgical procedure is performed to treat inflammatory bowel disease, polypoid syndrome, and granulomatous disease after medical therapeutic procedures have been unsuccessful. Ileostomy involves removal of the diseased portion of the bowel (small intestine) with the ileum used to form a stoma on the abdominal wall for bowel evacuation. A variety of surgical procedures may be used, depending on the extent and location of the affected portion of the bowel. An ileostomy with subtotal or total colectomy is performed on patients who are malnourished and have moderate to severe rectal disease. The Koch ileostomy provides continence without the use of appliances. Use of the Koch pouch procedure is contraindicated in many cases because of the length of the bowel that is lost with recurrence of disease in the pouch (Crohn's disease).

Colostomy

Permanent or temporary colostomies are performed for a variety of conditions. Temporary colostomies, used as palliative measures until the infant or child can undergo definitive surgical intervention, are performed for patients with the following circumstances: anorectal atresia (for decompression), Hirschsprung's disease and intestinal polyps, intussusception, granulomatous disease, and trauma. Permanent colostomies are performed for children with severe cases of Crohn's disease and multiple trauma. The sigmoid colostomy is most frequently performed. Temporary colostomies (e.g., transverse loop and double-barrel colostomies) are performed in children most often. In all types of colostomies, an intact portion of the colon is brought through an abdominal incision and is sutured to the abdominal wall to form a stoma.

CLINICAL MANIFESTATIONS

The response to the surgery should result in amelioration of symptoms associated with the primary disease. The child is left with an abdominal stoma through which bowel contents are emptied into an attached appliance or into an abdominal pouch (Kock's pouch). Although the child does not live with a normally functioning bowel after surgery, most children do well. If the child, adolescent, or parent learns to care properly for the colostomy or ileostomy, a life filled with educational, social, and athletic activities can be expected.

COMPLICATIONS RESULTING FROM SURGICAL INTERVENTION

1. Necrosis of colostomy (caused by inadequate blood supply)
2. Stricture formation
3. Retraction of the stoma
4. Prolapsed stoma
5. Herniation

6. Bleeding
7. Intestinal obstruction
8. Wound infection
9. Peritonitis
10. Spill-over of stool
11. Constipation bordering on obstruction
12. Nephrolithiasis
13. Fistula (if multiple fistulae or extensive undermining of subcutaneous tissue occurs, stoma must be excised and relocated elsewhere)
14. Convulsions (caused by electrolyte imbalances)

NURSING ASSESSMENT

1. Refer to "Gastrointestinal Assessment" in Appendix A.
2. Assess for abdominal distention, bowel sounds, tenderness and pain, and abdominal girth.

NURSING DIAGNOSES

Diarrhea
High risk for infection
Pain
Impaired tissue integrity
Knowledge deficit
Body image disturbance
Altered nutrition: less than body requirements
High risk for impaired skin integrity
Impaired home management maintenance
High risk for injury
Fluid volume deficit

NURSING INTERVENTIONS

Preoperative Care

1. Prepare infant, child, or adolescent and family for surgery.
   a. Provide age-appropriate explanations.
   b. Encourage ventilation of concerns.
   c. Introduce to age and sex-appropriate model who has undergone surgery to discuss pertinent and sensitive issues.
   d. Refer to local ileostomy support group.
   e. Demonstrate use of appliances.

2. Prepare child or adolescent and parents physically for procedures.
   a. Provide age-appropriate explanations before procedures, including description of sensations to be experienced.
   b. Explain use of cleansing enemas.
   c. Explain infusion of blood transfusions (to treat anemia).
   d. Explain infusion of hyperalimentation (to improve nutritional status).
   e. Explain infusion of albumin (to correct electrolyte imbalance).
   f. Explain administration of antibiotics (gentamicin or erythromycin to sterilize bowel).
   g. Explain insertion of Cantor tube night before surgery (to decompress stomach).
3. Prepare infant, child, or adolescent physically for surgery.
   a. Monitor infant's or child's response to enemas, laxatives, stool softeners (to evacuate bowel preoperatively).
   b. Monitor infant's or child's response to decompression of stomach and bowel (nasogastric tube [NG] and rectal tube).
   c. Provide nothing by mouth 12 hours before surgery.
   d. Provide only clear liquids 48 to 72 hours before surgery.
   e. Insert Foley catheter to decompress bladder.
   f. Administer antibiotics to sterilize bowel.
   g. Monitor vital signs q4 hr.
   h. Monitor for bowel complications (perforation or enterocolitis).
4. Promote and support optimal nutritional status.
   a. Compile dietary history, including food allergies.
   b. Monitor tolerance to food, noting type and amount.
   c. Monitor response to elemental feedings.
   d. Monitor response to low-residue, bland, high-protein, high-caloric diet.
   e. Monitor for signs of electrolyte imbalances—hypotension, tachycardia, oliguria, atonic muscles, general sense of confusion.

f. Monitor administration of total parenteral nutrition; observe child's or adolescent's response.
   (1) Maintain sterility of central line.
   (2) Record accurate input and output.
   (3) Obtain daily weights.
   (4) Monitor urinary specific gravity.
   (5) Check urinary glucose and acetone.
   (6) Obtain 24-hour urine sample for electrolytes, calcium, protein, phosphate, urea, nitrogen.
   (7) Monitor electrolyte balance.
g. Restrict intake of greasy, spicy, and lactose-containing foods.

5. Provide comfort and pain relief measures as indicated.
   a. Maintain bed rest during acute episode (decreased activity results in decreased peristalsis, decreased diarrhea, decreased pain).
   b. Provide diversional activities.
   c. Provide heating pad.
   d. Change position.
   e. Assess intensity, type, time, pattern of occurrence of pain, and child's response to pain relief measures.
   f. Monitor and observe child's response to analgesics and narcotics.
   g. Provide uninterrupted rest periods.

6. Promote skin integrity.
   a. Perineal care—apply A & D ointment or petroleum jelly to perineal area to prevent skin irritation or breakdown.
   b. Apply body moisturizers liberally.
   c. Provide sitz bath TID (for perianal or rectal fistulas or fissures).
   d. Provide foam mattress to prevent pressure sores.
   e. Change position q2 hr.

7. Promote and maintain hydration status.
   a. Record input and output.
   b. Record daily weights.
   c. Assess for signs of dehydration.
   d. Promote oral intake when appropriate.
   e. Monitor administration of elemental feedings or total parental nutrition.

8. Monitor and observe for child's or adolescent's response to and untoward side effects of medications.
9. Monitor, prevent, or report signs of potential or actual complications.
   a. Fistulas or fissures
   b. Hemorrhage
   c. Intestinal obstruction
   d. Liver abscess
   e. Ureteral obstruction
   f. Retroperitonitis
   g. Perforations
   h. Enterocolitis

Postoperative Care

1. Monitor child's response to surgery.
   a. Vital signs
   b. Intake and output (report any discrepancy)
   c. Dressing — amount of drainage, intactness
2. Monitor for signs and symptoms of complications.
   a. Stomal complications — prolapse, bleeding, excessive diarrhea, ribbonlike stools, failure to pass stool and flatus
   b. Sepsis
   c. Intestinal obstruction or constipation
   d. Prolapse of proximal segment
   e. Bleeding
   f. Increased stooling
   g. Infection
3. Promote return of peristalsis.
   a. Maintain patency of NG tube.
   b. Check functioning of suction machine.
   c. Irrigate with normal saline solution q4 hr and as needed.
   d. Check for placement of NG tube; auscultate and aspirate contents.
4. Promote and maintain fluid and electrolyte balance.
   a. Record intake per route (IV, NG, oral).
   b. Record output per route (urine, stool, NG drainage, emesis, stoma).
   c. Monitor for signs and symptoms of electrolyte imbalances.

  d. Consult with physician about disparities.
5. Alleviate or minimize pain and discomfort.
  a. Maintain patency of NG tube.
  b. Maintain position of comfort.
  c. Monitor child's response to administration of medications.
  d. Provide oral care (mouth can become dry with NG tube in place).
6. Provide stoma and skin care to promote healing and to prevent complications.
  a. Inspect stoma q4 hr for retraction, prolapse, or protrusion greater than 2 cm.
  b. Check for bleeding at stoma site.
  c. Check for obstruction—enlarged, pale, and edematous stoma.
7. Provide colostomy care (refer to institutional manual for specific technical and institutional procedure).
  a. Care of appliance
  b. Skin care
  c. Complications
   (1) Skin can become irritated by digestive enzymes.
   (2) Match adhesive to stoma size.
   (3) Apply protective cream to exposed area.
8. Protect child from infection.
  a. Provide Foley catheter care every shift.
  b. Change dressing as needed (perianal and colostomy).
  c. Monitor incision site.
  d. Refer to institutional procedure manual for care related to specific procedure.
  e. Change diaper frequently; diaper to avoid fecal contamination (as applicable).
  f. Perform pulmonary toilet q2-4 hr.
  g. Change position q2 hr (prevents atelectasis).
  h. Monitor for signs of systemic infection and local abscess.
9. Facilitate development of realistic adaptive body image.
  a. Encourage ventilation of feelings regarding stoma, outcome of surgery.

b. Encourage socialization through peer support groups.
c. Refer to community organizations.
d. Provide active problem-solving for concerns such as dress apparel and sexual activity.
10. Encourage and promote socialization with peers as a means to cope adaptively with impact of disease.
11. Modify adaptation of chronic sick role behavior by promoting socialization and normal daily activities.
12. Encourage ventilation of fears of body mutilation.

Home Care/Discharge Planning

1. Instruct child, parents, and family about ileostomy or Kock pouch care.
2. Instruct child or adolescent and parents to monitor and report signs of complications.
   a. Mechanical obstruction
   b. Peritonitis or wound infection
3. Instruct child or adolescent and parents about administration of total parental nutrition or NG feedings
4. Initiate referral to school nurse and teacher to promote continuity of care.
   a. Observations of child's response to condition
   b. Observations of untoward effects of medications and complications
   c. Observation of social interactions with peers and conduct in school
5. Refer to community organizations.
   a. Ostomy Association, Inc.
      201 Beverly Blvd.
      Los Angeles, CA 90052
      (213) 255-4681
   b. United Ostomy Association, Inc.
      36 Executive Park
      Suite 120
      Irvine, CA 92714-6744
      (714) 660-8624

BIBLIOGRAPHY

Adams D et al: Children with ostomies: comprehensive care planning, *Pediatr Nurs* 12(6):429, 1986.

Hagenah G, Harrigan J, Campbell M: Inflammatory bowel disease in children, *Nurs Clin North Am* 19(1):27, 1984.

Kibort P: Inflammatory bowel disease in childhood, *J Enterost Ther* 14(2):79, 1987.

Kirsner J, Shorter J: Recent developments in nonspecific inflammatory bowel disease, *N Engl J Med* 306:837, 1982.

Kodner I, Fry R: Inflammatory bowel disease, *Clin Symp* 34:3, 1982.

Michener W, Farmer R, Mortimer E: Long-term prognosis of ulcerative colitis with onset in childhood or adolescence, *J Clin Gastroenterol* 1:301, 1979.

Myer S: Overview of inflammatory bowel disease, *Nurs Clin North Am* 19(1):3, 1984.

Simmons M: Using the nursing process in treating inflammatory bowel disease, *Nurs Clin North Am* 19(1):11, 1984.

Sparacino L: Psychosocial considerations of the adolescent and young adult with inflammatory bowel disease, *Nurs Clin North Am* 19(1):41, 1984.

Swartz M: Beyond the scope: a nursing view of the extraintestinal bowel disease, *Gastroenterol Nurs* 12(1):3, 1989.

Thomas D: Bloody diarrhea in children, *Gastroenterol Nurs* 12(2):100, 1989.

Wilson C: The diagnostic work-up for the patient with inflammatory bowel disease, *Nurs Clin North Am* 19(1):51, 1984.

40 ❖ Iron Deficiency Anemia

PATHOPHYSIOLOGY

Iron deficiency anemia is the most common nutritional problem affecting children in the United States. Infants and children from lower socioeconomic strata are affected in particular. Iron deficiency anemia is the consequence of consuming insufficient iron to meet the infant's or child's nutritional requirements. Most often insufficient dietary intake results from consuming cow's milk and little or no solid foods during the first year of life. Other causes of iron deficiency anemia include depleted iron stores, blood loss, and, rarely, impaired absorption of iron. Fifty percent of the iron in breast milk is absorbed. Breast-milk iron is not absorbed as well as iron from animal sources; iron absorption from biosynthetic food ranges from 1% to 20%. Iron stores become depleted if the infant has not received iron-fortified milk and cereal by the age of 6 to 9 months. The normal values for iron are as follows: (1) serum iron—50 to 150 μg/dl; (2) serum ferritin—7 to 200 mg/ml; (3) free erythrocyte protoporphyrin—less than 3 μg/g hemoglobin; (4) total iron-binding capacity—250 to 400 μg/dl; and (5) percent saturation—greater than 15. Iron intake should be 2 mg/kg/day.

INCIDENCE

1. Three percent to 24% of infants 6 to 24 months of age have iron deficiency anemia.

2. Twenty-nine percent to 68% of infants 6 to 24 months of age are iron deficient.
3. Incidence of iron deficiency anemia in infants is highest in lower socioeconomic groups (35%).
4. Incidence of iron deficiency and iron deficiency anemia among adolescent girls is 11% to 17%.
5. Peak incidence for iron deficiency anemia occurs between 12 and 18 months of age.

CLINICAL MANIFESTATIONS

1. Pallor
2. Poor weight gain
3. Irritability
4. Easy fatigability; decreased concentration
5. Lethargy
6. Anorexia
7. Prone to infection
8. Porcelain-like skin color
9. Pica
10. Alterations in small bowel functioning

COMPLICATIONS

1. Poor muscular development (long-term)
2. Decreased attention span
3. Decreased performance on developmental tests

LABORATORY/DIAGNOSTIC TESTS

1. Free erythrocyte porphyrin level — increased
2. Serum iron concentration — decreased
3. Transferrin saturation — decreased
4. Serum ferritin concentration — decreased
5. Hemoglobin — decreased
6. Erythrocyte porphyrin — hemoglobin ratio (greater than 2.8 $\mu g/g$ is diagnostic for iron deficiency)

MEDICATIONS

1. Iron by mouth (po) (2 to 3 mg/kg) — ferrous sulfate, ferrous fumarate, ferrous succinate, ferrous gluconate
2. Vitamin C (ascorbic acid increases iron absorption) — must be administered simultaneously with iron

NURSING ASSESSMENT

Refer to "Cardiovascular Assessment" in Appendix A.

NURSING DIAGNOSES

Activity intolerance
Altered nutrition: less than body requirements
Knowledge deficit

NURSING INTERVENTIONS

1. Monitor child's therapeutic and untoward effects from iron therapy.
   a. Side effects (e.g., tooth discoloration) of oral therapy are infrequent.
   b. Instruct about measures to prevent tooth discoloration.
      (1) Take with fluids, preferably orange juice.
      (2) Rinse mouth after taking medication.
   c. Observe for side effects of intramuscular administration.
      (1) Staining of skin
      (2) Vomiting
      (3) Chills
      (4) Fever
      (5) Arthralgia
      (6) Urticaria
      (7) Pain at injection site
2. Instruct parents about appropriate nutritional intake.
   a. Reduce milk intake.
   b. Increase intake of meat and appropriate protein substitutes.
   c. Encourage inclusion of whole grains and green leafy vegetables in diet.
3. Gather information about dietary history and eating behaviors.
   a. Assess for factors contributing to nutritional deficiency—psychosocial, behavioral, and nutritional.
   b. Plan with parents an acceptable approach toward dietary habits.
   c. Refer to nutritionist for intensive evaluation and treatment if parents and child are noncompliant.

BIBLIOGRAPHY

Dallman P, Yip R: Changing characteristics of childhood anemia, *J Pediatr* 114(1):161, 1989.

Looker A et al: Iron status: prevalence of impairment in three Hispanic groups in the United States, *Am J Clinic Nutrit* 49:553, 1989.

Oski F, Stockman J: Anemia due to inadequate iron sources or poor iron utilization, *Pediatr Clin North Am* 27(2):237, 1980.

Oski F et al: Effect of iron therapy on behavior performance in nonanemic, iron-deficient infants, *Pediatrics* 71(6):877, 1983.

Sadowitz P, Oski F: Iron status and infant feeding practices in an urban ambulatory center, *Pediatrics* 72(1):33, 1983.

Yip R, Schwartz S, Deinard A: Screening for iron deficiency with the erythrocyte protoporphyrin test, *Pediatrics* 72(2):214, 1983.

41 ❖ Juvenile Rheumatoid Arthritis

PATHOPHYSIOLOGY

Juvenile rheumatoid arthritis is a chronic inflammatory disease that begins before the child is 16 years of age, affects the joints, and involves the connective tissue and the viscera. Although its cause is unknown, a genetic predisposition is thought to exist. It is the leading cause of disability in childhood; three quarters of children with generalized rheumatic disease have juvenile rheumatoid arthritis. Its diagnosis is based on the following criteria:

1. Objective evidence of arthritis (defined as joint swelling or joint limitation of motion, with heat, pain, or tenderness) in one or more joints must be documented. Pain or tenderness alone is not sufficient for a diagnosis of arthritis.
2. The arthritis must persist for at least 6 weeks in a given joint.
3. Other specific diseases that may cause or be associated with arthritis must be excluded.

Children diagnosed with juvenile rheumatoid arthritis are classified into one of three types according to their clinical manifestations: systemic-onset, pauciarticular-onset, and polyarticular-onset.

1. *Systemic-onset juvenile rheumatoid arthritis* is characterized by persistent intermittent fever (daily intermittent temperature elevations to 103° F [39.4° C] or more) with or without rheumatoid rash or other

organ involvement. Fever and the characteristic rash are considered typical. Systemic-onset juvenile rheumatoid arthritis is not associated with arthritis. Before a definite diagnosis can be made, objective arthritis must be present and may be pauciarticular or polyarticular.

2. *Pauciarticular-onset juvenile rheumatoid arthritis* is cumulative arthritis in one to four joints. Patients with systemic-onset juvenile rheumatoid arthritis are excluded from this category.

3. *Polyarticular-onset juvenile rheumatoid arthritis* is cumulative arthritis in five or more joints. Patients with systemic-onset juvenile rheumatoid arthritis are excluded from this category.

For classification purposes, joints are counted individually, with certain exceptions. The cervical spine is considered one joint. The carpal joints of each hand are counted as one joint, as are the tarsal joints of each foot. The metacarpophalangeal, metatarsophalangeal, proximal, distal, and interphalangeal joints are counted individually.

INCIDENCE

1. Slightly more common in females than males
2. Affects 250,000 children
3. Peak incidence—1 to 3 years and 8 to 12 years
4. Most common pediatric connective tissue disease
5. Rates of incidence: acute systemic—20%; single joint—30%; polyarticular or pauciarticular—50%

CLINICAL MANIFESTATIONS

Systemic-Onset Juvenile Rheumatoid Arthritis

1. Daily or twice-daily temperature elevations to 102.2° F (39° C) or higher, with rapid return to normal temperature
2. Temperature elevations, primarily in late afternoon or evening and preceded by chills
3. Irritability during temperature elevations
4. Salmon-colored macular rash on trunk and extremities; migratory, with no itching
5. Symmetric involvement of large and small joints, including cervical spine and temporomandibular joint
6. Extraarticular symptoms, including pericarditis, lymph-

adenopathy, hepatosplenomegaly (in one third of children)
7. Uveitis (iritis/iridocyclitis) — secondary complications include cataracts, glaucoma, visual loss, and blindness

Polyarticular-Onset Juvenile Rheumatoid Arthritis

1. Intermittent low-grade fever
2. Malaise and fatigue
3. Anorexia, weight loss
4. Morning stiffness, joint pain, and sluggishness with movement
5. Symmetric, asymmetric, or unilateral joint involvement
6. Tenderness, soft-tissue swelling in large and small joints
7. Large joints — affected first
8. Cervical spine — may be affected
9. Temporomandibular joint — affected, leading to impaired biting and shortness of mandible

Pauciarticular-Onset Juvenile Rheumatoid Arthritis

Type I

1. Primarily affects females, ages 1 to 4 years
2. Confined to one joint
3. Joints affected — knees, ankles, elbows
4. Painless swelling of joints
5. Iridocyclitis (25% of cases)
6. Poor weight gain, decreased appetite
7. Irritability, increased fatigue

Type II

1. Primarily affects boys 8 years old and older
2. Affects large joints of lower extremities
3. Possible heel pain and Achilles tendinitis
4. Sacroiliitis (in 90% of cases)
5. Iritis (in 20% of cases)
6. Low-grade fevers
7. Decreased appetite, poor weight gain

COMPLICATIONS

1. Flexion contractures of hip, knees, elbow
2. Dorsiflexion of proximal finger joints
3. Bilateral weakness of grip

4. Limitation of movement
5. Blindness
6. Leg-length discrepancy
7. Cardiopulmonary complications
8. Severe anemia
9. Renal, bone marrow, and liver toxicity to drugs

LABORATORY/DIAGNOSTIC TESTS

1. Erythrocyte sedimentation rate (ESR) — increased with acute systemic juvenile rheumatoid arthritis; normal with pauciarticular or polyarticular arthritis
2. Positive rheumatoid factor (pauciarticular only)
3. Positive antinuclear antibody (in 40% of cases)
4. Complete blood count (CBC) — systemic leukocytosis; 15,000 to 20,000 white blood cells (WBC) with acute systemic juvenile rheumatoid arthritis; thrombocytosis with normochromic or hypochromic anemia
5. Increased complement levels
6. Increased alpha globulins
7. Increased serum glutamic-oxaloacetic transaminase (SGOT) and increased serum glutamic-pyruvic transaminase (SGPT) (usually associated with salicylate therapy)
8. Culture of synovial fluid (to rule out other conditions)
9. Urinalysis (mild proteinuria accompanies increased fever)

MEDICATIONS

1. Nonsteroidal antiinflammatory drugs — used to control inflammation
   a. Aspirin — 3 g/m^2/24 hr by mouth (po) (to maintain serum salicylate level of 20 mg/dl)
   b. Indomethacin (Indocin) — has antiinflammatory effects similar to aspirin; used to treat moderate to severe juvenile rheumatoid arthritis during active phase; dosage — 2 mg BID or TID po; can be increased by 25 mg per week until therapeutic effect or maximal dose of 150 to 200 mg is achieved
   c. Tolmetin (Tolectin) — used for its analgesic, antiinflammatory, and antipyretic activity; acts in the same manner as aspirin and indomethacin
      (1) Initial dose — 20 mg/kg/day in divided dose po

  (2) Maintenance dose—15 to 30 mg/kg/day po
  d. Naproxen (Naprosyn)—used for antiinflammatory and analgesic effects in treatment of juvenile rheumatoid arthritis; dosage—10 mg/kg/day BID po
2. Gold salts—act by suppressing inflammation in the joint; dosage—1 mg/kg/week intramuscularly (IM) for 20 weeks, then same dose at 2- to 4-week intervals for as long as response is favorable
3. Penicillamine (D-Penicillamine)—action in treatment of juvenile rheumatoid arthritis not clearly understood; may act by inhibiting formation of collagen
  a. Initial dose—125 to 250 mg qd; dosage increased to 125 to 250 mg/day at 1- to 3-month intervals
  b. Maximum dose—1 to 1.5 g qd
4. Immunosuppressive drug (corticosteroid): Prednisone—used for antiinflammatory effects (glucocorticoid); inhibits phagocytosis and suppresses inflammatory reaction; used to suppress inflammatory immune responses in rheumatic disorders; dosage—2 mg/kg/24 hr po, then reduced to lowest effective maintenance dose; great deal of individual variation, with dosage based on child's condition

NURSING ASSESSMENT

Refer to "Neuromuscular Assessment" and "Skeletal Assessment" in Appendix A.

NURSING DIAGNOSES

Impaired physical mobility
Pain
Impaired home management maintenance
Altered growth and development
High risk for social isolation

NURSING INTERVENTIONS

1. Promote joint mobility, maintain strength, and prevent deformity of joints.
  a. Perform physical therapy exercises (range of motion [ROM]/passive range of motion [PROM])
  b. Patient should participate in physical activity exercise.

      (1) Avoid excessive strain on affected joints.
      (2) Take part in creative dance, bicycle riding, swimming, walking.
      (3) Avoid potentially straining activities—running, aerobics, jumping, kicking, excessive walking.
  c. Splint to prevent flexion contractures.
  d. Perform prone and active gluteal exercise with hip involvement.
  e. Cast with knee in severe flexion.
  f. Provide cervical collar for neck pain.
2. Provide pain relief measures as necessary.
  a. Tub bath for joint stiffness
  b. Heating pad to affected areas
  c. Crutches or other devices to avoid full weight bearing
3. Monitor child's responses to and untoward effects of medications.
  a. Nonsteroidal antiinflammatory agents (NSAIDs) –aspirin, indomethacin, tolmetin, naproxen
  b. Gold salt injections
  c. Penicillamine
  d. Immunosuppressive drugs (corticosteroids)
4. Collaborate with physical therapist in reinforcement and continuation of exercise and treatment program.
5. Prepare child preoperatively for procedures and surgeries as indicated for treatment of condition. They may include the following.
  a. Diagnostic biopsy
  b. Synovectomy
  c. Capsulotomy
  d. Soft-tissue release
  e. Osteotomy
  f. Arthrodesis
  g. Epiphysiodesis
  h. Arthroplasty
  i. Total joint or hip replacement
6. Provide emotional support to child and family as indicated during hospitalization.

Home Care

1. Encourage compliance with treatment plan.
  a. Follow-up home visits and calls

    b. Evaluation at clinic
2. Coordinate and manage long-term follow-up.
    a. Monitor adherence to medical regimen.
    b. Monitor compliance with consultation referrals.

BIBLIOGRAPHY

Baum J: Juvenile arthritis, *Am J Dis Child* 135:557, 1981.

Brewer E et al: Current proposed revision of JRA criteria, *Arthritis Rheum* 20(suppl 2):195, 1977.

Calabro J: Juvenile rheumatoid arthritis, *Clin Pediatr Med Surg* 5(1):57, 1988.

Dykstra D et al: Pediatric rehabilitation. Joint and connective tissue diseases, part 5, *Arch Phys Med Rehab* (Supplement) 70(5-5): Study Guide Issue: S 179, 1989.

Hughes J, ed: *Synopsis of pediatrics,* St. Louis, 1984, Mosby–Year Book.

Lovell D et al: Development of a disability measurement tool for juvenile rheumatoid arthritis: the Juvenile Arthritis Functional Assessment Scale, *Arthritis Rheum* 32(11):1390, 1989.

Miller J: *Juvenile rheumatoid arthritis,* Littleton, Mass, 1979, John Wright-PSG.

Neuberger J, Neuberger G: Epidemiology of the rheumatic diseases, *Nurs Clin North Am* 19(4):713, 1984.

Page-Goertz S: Even children have arthritis, *Pediatr Nurs* 15(1):11, 1989.

Rennebohm R, Correll J: Comprehensive management of juvenile rheumatoid arthritis, *Nurs Clin North Am* 19(4):647, 1984.

Techner D et al: Gait deviations in patients with juvenile rheumatoid arthritis, *Phys Ther* 67(9):1335, 1987.

Ungerer J et al: Psychosocial functioning in children and young adults with juvenile arthritis, *Pediatrics* 81(2):195, 1988.

Varni J, Wako G, Katz E: A cognitive-behavioral approach to pain associated with pediatric chronic disease, *J Pain Sympt Manag* 4(4):238, 1989.

42 ❖ Kawasaki Disease

PATHOPHYSIOLOGY

Also known as mucocutaneous lymph node syndrome, Kawasaki disease is a triphasic, acute febrile exanthematous illness of children. Although its cause is still unknown, it has been associated with infectious agents, immunologic processes, and genetic susceptibility. Its pathophysiology is undescribed, and its treatment is undetermined. The effects of this disease occur in three phases (acute, subacute, and convalescent) and are described in "Clinical Manifestations."

INCIDENCE

1. Myocardiopathy with congestive heart failure (CHF) develops in 10% of the cases.
2. Major complications occur in 20% of the cases.
3. Mortality is 2%.

CLINICAL MANIFESTATIONS

Acute Phase (10 to 14 days)

For the diagnosis of Kawasaki disease, the child must meet five of the first six principal criteria.

1. Abrupt onset of fever, which is remittent and typically high, lasts more than 5 days, and is unresponsive to antibiotic therapy
2. Conjunctival infection lasting 3 to 5 weeks, with no exudate or corneal scarring

3. Oropharyngeal manifestations, with erythematous, fissuring lips and oropharynx and hypertrophic papillae of the tongue ("strawberry tongue")
4. Indurative edema of the extremities, with erythematous palms and soles and fusiform swelling of the digits
5. Erythematous body rash on day 5 of illness—rash is typically macular but ranges from scarlatiniform, papular, discrete raised urticarial plaques to morbilliform. It begins on the extremities, spreads to the trunk, and is often pruritic.
6. Cervical lymphadenopathy, which is usually unilateral, is greater than 1.5 cm in size, and "melts away" as the fever subsides
7. Associated features—pyuria and urethritis, diarrhea, aseptic meningitis, irritability and lability of mood, severe lethargy, and hepatic dysfunction lasting from 7 to 10 days
8. Acute pericarditis and acute perivascularitis of coronary arteries and aorta, with intimal inflammatory infiltrate

Subacute Phase (10 to 25 Days)

1. Anorexia
2. Irritability
3. Arthritis—most commonly in large joints (knees, hips, elbows)
4. Arthralgia caused by joint fluid
5. Desquamation of the extremities, beginning at the digits and then peeling off in sheets from the palms and soles
6. Panvasculitis of coronary arteries and formation of aneurysms; intimal inflammation and thrombosis formation may lead to stenosis or obstruction.

Convalescent Phase (25 to 60 Days)

1. Signs of illness have subsided.
2. Deep transverse groove is across the fingers and toenails ("Bow's lines").
3. Disease is usually self-limiting.

COMPLICATIONS

1. CHF
2. Aneurysms
3. Coronary thromboses

LABORATORY/DIAGNOSTIC TESTS

1. Electrocardiogram (ECG) — used to detect cardiac arrhythmias
2. Echocardiograms — used to assess cardiac enlargement and contractility of the ventricles
3. Complete blood count (CBC) — slight anemia elevated WBC (first phase)
4. Platelet count (elevated); ESR elevated
5. C reactive protein elevated
6. SGOT elevated
7. SGPT elevated
8. Serum albumin decreased
9. IgA, IgG, and IgM elevated
10. Abdominal ultrasound to assess enlargement of internal organs

MEDICATIONS

1. Aspirin therapy
   a. 80 to 100 mg/kg/day (first 14 days or until fever controlled)
   b. 10 mg/kg/day given 14 to 35 days and at least for 3 months up to 1 year after onset
2. Gamma globulin (IVGG) 400 mg — 2 g IV; dosage and frequency vary based on severity of conditions; decreases inflammation of blood vessels
3. Persantine — 4 mg/kg/day TID for treatment of coronary aneurysms

NURSING ASSESSMENT

1. Refer to "Cardiovascular Assessment" in Appendix A.
2. Baseline assessment includes the signs and symptoms of the following:
   a. Dehydration
   b. Erythematous body rash

NURSING DIAGNOSES

High risk for infection
Impaired tissue integrity
Fatigue
Altered nutrition: less than body requirements
High risk for injury
High risk for decreased cardiac output

Pain
High risk for altered skin integrity
Impaired physical mobility
Activity
Impaired home maintenance management

NURSING INTERVENTIONS

1. Monitor child's clinical status.
   a. Rectal temperature q2 hr
   b. Skin turgor, mucous membranes, and anterior fontanel q4 hr
   c. Strict record of intake and output
   d. Specific gravity every shift
   e. Measurement of stools
   f. Oral mucous membranes
   g. Erythematous body rash
   h. Blood pressure q2 hr
2. Institute measures to lower fever.
   a. Medicate with antipyretics; monitor child's response to medications.
   b. Provide tepid sponge baths for temperatures greater than 102.2° F (39° C).
   c. Offer cool fluids q2 hr.
   d. Assess which fluids (such as Popsicles and Jello) child prefers.
   e. Monitor intravenous (IV) therapy, if applicable, q1-2 hr, checking for infiltration or complications (see institutional procedures manual for IVs).
   f. Maintain seizure precautions because 3% to 5% of children between 6 months and 3 years of age may develop seizures when they have temperatures as low as 101.8° F (38.8° C) if the temperature rises rapidly (as it does with Kawasaki disease).
   g. Explain unusual nature of temperature to parents in terms of its intermittent pattern, duration, and resistance to antipyretics; anticipatory guidance will prevent parental anxiety about the unusual nature of the fever.
3. Monitor child for cardiac complications.
   a. Use cardiac monitor as ordered during acute and subacute phases; report any arrhythmias to physician.

  b. Explain the purpose of the ECG and the aberrations caused by child's movement to the parents and the child.
  c. Allow child to change his or her own electrodes during daily bath.
  d. Allow child to put electrodes on doll.
4. Provide comfort measures for the child to ease discomfort of condition.
  a. Perform oral hygiene q2 hr with toothette and hydrogen peroxide normal saline solution.
  b. Apply petroleum jelly to lips q2 hr; children may apply it to themselves or put it on a doll first.
  c. Avoid soaps, ointments, and lotions on skin; keep skin clean, dry, and exposed to air.
  d. Cool, moist compresses may be applied to itching areas.
  e. Provide a sheepskin for child to lie on.
  f. Discourage scratching through diversional activities; for young children, soft, loose mittens may be helpful.
  g. Encourage bed rest and elevation of extremities until swelling has subsided.
  h. Teach parents how to hold and comfort the child who has an IV and electrodes in place.
  i. Keep stimulation to a minimum.
  j. Explain to parents that tactile stimulation may be irritating, but a soothing voice may provide security.
  k. Provide dim lights.
  l. Provide quiet music.
5. Provide and promote the child's nutritional status.
  a. Provide comfort measures for mouth (see number 4).
  b. Begin with bland foods in small amounts.
  c. Encourage parents to bring in favorite foods from home, and assess for favorite foods in hospital.
  d. Avoid hot, spicy foods.
  e. Offer high-calorie liquids.
6. Prevent contractions related to imposed restrictions and range of motion (ROM) limitations.
  a. Perform passive range of motion (PROM) exercises to edematous extremities q2-4 hr when child is on bed rest; teach parents how to do the exercises, and explain their importance to them.

    b. When child is able, use active ROM, making it a game for the child.

    c. Place IVs in a position that allows maximal movement.

    d. Elevate extremities as necessary.

7. Alleviate anxiety caused by all of the invasive procedures for diagnostic tests and by pain, a new environment, strange people, knowledge deficit, therapeutic play, and age-related fears.

    a. Provide play therapy during all phases of illness and for each new procedure (i.e., ECGs, needle play); base therapy on child's developmental level.

    b. Explain each procedure at child's and parents' cognitive levels; explain risk before procedure for toddlers and preschoolers. Allow enough time for them to ask questions.

    c. Suggest ways for parents to support their child during hospitalization and procedures (e.g., holding the child after the procedure).

    d. Assure the child that the procedure is not being done because the child is "bad."

    e. Consult parents and child about preferences among "quiet" toys and activities during acute phase of illness; encourage parents and volunteers to play with child, allowing for rest periods and then passive participation.

    f. Explain the meaning of the presence of swollen lymph nodes to parents.

8. Provide emotional support to parents.

    a. Provide and reinforce explanations to parents about procedures.

    b. Encourage use of preexisting support systems (e.g., relatives, friends, clergy).

    c. Encourage ventilation of feelings.

    d. Provide for physical comforts (e.g., sleeping arrangements, bathing).

Home Care

Instruct parents about long-term management.

1. Instruct parents and child, in a developmentally appropriate manner, about the importance of follow-up care,

including ECGs, echocardiograms, and chest x-ray examinations every 3 months for 1 year. Two thirds of coronary thromboses and aneurysms regress after 1 year.
2. Instruct parents verbally and with written reinforcement about the signs and symptoms of cardiac complications (i.e., aneurysms and coronary thromboses); tell them to contact the physician immediately if the child has any of these signs and symptoms.
3. Instruct the parents about the importance of anticoagulant therapy such as aspirin. Explain to parents the rationale about why some children with Kawasaki disease may need to have a coronary artery bypass graft performed.

BIBLIOGRAPHY

Kitamura S et al: Surgery for coronary heart disease due to mucocutaneous lymph node syndrome (Kawasaki disease), *Am J Cardiol* 51(2):444, 1983.

L'Orange C, Werner-McCullough D: Kawasaki disease: a new threat to children, *Am J Nurs* 83(4):558, 1983.

Lux K: New hope for children with Kawasaki disease, *J Pediatr Nurs* 6(3):159, 1991.

Lynch MH, Gray JL: Kawasaki disease: would you know it if you saw it? and what would you do about it? *Pediatr Nurs* 8(2):96, 1982.

McEnhill M, Vitale K: Kawasaki disease: new challenges in care, *MCN: Am J Maternal-Child Nurs* 14(6):406, 1989.

Nash D: Kawasaki disease: application of the Roy Adaptation Model to determine interventions, *J Pediatr Nurs: Nurs Care Child Fam* 2(5):308, 1987.

Terai M et al: Coronary arterial thrombi in Kawasaki disease, *J Pediatr* 6(1):75, 1988.

43 ❖ Lead Poisoning

PATHOPHYSIOLOGY

Lead poisoning refers to the excessive accumulation of lead in the blood. The diagnosis of lead poisoning is made when the child has two or more of the following conditions:

- Serum lead levels equal to or greater than 70 μg/dl, with or without symptoms
- Erythrocyte protoporphyrin equal to or greater than 250 μg/dl whole blood and serum lead equal to or greater than 50 μg/dl, with or without symptoms
- Erythrocyte protoporphyrin level greater than 109 μg/dl, with elevated serum iron level (≥30 ug/dl) and symptomatic
- Serum lead levels greater than 49 μg/dl and symptomatic

Younger children absorb a greater proportion of lead because of their greater intake of dietary fat and their decreased intake of calcium and iron. Excessive amounts of absorbed lead accumulate in the blood, bones, and soft tissue. Soft-tissue absorption is of great concern because it can result in reversible renal failure and central nervous system (CNS) toxicity. Late signs of lead toxicity include coma, stupor, convulsions, and death. Lead poisoning is considered chronic if the lead has been accumulated over a period of time greater than 3 months. Lead interferes with heme synthesis and has a toxic effect on the red blood cells, resulting in a decrease in the number of red blood cells and the amount of hemoglobin in cells, leading to an anemic state.

Lead can be ingested from household utensils, ceramics and pottery, printed materials, and auto emissions. Cracked paint from the walls of old homes (lead-based paint is the most "high-dose" source of lead and is the most common and serious cause of lead poisoning) and toys are other sources of lead. Lead can be found in evaporated milk, fruit juices, and various food products because it is absorbed from the solder of cans. A high incidence of lead poisoning is associated with pica eaters.

INCIDENCE

1. Peak age of incidence is 2 to 3 years.
2. Children between ages 1 and 6 years who live in poorly maintained housing are at a high risk.
3. Rate of incidence is 140 per 100,000 children.

CLINICAL MANIFESTATIONS

1. Nonspecific symptoms—anorexia, malaise, headache, constipation, diarrhea, nausea, failure to thrive, abdominal pain
2. Lead lines in gums around teeth
3. Nausea and vomiting
4. Tachycardia
5. Hypertension or hypotension
6. Lacrimation
7. Nasal congestion
8. Sneezing
9. Muscle pains
10. Renal toxicity

Symptoms of Chronic Lead Poisoning

1. Increased incidence of learning disorders
2. Behavioral disorders
3. Perceptual deficits
4. Hyperactivity, decreased attention span

COMPLICATIONS

1. Cerebral edema
2. CNS toxicity—persistent vomiting, irritability, clumsiness, ataxia, loss of developmental skills

3. Severe and permanent brain damage—occurs in 80% of children who develop severe and acute encephalopathy
4. Late signs—stupor, coma, convulsions, and death

LABORATORY/DIAGNOSTIC TESTS

1. Blood lead levels— ≥ 70 µg/dl (measures level of lead absorption)
2. Erythrocyte protoporphyrin—50 to 249 µg/dl indicates iron deficiency; ≥ 300 µg/dl indicates lead toxicity (measures adverse effect of lead on heme synthesis)
3. Complete blood count (CBC)
4. Serum iron
5. Total nonbinding capacity
6. Serum ferritin
7. Flat plate x-ray examination of abdomen (indicates ingestion of lead if positive)
8. Radiogram of long bone (increased density at metaphyses of radius, ulna, femur, tibia, and fibula)
9. Edetate calcium disodium (CaEDTA) mobilization test (provides an indication of the potentially mobile amount of lead [Pb] in the body; indicates whether chelation therapy will be useful)—ratio (µg Pb/mg edetate calcium disodium) >1 indicative of an increase five times that of the mobile fraction of total body lead burden
10. δ-Aminolevulinic acid (ALA) in urine (increased excretion in urine [≥ 3 mg/m] is abnormal)
11. Coproporphyrin (coproporphyrin III) in urine (increased excretion >100 µg/dl is associated with increased serum lead levels)
12. 24-hr urine (determines amount of lead excreted)

MEDICATIONS

1. Dimercaprol (BAL)—4 mg/kg/dose intramuscularly (IM) q4 hr for 3 to 7 days; chelates with lead and removes lead from red blood cells (RBCs), resulting in decreased serum lead levels; administered alone before first dose of edetate calcium disodium, then used in combination with edetate calcium disodium q4 hr
2. Edetate calcium disodium—administered for 5 to 7 days,

50 to 75 mg/kg/24 hr q4 hr IM; chelates with increased accumulation of lead and excreted in urine

3. Penicillamine—30 to 40 mg/kg/24 hr by mouth (po); administered after parenteral course of edetate calcium disodium when serum lead levels remain increased; administered for 3 to 6 months after initial chelation therapy

NURSING ASSESSMENT

Refer to "Neuromuscular Assessment" in Appendix A.

NURSING DIAGNOSES

Activity intolerance
Pain
High risk for injury
Knowledge deficit
Fluid volume deficit
Altered nutrition: less than body requirements
Altered thought process

NURSING INTERVENTIONS

1. Monitor child's neurologic status, and report the following.
   a. Changes in level of consciousness (LOC)
   b. Twitching or seizure activity
   c. Complaint of headaches
   d. Projectile vomiting
   e. Pupillary response
   f. Fontanels
2. Monitor child's vital signs, and report the following.
   a. Increased apical pulse
   b. Decreased or increased blood pressure
3. Monitor input and output.
   a. Record urinary and stool output.
   b. Monitor fluid restrictions.
4. Monitor child's reaction to chelation therapy.
   a. Dimercaprol
      (1) Fever (occurs in 30% of children)
      (2) Local pain, gluteal abscess, and skin sensitivity (if not given deep IM)

Table 6. Summary of Recommended Follow-up

Frequency	Diagnostic category						
	Class IV*	Class III†	Class II	Class Ia: with iron deficiency anemia	Class Ib	Class I: age 12-36 months	Class I: age 36 months
1-2 weeks	XX‡						
4 weeks		XX					
6 weeks	X (in summer)	X (in summer)					
3 months	X (after 6 months stable)		XX	Arrange treatment of iron deficiency	X (until blood lead normal)	XX	
1 year		X (after first year of follow-up)		Follow as group 1		X	X

From Centers for Disease Control: Increased lead absorption and lead poisoning in young children, *J Pediatr* 87 (11), 1975.

*After hospitalization has been completed.

†Symptomatic or treated patients in group III should be followed as group IV.

‡X, Minimal; XX, optimal.

      (3) Increased blood pressure, tachycardia (may occur within few minutes of administration and last several hours)

      (4) Decreased urinary output

      (5) Garliclike odor to breath

      (6) Nausea and/or vomiting

      (7) Headache

      (8) Burning sensation of lips, mouth, and throat

  b. Edetate calcium disodium

      (1) Decreased blood pressure (20 to 30 minutes after infusion)

      (2) Symptoms of hypocalcemia—paresthesia of lips, tongue, fingers, and feet, carpopedal spasm, seizures, Chvostek's and Trousseau's signs

      (3) Decreased urinary output

      (4) Pain, erythema, dermatitis at infusion site

  c. Penicillamine

      (1) Sensitivity reactions

      (2) Anorexia, nausea, vomiting

Home Care

1. Instruct parents to identify and remove lead hazards from environment(s) in which child spends considerable time before he or she is discharged for home.
   a. Scrape off and remove all readily accessible lead-based paint.
   b. Regularly sweep and mop.
   c. Remove toys with lead-based paint and earthenware.
2. Instruct parents about supervising child more closely if he or she is a pica eater.
3. Instruct and counsel parents about recommended follow-up services (Table 6).

BIBLIOGRAPHY

Barker P, Lewis D: Management of lead exposure in pediatric populations, *Nurse Pract: Am J Prim Health Care* 15(12):8, 1990.

Brown M, Bellinger D, Matthews J: In utero lead exposure, *MCN: Am J Maternal-Child Nurs* 15(2):94, 1990.

Centers for Disease Control: Preventing lead poisoning in young children, *J Pediatr* 93:709, 1978.

Clark M et al: Interaction of iron deficiency and lead and the hematologic findings in children with severe lead poisoning, *Pediatrics* 81(2):247, 1988.

Coppens N et al: The relationship between elevated lead levels and enrollment in special education, *Com Fam Health* 12(4):39, 1990.

Langer B, Modrcin-McCarthy M: Lead poisoning: an ongoing pediatric nursing concern, *Issues Compr Pediatr Nurs* 4(3):23, 1980.

Ritz E et al: Lead and the kidney, *Adv Nephrol* 17:241, 1988.

Rudner N: Children with elevated lead levels, *J Pediatr Health Care* 2(1):46, 1988.

Sachs H et al: Lead poisoning without encephalopathy, *Am J Dis Child* 133:786, 1979.

44 ❖ Leukemia, Childhood

PATHOPHYSIOLOGY

Acute lymphoid, or lymphocytic, leukemia (ALL) is a cancer of the tissues that produce white blood cells (leukocytes). Excessive amounts of immature or abnormal leukocytes are manufactured, and they invade various organs of the body. The leukemic cells invade the bone marrow, displacing the normal cellular elements. As a result, anemia develops, and insufficient numbers of red blood cells are produced. Bleeding occurs as a result of decreased circulating numbers of platelets. Infections occur more frequently because of the decreased number of leukocytes. Invasion of leukemic cells in the vital organs causes hepatomegaly, splenomegaly, and lymphadenopathy.

Acute nonlymphoid leukemia (ANLL) includes the following types of leukemia: acute myeloblastic leukemia, acute monoblastic leukemia, and acute myelocytic leukemia. Bone marrow dysfunction occurs, resulting in decreased numbers of red blood cells, neutrophils, and platelets. Leukemic cells infiltrate lymph nodes, spleen, liver, bones, and the central nervous system, as well as the reproductive organs. Chloromas or granulocytic sarcomas are found in some children.

INCIDENCE

ALL

1. ALL is the most common type of childhood cancer, accounting for one third of all cases of cancer in white children.
2. Highest incidence is in children between the ages of 3 and 5 years.
3. Females have a better prognosis overall than males.
4. Blacks have less frequent remissions and a lower median survival rate.
5. Testicular involvement occurs in 10% of males.

ANLL

1. There is no peak age of incidence.
2. ANLL accounts for 25% of all cases of childhood leukemia.
3. Risk of the disorder increases for children with congenital chromosome disorders such as Down syndrome.
4. It is more difficult to induce remission than in children with ALL (70% remission rate).
5. Remission is briefer than in children with ALL.
6. Fifty percent of children undergoing bone marrow transplantation have a prolonged remission.

CLINICAL MANIFESTATIONS

ALL

1. Evidence of anemia, bleeding, and/or infections
   a. Fever
   b. Fatigue
   c. Pallor
   d. Anorexia
   e. Petechiae and/or hemorrhage
   f. Bone and joint pain
   g. Vague abdominal pain
   h. Weight loss
   i. Enlargement and fibrosis of organs of the reticuloendothelial system—liver, spleen, and lymph glands
2. Increased intracranial pressure resulting from infiltration of the meninges
   a. Pain and stiffness of the neck
   b. Headache

    c. Irritability
    d. Lethargy
    e. Vomiting
    f. Papilledema
    g. Coma
3. Central nervous system symptoms related to site of involvement in the system
    a. Lower-extremity weakness
    b. Difficulty voiding
    c. Learning difficulties, especially with math and memorization (late side effect of therapy)

ANLL

1. Gingival hypertrophy
2. Chloroma of spine (mass lesion)
3. Perirectal necrotic or ulcerous lesions
4. Hepatomegaly and splenomegaly in less than 50% of children
5. Same clinical manifestations as in patient with ALL (see section on ALL)

COMPLICATIONS
ALL

1. Bone marrow failure
2. Infections
3. Hepatomegaly
4. Splenomegaly
5. Lymphadenopathy

ANLL

1. Bone marrow failure
2. Infections
3. Disseminated intravascular coagulation (DIC)
4. Splenomegaly
5. Hepatomegaly

LABORATORY/DIAGNOSTIC TESTS

1. Complete blood count (CBC) — children with CBC count less than 10,000/mm^3 at time of diagnosis have the best prognosis. A white blood count of more than 50,000/mm^3 is an unfavorable prognostic sign in a child of any age.

2. Lumbar puncture: to assess CNS involvement.
3. Chest x-ray examination detects mediastinal involvement.
4. Bone marrow aspiration—a finding of 25% blast cells confirms the diagnosis.
5. Bone scan or skeletal survey assesses bone involvement.
6. Renal, liver, and spleen scans assess leukemic infiltrates.
7. Platelet count indicates clotting capacity.

MEDICATIONS

Drug protocols vary according to the type of leukemia and the type of drug regimen to which the child is assigned. The process of inducing remission in the child consists of three phases: induction, consolidation, and maintenance. During the induction phase (for approximately 3 to 6 weeks) the child receives a variety of chemotherapeutic agents to induce remission. The intensive period is extended for 2 to 3 weeks during the phase of consolidation to combat involvement of the central nervous system (CNS) and other vital organs. Maintenance therapy is administered for several years after diagnosis to sustain remission. The medications used to treat childhood leukemias follow.

Prednisone

Prednisone is primarily used for its potent antiinflammatory effects in disorders involving many organ systems. It is used for treatment of acute childhood leukemias.

Side effects

1. Fluid and electrolyte disturbances—sodium retention, fluid retention, congestive heart failure in susceptible patients, potassium loss, hypertension
2. Musculoskeletal—muscle weakness, osteoporosis, pathologic fracture of long bones
3. Gastrointestinal—peptic ulcer with possible hemorrhage, pancreatitis, abdominal distention
4. Dermatologic—impaired wound healing, petechiae and ecchymoses, facial erythema
5. Neurologic—increased intracranial pressure with papilledema, convulsions, vertigo, and headache

6. Endocrine — development of cushingoid state, manifestations of latent diabetes mellitus
7. Ophthalmic — posterior subcapsular cataracts
8. Metabolic — negative nitrogen balance resulting from protein catabolism

Dosage. Dosage should be individualized according to the severity of the disease and the response of the patient, rather than by strict adherence to the ratio indicated by age or body weight.

Vincristine (Oncovin)

Vincristine is an antineoplastic that inhibits cell division during metaphase. It is used with cyclophosphamide (Cytoxan) in treatment of ALL.

Side effects

1. Neuromuscular — peripheral neuropathy, nerve pain, paresthesias of hands and feet, loss of deep tendon reflexes
2. Hematologic — thrombocytopenia, anemia, leukopenia
3. Gastrointestinal — stomatitis, anorexia, nausea, vomiting, diarrhea
4. Other — convulsions, hyperkalemia, hyperuricemia

Dosage. Refer to treatment protocol for dosage.

Asparaginase

Asparaginase decreases the level of asparagine (an amino acid necessary for tumor growth). It is used in the treatment of ALL.

Side effects

1. Allergic manifestations — most serious side effects of asparaginase; are lessened by the addition of mercaptopurine, cytosine arabinoside, and other immune suppressants
   a. Chills and fever within 1 minute of administration
   b. Skin reactions
   c. Respiratory distress
   d. Hypotension
   e. Substernal pain

    f. Nausea and vomiting
    g. Anaphylaxis
2. Liver toxicity with attendant jaundice, hypoalbumine-
   mia, and occasional depression of clotting factor
3. Pancreatitis
4. Diabetes mellitus
5. Disturbances of calcium metabolism

Dosage. The dosage of asparaginase is highly individualized.

Methotrexate (Amethopterin)

Methotrexate is classified as an antimetabolite. It interferes
with folic acid metabolism. Folic acid is essential to the
synthesis of the nucleoproteins required by rapidly multiplying cells. Methotrexate is used in the treatment of ALL.

In the presence of infection, methotrexate should be
used with caution. Therapy with other bone marrow de-
pressants should also be avoided unless the condition of
the patient warrants its use. It can be given orally, intramuscularly (IM), IV, or intrathecally.

Side effects

1. Skin reactions — generalized erythematous rash, urticaria, acne, pruritus
2. Occasional alopecia
3. Oral and gastrointestinal (GI) tract ulcerations
4. Chills
5. Fever
6. Vomiting
7. Diarrhea
8. Cystitis
9. Bone marrow depression (with occasional hemorrhage
   or septicemia)
10. Liver toxicity
11. Pneumonitis

Mercaptopurine (Purinethol)

Mercaptopurine interferes with the synthesis of nucleic
acid, which is especially needed when the cells are growing
and multiplying rapidly.

The primary effects of mercaptopurine occur in tissues in which there are rapid cellular growth and a high rate of nucleic metabolism (e.g., bone marrow and gastric epithelium). There is a reduction in leukocyte, thrombocyte, and reticulocyte formation. It is used in the treatment of ALL.

Side effects

1. Anorexia
2. Nausea and vomiting
3. Diarrhea (sometimes bloody) caused by injury to GI epithelium
4. Degenerative liver changes with jaundice with very large doses
5. Bone marrow depression

Dosage. Mercaptopurine is administered by mouth (po) only. Refer to treatment protocol for dosage.

Cytarabine (Cytosar; Cytosine Arabinoside)

Cytarabine is currently indicated for induction of remission in patients with acute granulocytic leukemia. Cytarabine is a potent bone marrow suppressant. Patients receiving this drug must be under close medical supervision and, during induction therapy, should have leukocyte and platelet counts performed frequently. The treatment is modified or suspended when the drug-induced depression has resulted in a platelet count less than 50,000 or a polymorphonuclear granulocyte count less than 1000/mm^3.

Side effects

1. Nausea and vomiting
2. Leukopenia, thrombocytopenia, bone marrow suppression
3. Anemia
4. Rash
5. Anorexia
6. Bleeding (all sites)
7. Diarrhea
8. Oral inflammation or ulceration
9. Megaloblastosis
10. Hepatic dysfunction

Dosage. Cytarabine is not active orally. It may be given by IV infusion or injection. It must be stored in a refrigerator until reconstituted.

Allopurinol (Zyloprim)

Allopurinol inhibits the production of uric acid by blocking the biochemical reactions that immediately precede uric acid formation. The result is a lowering of blood and urinary uric acid levels. It is given prophylactically to prevent tissue urate deposits or renal calculi in patients with leukemia who are receiving chemotherapy with a resultant elevation of serum uric acid. Allopurinol also inhibits the oxidation of mercaptopurine, therefore necessitating the use of smaller doses of mercaptopurine (one fourth to one third of the regular dose).

Side effects

1. Occasional liver toxicity
2. Asymptomatic increase in serum glutamic-oxaloacetic transaminase (SGOT) and serum glutamic-pyruvic transaminase (SGPT)

Dosage. Allopurinol is administered po. Refer to treatment protocol for dosage.

Cyclophosphamide (Cytoxan)

A potent antitumor agent of the nitrogen mustard group and an alkylating agent, the exact mechanism of action of cyclophosphamide has not been determined. In contrast to other mustard compounds, it is inert when placed in direct contact with bacteria, leukocytes, and most tumor cells in culture. Cyclophosphamide is used in the treatment of ALL and acute monocytic leukemia.

Side effects

1. Nausea and vomiting
2. Anorexia
3. Alopecia (occurs in at least 50% of patients)
4. Leukopenia (decreased white blood count [WBC])
   a. An expected effect
   b. Ordinarily a guide to therapy
   c. Child susceptible to bacterial infection

5. Sterile hemorrhagic cystitis (bladder mucosa may be injured by some active mustard derivatives that are excreted in the urine)

   Dosage. Cyclophosphamide is administered IV, intravenous fast drip (IVFD), po, or IM.

Daunorubicin (Daunomycin)

Daunorubicin binds to DNA. It is used to inhibit cell division during the treatment of acute leukemia.

Side effects

1. Sclerosing of vein—use two-needle technique (mix with one needle and dispose of that needle; administer with new needle).
2. Nausea and vomiting (soon after administration)
3. Bone marrow depression
4. Cardiac dysrhythmia and death (rare); occurs at total dose >650 mg/m^2.

   Dosage. Administer IV push. Refer to treatment protocol for dosage.

NURSING DIAGNOSES

Activity intolerance
High risk for infection
Fluid volume excess
Impaired tissue integrity
High risk for injury
Body image disturbance
Anxiety
High risk for decreased cardiac output
High risk for fatigue
Altered growth and development
Altered family processes

NURSING ASSESSMENT

Refer to cardiovascular, respiratory, and neurologic assessments.

NURSING INTERVENTIONS

1. Monitor child for reactions to medications (Table 7).
2. Monitor for signs and symptoms of infection.
   a. *Fever* is the most important sign of infection.

Text continued on p. 285.

Table 7. Nursing Interventions Related to the Child Undergoing Chemotherapy and Radiotherapy

Responses to chemotherapy and radiotherapy	Nursing interventions
Diarrhea	Offer fluids po.
	Perform skin care to buttocks and perineal area.
	Monitor effectiveness of antidiarrheal medications.
	Avoid high cellulose foods and fruit.
	Offer small, frequent feedings; include child's favorites if possible.
	Decrease or eliminate meat.
	Observe for signs of dehydration.
	Monitor IV infusions.
Anorexia	Monitor input and output.
Nausea and vomiting	Offer small, frequent feedings of *any bland foods* high in nutrients and calories.
	Consult with child and parents to develop meal plan that incorporates child's likes and dislikes.
	Maintain adequate fluid intake, using Popsicles, ice cream, gelatin, noncarbonated beverages.
	Obtain daily weights.
	Observe for dehydration.
	Monitor side effects of antiemetics (e.g., chlorpromazine [Thorazine], promethazine [Phenergan], hydroxyzine pamoate [Vistaril], diphenhydramine [Benadryl]).

Table 7. Nursing Interventions Related to the Child Undergoing Chemotherapy and Radiotherapy—cont'd.

Responses to chemotherapy and radiotherapy	Nursing interventions
Fluid retention	Monitor input and output.
	Obtain daily weights.
	Evaluate for respiratory distress and edema.
	Provide frequent changes of position.
	Monitor side effects of diuretics.
Hyperuremia	Monitor input and output.
	Encourage fluid intake (how many ml/24 hr).
	Provide skin care to decrease itching.
	Monitor serum creatinine and uric acid levels.
	Monitor side effects of allopurinol.
Chills and fever	Monitor vital signs and frequency of symptoms.
	Evaluate source of symptoms (e.g., tumor or infection).
	Monitor side effects of antipyretics.
	Provide comfort measures such as blankets and tepid sponge baths.
Stomatitis and mouth ulcers	Provide comfort measures such as frequent mouth rinses, use of mouth swabs, and hard candy.
	Avoid hard-bristle toothbrush.
	Avoid glycerine swabs.
	Avoid hard foods that require excessive chewing

Continued.

Table 7. Nursing Interventions Related to the Child
Undergoing Chemotherapy and Radiotherapy—cont'd.

Responses to chemotherapy and radiotherapy	Nursing interventions
	and foods that are acid or spicy.
	Avoid hot foods.
Cardiotoxicity (doxorubicin and daunorubicin)	Monitor changes in electrocardiogram (ECG) and vital signs.
	Observe for signs and symptoms of congestive heart failure.
Hemorrhagic cystitis (cyclophosphamide)	Encourage frequent voiding after drug administration.
	Offer oral fluids in *large amounts.*
	Monitor IV fluids.
	Encourage voiding before sleep.
Alopecia	Prepare child and family for hair loss.
	Reassure child and family that hair loss is temporary.
	Prepare child and family for hair regrowth that differs in color and texture from former hair.
	Arrange for another child in same developmental stage to visit child and talk about the experience.
	Suggest use of scarf, hat, wig before hair loss as a transition measure.
	Wash scalp frequently to prevent cradle cap.
Pain	Evaluate child's verbal and nonverbal behavior for evidence of pain.

Table 7. Nursing Interventions Related to the Child Undergoing Chemotherapy and Radiotherapy—cont'd.

Responses to chemotherapy and radiotherapy	Nursing interventions
	Note cultural aspects affecting pain behavior.
	Use age-appropriate terminology when asking child about pain experience.
	Monitor vital signs.
	Evaluate sleep patterns that may be altered by pain.
	Monitor side effects of analgesics and narcotics.
	Offer approaches to deal with pain such as hypnosis, biofeedback, relaxation techniques, imagery, distraction, cutaneous stimulation, and desensitization.
Leukopenia	Observe for signs and symptoms of infection and inflammation.
	Monitor vital signs.
	Screen visitors for contagious disease and infections.
	Monitor white blood cell count and differential.
	Ensure that good hygienic measures are maintained.
	Prevent breaks in the skin integrity (e.g., keep nails short and prevent injuries).
Thrombocytopenia	Observe for signs and symptoms of bleeding (petechiae and/or hemorrhage).
	Monitor vital signs.
	Monitor platelet count.
	Prevent injury or trauma to body.

Continued.

Table 7. Nursing Interventions Related to the Child Undergoing Chemotherapy and Radiotherapy—cont'd.

Responses to chemotherapy and radiotherapy	Nursing interventions
	Avoid rectal temperatures.
	Avoid injections.
	Monitor platelet transfusions.
	Provide pressure on bleeding sites.
Anemia and/or fatigue	Evaluate signs and symptoms of anemia.
	Monitor CBC and differential.
	Provide for periods of rest and sleep.
	Encourage quiet play activities.
Increased risk of fractures	Avoid weight bearing on affected limb.
	Prevent accidents and injuries.
	Encourage nonambulatory play activities.
Delayed physical and sexual development	Provide anticipatory guidance to parents about child's growth retardation, skeletal deformities, and delayed sexual development.
	Discuss possibility of sterility with child and family.
Chromosomal damage	Provide patient and family teaching about effects of radiation and chemotherapy on cells.
	Provide genetic counseling.
Hypersensitivity to the medication, resulting in anaphylactic shock	Have the following medications available: hydrocortisone, epinephrine, and diphenhydramine (Benadryl).

Table 7. Nursing Interventions Related to the Child
Undergoing Chemotherapy and Radiotherapy — cont'd.

Responses to chemotherapy and radiotherapy	Nursing interventions
Phlebitis and necrosis of tissue, resulting from infiltration of IV infusion	Observe for dyspnea, restlessness, and urticaria.
	Avoid vesicant agents near a joint.
	Stop IV flow if infiltration is suspected.
	Tissue may be treated with drug-specific antidote and hydrocortisone.
	Apply cold compress to site.
	Continue to observe site for signs of inflammation and necrosis.
	Grafting and surgical excision may be indicated if necrosis results.

b. Treat all of the patients as if they are neutropenic
   until results of tests are obtained. Isolate them from
   other clinic patients, especially those children with
   infectious diseases, particularly chicken pox.
c. Have the child wear a mask if he or she is around
   other people and is severely neutropenic (WBC less
   than 1000).
d. Be aware that if the child is neutropenic, he or she
   may not receive chemotherapy. The child may receive
   IV antibiotics if a fever is also present. NOTE: More
   patients die from infection than from their disease.
3. Monitor for signs and symptoms of hemorrhaging.
   a. Check skin for bruising and petechiae.
   b. Check for nosebleeds and bleeding gums.
   c. If an injection is given, apply pressure to the site for
      longer than usual (approximately 3 to 5 minutes) to
      be sure bleeding has stopped. Check back to be sure
      bleeding has not restarted.

4. Monitor for signs and symptoms of complications.
   a. Radiation somnolence—beginning 6 weeks after receiving craniospinal radiation, children exhibit great fatigue and anorexia for approximately 1 to 3 weeks. Parents often worry about relapse at this time and need to be reassured.
   b. CNS symptoms—these symptoms—headache, blurred or double vision, vomiting—can indicate CNS leukemic involvement.
   c. Respiratory symptoms—these symptoms—coughing, lung congestion, dyspnea—may indicate pneumocystitis or other respiratory infection.
   d. Cell lysis—rapid cell lysis after chemotherapy can affect blood chemistries, causing increased calcium and potassium.
5. Monitor for concerns and anxiety about the diagnosis of cancer and its related treatments; monitor for emotional responses such as anger, denial, and grief.
   a. All interventions are based on the child's level of psychologic development.
   b. Provide emotional support, stress reduction techniques, and anxiety management.
   c. Encourage verbalization of concerns and fears (child's and family's).
   d. Individualize patient's and family's education to each patient and family and to each specific phase of the disease.
   e. Provide anticipatory guidance related to side effects of therapy and special needs of each child according to his or her developmental level.
   f. Perform behavioral interventions using relaxation, guided imagery, and hypnosis.
6. Monitor disruptions in family functioning.
   a. All interventions are based on the family's cultural, religious, educational, and socioeconomic background.
   b. Involve siblings as much as possible because they have many concerns and feelings about the changes in the child and the family's functioning.
   c. Consider the possibility that siblings feel self-blame and guilt.

    d. Encourage family unity by having 24-hour visitation privileges for all family members.

Home Care/Discharge Planning

The interventions identified for acute care management apply for long-term care as well.

BIBLIOGRAPHY

Bossert E, Martinson I: Kinetic family drawings revised: a method of determining the impact of cancer on the family as perceived by the child with cancer, *J Pediatr Nurs* 5(3):204, 1990.

Bosworth T: Leukemia through a teenager's eyes, *MCN: Am J Maternal-Child Nurs* 14(2):93, 1989.

Gallagher J: Acute lymphocytic leukemia treatment: effects on learning, *J Pediatr Health Care* 3(5):257, 1989.

Hockenberry M, Coody D, Bennett B: Childhood cancers: incidence, etiology, diagnosis and treatment, *Pediatr Nurs* 16(3):239, 1990.

Hydzik C: Late effects of chemotherapy: implications for patient management and rehabilitation, *Nurs Clin N Am* 25(2):423, 1990.

Hymovich D: A theory for pediatric oncology nursing practice and research, *J Pediatr Oncol Nurs* 7(4):131, 1990.

Lange B et al: Home care involving methotrexate infusions for children with acute lymphoblastic leukemia, *J Pediatr* 112(3):429, 1988.

Munet-Vilaro F, Vessey J: Children's explanation of leukemia: a Hispanic perspective, *J Pediatr Nurs* 5(4):274, 1990.

Peckham V et al: Educational late effects in long-term survivors of childhood acute lymphocytic leukemia, *Pediatrics* 81(1):127, 1988.

Pfaff V, Smith L, Grouan D: The effects of music-assisted relaxation on the distress of pediatric cancer patients undergoing bone marrow aspirations, *Child Health Care* 18(4):232, 1989.

Rhoades A: A minor's refusal of treatment, *MCN: Am J Maternal-Child Nurs* 15(4):261, 1990.

Ruccione K: Acute leukemia in children — current perspectives, *Issues Compr Pediatr Nurs* 6(5/6):329, 1983.

Sabio H: Advances in the diagnosis and treatment of hematologic malignancies, *J Pediatr Oncol Nurs* 7(2):69, 1990.

Stutzman H: Explaining leukemia to classmates, *J Assoc Pediatr Oncol Nurses* 2(1):15, 1985.

Suderman J: Pain relief during routine procedures for children with leukemia, *MCN: Am J Maternal-Child Nurs* 15(3):163, 1990.

Waskerwitz M et al: An overview of cancer in children in the 1980's, *Nurs Clin North Am* 20(1):5, 1985.

45 ❖ Meningitis

PATHOPHYSIOLOGY

Meningitis is an acute inflammation of the meninges. The organisms responsible for bacterial meningitis invade the area either directly as a result of a traumatic injury or indirectly when they are transported from other sites in the body to the cerebrospinal fluid (CSF). A variety of organisms can invade the central nervous system and produce an inflammation of the meninges. In neonates, the primary organisms responsible are gram-negative enteric bacilli, gram-negative rods, and Group B streptococci. In children 3 months to 5 years of age, the primary organism responsible for meningitis is *Haemophilus influenzae* type b. Meningitis in older children is usually the result of a *Neisseria meningitidis* infection or a staphylococcal infection.

Aseptic meningitis is usually caused by a virus and affects young adults more often than children. Older children usually manifest a variety of nonspecific prodromal signs and flulike symptoms that last for 1 to 2 weeks. Although fatigue and weakness may last for a number of weeks, sequelae are uncommon. The child is evaluated and treated as a patient with bacterial meningitis until it is ruled out. Viral meningitis usually requires only a brief hospitalization, with supportive care at home the primary intervention.

Otitis media, sinusitis, or respiratory infections may be the initial site of infection. In addition, a predisposition

288

resulting from an immune deficiency increases the likelihood of this disorder. Once the meninges are infected, the
organisms are spread through the cerebrospinal fluid (CSF)
to the brain and adjacent tissues. Prognosis varies, depending on a variety of factors. Neonatal meningitis has
a high mortality rate and an increased incidence of neurologic sequelae. Bacterial meningitis results in a large
number of patients having behavioral changes, motor
dysfunction, and cognitive changes such as perceptual
deficits.

INCIDENCE

1. More males than females have meningitis.
2. Peak incidence is at 6 to 12 months of age.
3. Highest rate of morbidity is from birth to 4 years
   of age.

CLINICAL MANIFESTATIONS

Neonates

1. Subnormal temperature
2. Fever
3. Pallor
4. Lethargy
5. Irritability
6. Poor feeding
7. Seizures

Later symptoms associated with poor prognosis

1. Bulging fontanels
2. Opisthotonus

Infants and Young Children

1. Lethargy
2. Irritability
3. Pallor
4. Anorexia
5. Nausea and vomiting
6. Increased crying
7. Insistence on being held
8. Increased intracranial pressure (ICP)
9. Increased head circumference

Older Children

1. Headache
2. Fever
3. Vomiting
4. Irritability
5. Photophobia
6. Spinal and nuchal rigidity
7. Positive Kernig's sign
8. Positive Brudzinski's sign
9. Opisthotonic posturing
10. Petechiae (*H. influenzae* and meningococcal meningitis)
11. Septicemia
12. Shock
13. Disseminated intravascular coagulation (DIC)
14. Confusion
15. Seizures

COMPLICATIONS

1. Deafness
2. Blindness
3. Subdural effusions
4. Increased secretion of antidiuretic hormone (ADH)
5. Developmental delay
6. Hydrocephalus
7. Cerebral edema

LABORATORY/DIAGNOSTIC TESTS

1. Lumbar puncture and culture of CSF with the following results
   a. Increased white blood count (WBC)
   b. Glucose level — decreased (bacterial); normal (viral)
   c. Protein — high (bacterial); slightly elevated (viral)
   d. Pressure — increased
   e. Identification of causative organism — meningococcal, gram-positive (streptococci, staphylococci, pneumococci, *H. influenzae*), or viral (coxsackievirus, ECHO virus)
   f. Lactic acid — elevated (bacterial)
   g. Serum glucose — elevated
2. Blood culture — to identify causative organism
3. Urine culture — to identify causative organism

4. Nasopharyngeal—to identify causative organism
5. Computed tomography (CT) scan—to identify abscess, subdural effusion, or hydrocephalus
6. Serum electrolytes—elevated if child dehydrated; increased serum sodium (Na^+); decreased serum potassium (K^+)
7. Urine osmolarity—increased with increased secretion of ADH

MEDICATIONS

1. Antibiotics—used to treat infection; choice of antibiotics dependent on identification of causative organism
2. Anticonvulsants—phenobarbital; for convulsions, status epilepticus: 16 to 100 mg IM; 5 to 10 mg/kg up to 20 mg/kg/24 hr IV: long-term management: 3 to 5 mg/kg/24 hr po.

NURSING ASSESSMENT

Refer to "Neuromuscular Assessment" in Appendix A.

NURSING DIAGNOSES

High risk for infection
Sensory/perceptual alterations
Fluid volume deficit
Pain
Altered nutrition: less than body requirements
High risk for injury
Diversional activity deficits
Sleep pattern disturbance
Knowledge deficit

NURSING INTERVENTIONS

1. Monitor infant's or child's vital signs and neurologic status as often as q2 hr.
   a. Temperature, respiratory rate, apical pulse
   b. Level of consciousness (LOC)
   c. Kernig's sign
   d. Brudzinski's sign
   e. Pupils equal, react to light (PERL)
2. Monitor child's hydration status; observe for signs of hydration.
   a. Decreased skin turgor

      b. Increased urinary output
      c. Increased urinary osmolarity
      d. Signs and symptoms of hyponatremia
      e. Increased urinary specific gravity
      f. Input and output
      g. Daily weights

3. Monitor child for seizure activity (see Chapter 64, "Seizure Disorders").
4. Institute isolation procedures with respiratory precautions to protect others from infectious contact; keep child in isolation for 24 hr after antibiotics are started.
5. Monitor the IV infusion and the side effects of medications.
      a. Antibiotics — the usual course of antibiotic treatment is 10 to 14 days; culture results and clinical response will be continually reassessed and will indicate need for changes in antibiotic therapy (see "Medications").
      b. Anticonvulsants.
6. Provide comfort measures in an environment that is quiet and has minimal stressful stimuli.
      a. Avoid bright lights and noise.
      b. Avoid excessive manipulation of the child.
7. Position child with head of bed slightly elevated to decrease cerebral edema; monitor administration of fluids.
8. Reduce fever through the use of tepid sponge baths or hypothermia mattress.
9. Support child emotionally when he or she undergoes a lumbar puncture and other tests.
      a. Provide age-appropriate explanations before procedures.
      b. Restrain child to prevent occurrence of injury.
10. Provide emotional support to family.
      a. Provide and reinforce information about condition and hospitalization.
      b. Encourage ventilation of feelings of guilt and self-blame.
      c. Encourage use of preexisting support.
      d. Provide for physical comforts (e.g., sleeping arrangements, hygiene needs).

11. Provide age-appropriate diversional activities (see Appendix B, *Growth and Development*).

Home Care

1. Instruct parents about administration of medications, and monitor for side effects.
2. Instruct parents to monitor for long-term complications and their signs and symptoms.

BIBLIOGRAPHY

Friedman A, Fleisher G: Meningitis: update of recommendations for the neonate, *Clin Pediatr* 19(6):395, 1983.

Fulginiti VA: Treatment of meningitis in the very young infant, *Am J Dis Child* 70:43, 1983.

Gaddy DS: Meningitis in the pediatric population, *Nurs Clin North Am* 15(1):83, 1980.

Saez-Llorens X, McCracken GH Jr: Bacterial meningitis in neonates and children, *Infect Dis Clin North Am* 4(4):623, 1990.

Spaniolo A et al: Case study of a child with meningococcemia, *J Pediatr Nurs* 1(6):396, 1986.

Stutman H et al: Bacterial meningitis in children: diagnosis and therapy. A review of recent developments, *Clin Pediatr* 26(9):431, 1987.

Swanwick T: Meningitis and the child, *Nursing*, 3(46):8, 1989.

Vallejo JG, Kaplan SL, Mason EO Jr: Treatment of meningitis and other infections due to ampicillin-resistant *Haemophilus influenzae* type b in children, *Review Infect Dis* 13(2):197, 1991.

Wink D: Bacterial meningitis in children, *Am J Nurs* 84:456, April 1984.

46 ❖ Muscular Dystrophy

PATHOPHYSIOLOGY

Muscular dystrophy is a disorder that results in bilateral and symmetrical wasting of the voluntary muscles. The muscles hypertrophy, and the muscle tissue is replaced with both connective tissue and fatty deposits. Types of muscular dystrophy include: Duchenne, Becker's, limb-girdle, congenital, ocular, and facioscapulohumeral. The onset of sex-linked recessive types (Duchenne, limb-girdle, congenital) is earlier than that of dominant types (facio-scapulohumeral, ocular). Initially seen symptoms include gait abnormality and clumsiness. Muscles of the hands, feet, tongue, palate, and mastication are rarely affected. Mild to moderate retardation is not unusual. Children affected with muscular dystrophy rarely live beyond 20 years of age.

Duchenne Muscular Dystrophy

1. Duchenne muscular dystrophy is transmitted as a sex-linked recessive gene.
2. It is characterized by progressive involvement of voluntary muscles.
3. It runs a rapid course.
4. Onset of symptoms occurs between 3 and 10 years of age.
5. Death occurs approximately 10 to 15 years after onset.

INCIDENCE

1. Duchenne muscular dystrophy affects males (X-linked recessive).

2. Duchenne muscular dystrophy accounts for approximately 50% of all cases.
3. Becker's muscular dystrophy affects males.
4. Facioscapulohumeral muscular dystrophy affects both sexes equally.
5. Limb-girdle and ocular muscular dystrophies affect either sex (autosomal recessive).
6. Approximately 50% of the sisters of boys with muscular dystrophy will be carriers, and one half of their offspring will inherit the disease.
7. Approximately 50% of children with muscular dystrophy can be characterized as having normal personalities.

CLINICAL MANIFESTATIONS OF DUCHENNE MUSCULAR DYSTROPHY

Symptoms are related to the voluntary muscles that are affected. The most frequently occurring symptoms are as follows:
1. Difficulty lifting arms above head
2. Waddling gait
3. Poor balance
4. Gowers' sign—"walking up legs" from sitting to standing position
5. Difficulty climbing stairs
6. Difficulty rising to standing position
7. Difficulty running
8. Flat smile
9. Flat affect

LABORATORY/DIAGNOSTIC TESTS

1. Electromyogram (EMG)—demonstrates less electrical activity in affected muscles
2. Muscle biopsy—diagnostic; indicates presence of fat
3. Creatine phosphokinase (CPK)—increased

NURSING ASSESSMENT

Refer to "Neuromuscular Assessment" in Appendix A.

NURSING DIAGNOSES

Impaired physical mobility
Altered growth and development

Altered nutrition: less than body requirements
Impaired home maintenance management
Altered family processes
Diversional activity deficit
Self-care deficit: bathing/hygiene
                   dressing/grooming, feeding,
                   toileting
Low self-esteem: chronic

NURSING INTERVENTIONS

Long-Term Management/Home Care

1. Promote optimal muscular functioning.
   a. Reinforce physical therapy exercise regimen.
   b. Discourage inactivity and promote rest (inactivity promotes progression of disease).
2. Promote self-care activities as a means of enhancing child's sense of independence and self-sufficiency.
   a. Investigate and recommend use of adaptive devices as appropriate.
   b. Provide recommendations for home adaptations (e.g., grab bars, overhead slings, raised toilets).
   c. Recommend use of adaptive equipment as necessary (e.g., braces to prevent slumping and to facilitate standing).
3. Assist parents in expressing and working through feelings of guilt, resentment, and anger.
4. Encourage parents, in collaboration with the child, to select realistic goals for achievement and living.
5. Provide support for child and family as they cope with disease.
   a. Refer to social worker or psychologist.
   b. Refer to Muscular Dystrophy Association.
   c. Refer to parent support group.
   d. Refer to peer support group.
6. Provide information and make referrals about available educational resources.
   a. Encourage child to attend school.
   b. Refer parents to educational specialist.
7. Encourage and support parents' seeking genetic counseling.

8. Encourage parents and siblings to mourn (loss of the "perfect child") and to learn to cope.
   a. Refer to parent and sibling support group.
   b. Refer to counselor or therapist as needed.
   c. Encourage use of support systems (family and friends) to ventilate feelings.
9. Provide information, and assess long-term care needs pertaining to:
   a. Scoliosis
   b. Pulmonary and cardiac problems.

BIBLIOGRAPHY

Bach JR, Campagnolo DI, Hoeman S: Life satisfaction of individuals with Duchenne muscular dystrophy using long-term mechanical ventilatory support, *Am J Phys Med Rehab* 70(3):129, 1991.

Cole C et al: Parental testing for Duchenne and Becker muscular dystrophy, *Lancet* 1(8580):262, 1988.

Conway B. In Carini S, Owen S: *Neurological and neurosurgical nursing,* ed 7, St. Louis, 1978, Mosby–Year Book.

Fenichel GM et al: A comparison of daily and alternate-day prednisone therapy in the treatment of Duchenne muscular dystrophy, *Arch Neurol* 48(6): 575, 1991.

Greenberg CR et al: Three years' experience with neonatal screening for Duchenne/Becker muscular dystrophy: gene analysis, gene expression, and phenotype prediction, *Am J Med Genet* 39(1):68, 1991.

Smith RA et al: Assessment of locomotor function in young boys with Duchenne musuclar dystrophy, *Muscle and Nerve* 14(5):462, 1991.

Thompson R, O'Quinn S: *Developmental disabilities: etiologies, manifestations, diagnoses, and treatments,* New York, 1979, Oxford University Press.

47 ❖ Nephrotic Syndrome

PATHOPHYSIOLOGY

Nephrotic syndrome is the clinical state caused by increased glomerular permeability to plasma proteins, resulting in (1) proteinuria >50 mg/kg/day, (2) proteinemia <6 g/day, and (3) albuminemia <3 g/day. The loss of protein causes decreased plasma osmotic pressure and increased hydrostatic pressure, resulting in the accumulation of fluids in interstitial spaces and abdominal cavities. The decrease in vascular fluid volume stimulates the renin-angiotensin system, resulting in secretion of antidiuretic hormone (ADH) and aldosterone. Tubular reabsorption of sodium (Na^+) and water is increased, expanding the intravascular volume.

Nephrotic syndrome is the pathologic outcome of various causes that alter glomerular permeability. These causes can be categorized into three basic types: congenital, idiopathic, and secondary (see box on facing page). Nephrotic syndrome is classified according to the clinical findings and the microscopic examination of renal tissue. Based on clinical classification, the syndrome types differ according to the course of the disease, treatment, and prognosis. These types are minimal-change nephrotic syndrome, focal glomerular sclerosis, and diffuse proliferative glomerulonephritis. The mortality rate is low; morbidity is related to the underlying pathology and response to treatment. Only 5% to 10% of children will progress to end-stage renal disease.

Causes of Nephrotic Syndrome

Congenital

> Finnish type (inherited)
> Syphilitic or cytomegaloviral

Idiopathic

> Most frequent type
> Accounts for 80% of diagnostic cases
> May appear at any age but increased prevalence at younger age

Secondary

> Postinfectious glomerulonephritis
> Systemic disease
> Hemolytic-uremic syndrome
> Diabetes mellitus
> Renal vein thrombosis
> Alport's syndrome
> Allergic nephrosis—after bee sting, pollen inhalation, or immunization procedure
> Toxic nephrosis—drugs and heavy metals
> Rare cases—sickle cell anemia, hypoproteinemia

Prognosis is poor in children who do not respond to treatment.

INCIDENCE

1. One half of the children diagnosed with idiopathic nephrosis are less than 4 years old.
2. Two thirds of the children diagnosed with idiopathic nephrosis are less than 5 years old.
3. Boys are affected twice as often as girls.
4. Nephrotic syndrome occurs in 16 per 100,000 children.
5. Congenital nephrotic syndrome accounts for more than 95% of the cases diagnosed in children less than 1 year old.
6. Siblings infrequently are affected (congenital nephrotic syndrome).

7. Idiopathic nephrotic syndrome has a 5% to 6% mortality rate.

CLINICAL MANIFESTATIONS

1. Proteinuria (index of disease activity)
2. Pitting edema (lasting from several days to weeks); periorbital edema in morning; dependent edema in evening
3. Lethargy and irritability
4. Ascites, pleural effusion (can cause dyspnea if becomes severe)
5. Pallor caused by fluid retention
6. Increased weight gain (occurs slowly)
7. Diarrhea, anorexia, and poor intestinal absorption caused by edema of intestinal tract
8. Dark, frothy urine; decreased urinary output

COMPLICATIONS

1. End-stage renal disease
2. Hypercoagulability
3. Pneumonia
4. Chicken pox and rubeola
5. Peritonitis
6. Cellulitis
7. Untoward side effects from steroids
8. Infection

LABORATORY/DIAGNOSTIC TESTS

1. Urine protein (increased; 300 to 1000 mg protein/dl; 3+ or 4+)
2. Increased urinary creatinine and urea clearances
3. Urinalysis—hyaline and granular casts, transient hematuria
4. Serum albumin (decreased)
5. Serum electrolytes (sodium [Na^+], potassium [K^+], chlorine [Cl^-] normal)
6. Complete blood count (CBC); hemoglobin (Hb); hematocrit (Hct) (normal or elevated because of erythrocytosis, hemoconcentration)
7. Sedimentation rate (increased because of distorted serum protein)

8. Decreased protein-bound iodine
9. Decreased thyroxin
10. Total hemolytic complements B and C (normal)
11. Serum pH (metabolic alkalosis is a result of diuretic use)
12. Serum calcium (decreased)
13. Serum cholesterol (increased 450 to 1500 mg/100 ml)
14. Renal biopsy (diagnostic; not routinely done)

MEDICATIONS

1. Prednisone or prednisolone (one of many drug regimens) — has antiinflammatory effects; inhibits phagocytosis and suppresses other clinical manifestations of inflammation; used in the treatment of nephrotic syndrome to induce remission
   a. 2 mg/kg/day in three or four divided doses by mouth (po) until urine is protein free for 5 days
   b. If no remission — 4 mg/kg (maximum of 120 mg) po qod for 28 days
   c. Maintenance dose — 2 mg/kg/day (up to 80 mg/day) po qod; gradually reduce over 2 to 4 months
2. Cytotoxic therapy (immunosuppressive) for patients resistant to steroid therapy
   a. Cyclophosphamide (Cytoxan) — 2.5 to 3 mg/kg/day for 8 weeks
3. Antibiotics (penicillin) — administered prophylactically or therapeutically
4. Diuretics — used to induce diuresis
   a. Furosemide (Lasix) — administered po or intravenously (IV) 0.5-2 mg/kg/dose
   b. Chlorothiazide — 20 mg/kg/24 hr
   c. Spironolactone — 3 mg/kg/24 hr
5. Salt-poor albumin (1 to 2 g/kg/day)
6. Calcium and vitamin D

NURSING ASSESSMENT

Refer to "Renal Assessment" in Appendix A.

NURSING DIAGNOSES

Altered tissue perfusion
High risk for injury

Fluid volume excess
Altered nutrition: less than body requirement
Impaired skin integrity
High risk for infection
Knowledge deficit

NURSING INTERVENTIONS

1. Monitor child's clinical status.
   a. Report changes to physician.
   b. Monitor urine for proteinuria and hematuria (indicates progression of disease).
2. Monitor and control edema; prevent complications.
   a. Assess edematous areas for changes in condition.
   b. Promote bed rest during periods of severe edema and periods of rapid weight loss during diuresis.
3. Monitor child's therapeutic response to and untoward effects of medications.
   a. Accurate input and output
   b. Daily weights
   c. Signs of electrolyte imbalance—hypokalemia, hyponatremia (diuretics)
   d. Prednisone side effects
   e. Cyclophosphamide side effects
4. Encourage and support nutritional intake and status.
   a. Provide diet high in calories and protein (to minimize negative nitrogen balance).
   b. Decrease sodium.
   c. Avoid selected foods; provide no salty fish, meats, and potato chips, and restrict milk and bread.
   d. Provide calcium supplements (to decrease osteoporosis).
5. Provide skin care to maintain integrity and suppleness.
   a. Bathe frequently.
   b. Dry the moist areas of skin (e.g., folds of skin, male genitalia).
   c. Position child so edematous areas are not in contact with anything.
6. Monitor and prevent complications.
   a. Circulatory disturbance (e.g., hypovolemia resulting from protein and fluid loss)

    b. Signs of infection (may be masked by steroids)
    c. Complications from steroids—gastrointestinal (GI) bleeding, decreased resistance to infection, hypertension, increased intracranial pressure (ICP)
    d. Cellulitis
    e. Peritonitis (may result when ascites is present)
    f. Pneumonia (caused by compression of lung by pleural effusion and diaphragm)
    g. Chicken pox and rubeola
    h. Hypercoagulability (from femoral vein or arterial puncture)
7. Provide emotional support to parents.
    a. Encourage ventilation of concerns.
    b. Provide and reinforce information about child's condition and hospitalization.
    c. Encourage use of previous sources of support.
    d. Provide for physical comfort (e.g., sleeping arrangements, bathing).
8. Provide age-appropriate activities and toys for child (see Appendix B, *Growth and Development*).
9. Alleviate or minimize child's anxiety during hospitalization.
    a. Provide age-appropriate explanations before procedures.
    b. Provide play therapy.
    c. Incorporate home routines into hospitalization (e.g., bedtime routine).

Home Care

1. Provide child and parents instruction about disease process.
2. Instruct child and parents about therapeutic and untoward effects of medications.
3. Inform school teacher and school nurse about limits on child's activities and diet.
4. Provide parents written instructions to enhance compliance.
    a. Diet
    b. Prevention of infection
    c. Skin care

    d. Administration of medications
    e. Activity restrictions
    f. Follow-up visits
5. Provide parents information about infection control.

BIBLIOGRAPHY

Brodehl J, Ehrich J: Short versus standard prednisone therapy for critical treatment of idiopathic nephrotic syndrome in children, *Lancet* 1:380, 1988.

Habib R, Gubler M: Focal glomerular sclerosis associated with idiopathic nephrotic syndrome in children. In Rubin M, Burratt M, eds: *Pediatric nephrology*, Baltimore, 1975, Williams & Wilkins.

Hutt M: Proteinuria and the nephrotic syndrome. In Schrier R, ed: *Renal electrolyte disorders*, Boston, 1976, Little, Brown & Co.

Rance C, Arbrus G, Bulfe J: Management of the nephrotic syndrome in children, *Pediatr Clin North Am* 23(4):735, 1976.

Warshaw B, Hymes C: Daily single-dose and daily reduced-dose prednisone therapy for children with the nephrotic syndrome, *Pediatrics* 83:694, 1989.

Wynn S et al: Long term prognosis for children with nephrotic syndrome, *Clin Pediatr* 27(2):63, 1988.

Yu E et al: Encephalopathy associated with steroid treated nephrotic syndrome, *Int J Pediatr Nephrol* 8(3):135, 1987.

48 ❖ Neuroblastoma

PATHOPHYSIOLOGY

Neuroblastoma is an embryonal tumor that arises from the neural crest. It may originate from the adrenal gland or the sympathetic ganglia. The cause of neuroblastoma is unknown. The chest and neck are common sites for it. The neuroblastoma cells can synthesize and metabolize catecholamines.

Staging Procedure

Staging refers to the determination of the exact extent of the disease at the time of diagnosis. Stage I refers to localization of the tumor, whereas Stage IV involves metastases. There is a high rate of spontaneous regression in children less than 2 years of age whether the child is diagnosed with Stage I or Stage IV disease. Two major types of staging systems are currently used in pediatric practice: (1) the TNM method of classification, which is based on the anatomic factors present; and (2) stage grouping, which uses both anatomic and biologic variables.

Staging can be achieved by three methods:

1. Clinical diagnostic staging, which is noninvasive and relies on physical examination and diagnostic studies
2. Surgical evaluation staging, which uses biopsy results
3. Postoperative (pathologic) treatment staging, which relies on the histologic examination of cancer tissue after its surgical removal

INCIDENCE

1. Neuroblastoma accounts for 10% of childhood cancers.
2. It causes 15% of childhood deaths related to cancer.
3. Ninety percent occurs in children less than 5 years of age.
4. Two thirds of the children have metastatic disease at the time of diagnosis.
5. The 2-year survival rate for Stage IV children is 10%.
6. Prognosis is good for children less than 2 years of age.

CLINICAL MANIFESTATIONS

1. Symptoms related to neck and chest mass
   a. Exophthalmos
   b. Ptosis
   c. Anhidrosis
   d. Miosis
   e. Heterochromia (irises of different colors)
   f. Respiratory dysfunction
   g. Neck and facial edema
   h. Cough
2. Symptoms related to bone marrow involvement
   a. Anemia
   b. Bleeding
   c. Infection
3. Symptoms related to abdominal mass
   a. Anorexia
   b. Altered bowel and/or bladder function
   c. Abdominal pain
4. Neurologic symptoms and paralysis resulting from pressure of mass on spinal column
5. Symptoms related to olfactory mass
   a. Nasal obstruction
   b. Epistaxis
6. Symptoms related to cervical and thoracic mass
   a. Ataxia
   b. Myoclonus
   c. Opsoclonus

General Symptoms

1. Profuse diarrhea
2. Weight loss
3. Irritability

4. Fatigue
5. Lethargy
6. Anorexia
7. Palpable mass

COMPLICATIONS

1. Increased intracranial pressure (ICP)
2. Hydrocephalus
3. Papilledema
4. Tracheal decomposition
5. Hydronephrosis
6. Spinal cord decomposition, resulting in paralysis
7. Bladder obstruction
8. Bowel obstruction
9. Pathologic fractures
10. Cerebral ataxia

LABORATORY/DIAGNOSTIC TESTS

1. Complete blood count (CBC) — to detect anemia caused by many secondary factors (e.g., hemorrhage, disseminated intravascular coagulation [DIC])
2. White blood count (WBC) — decreased because of bone marrow and secondary infection
3. Urinary vanillylmandelic acid (VMA)/hemavanitic acid (HVA) — elevated because of increased secretion of catecholamines from adrenal medulla
4. X-ray studies of chest, skull, and long bones — to detect metastases
5. Intravenous pyelogram (IVP), including inferior vena cava — to detect extent of disease
6. BMA — to assess extension of tumor to the marrow
7. Ferritin level — elevated levels indicate poor prognosis

MEDICATIONS

Antineoplastics

Used in various combinations and schedules.

1. Cyclophosphamide (Cytoxan) — blocks the synthesis of DNA, RNA, and protein; also has significant immunosuppressive activity
2. Vincristine sulfate (Oncovin) — inhibits cell division during metaphase

3. VM-26
4. Cisplatin
5. Melphalan
6. Doxorubicin
7. Dimethyltriazenoimidazole carboxamide (DTIC)

Radiation

1. 1800 rads—infants
2. 3500-4000 rads—child for 2 to 4 weeks depending on child's age

NURSING ASSESSMENT

Refer to nursing assessment of involved site (see Appendix A).

NURSING DIAGNOSES

High risk for injury
High risk for infection
Fluid volume excess
Activity intolerance
Pain
Knowledge deficit
Social isolation

NURSING INTERVENTIONS

Preoperative Care

1. Observe for signs and symptoms related to location of tumor.
2. Monitor child's clinical status.
   a. Monitor vital signs.
   b. Monitor for signs of ICP.
   c. Assess neurologic status.
   d. Obtain abdominal and cranial measurements.
3. Monitor for signs of infection.
   a. Drainage
   b. Decreased WBC (provide reverse isolation)
   c. Pneumonia
   d. Fever (initiate cooling measures)
4. Prepare child for staging with age-appropriate explanations (see Appendix B, *Growth and Development*).

5. Provide emotional support to parents.
   a. Encourage expression of feelings.
   b. Provide for physical comforts (sleeping and hygiene).
   c. Encourage use of preexisting support systems.
6. Provide and reinforce information given to parents.
7. Prepare and support child during collection of laboratory data.

Postoperative Care

1. Monitor child's clinical status.
   a. Vital signs
   b. Abdominal girth
   c. Neurologic status
2. Maintain child's fluid and electrolyte status.
   a. Assess for signs and symptoms of fluid overload.
   b. Record input and output.
   c. Monitor rate of IV infusion.
   d. Monitor for signs of electrolyte imbalance.
3. Promote and maintain respiratory function.
   a. Increase head of bed (HOB) to semi-Fowler's position.
   b. Perform chest physiology.
   c. Turn, cough, and deep breathe.
   d. Change position q3 hr.
4. Monitor for signs of infection.
   a. Drainage
   b. Decreased WBC (provide reverse isolation)
   c. Chest sounds
   d. Fever
5. Provide pain relief measures.
   a. Maintain position of comfort.
   b. Provide environmental management (decreased noise, dim lights)
   c. Provide analgesics and narcotics as necessary.
6. Manage side effects of radiotherapy and chemotherapy.
   a. Nausea and vomiting
      (1) Administer antiemetic 20 minutes before treatment.
      (2) Administer drug at bedtime or on empty stomach.

(3) Observe for signs and symptoms of dehydration.
  b. Myelosuppression
    (1) Observe for transfusion reactions.
    (2) Encourage quiet activities when prone to infection or bleeding.
    (3) Protect IV from dislodging.
  c. Infection
    (1) Check for potential sites of infection (e.g., needle puncture sites or mucosal ulcers).
    (2) Prevent skin breakdown.
    (3) Provide meticulous care of skin, especially mouth and perianal area.
7. Provide emotional support to child.
  a. Encourage age-appropriate activities (see Appendix B, *Growth and Development*).
  b. Encourage age-appropriate means for ventilation of feelings.
  c. Encourage interactions with age-appropriate mates.
8. Provide emotional support to family (see "Preoperative Care").

Home Care/Discharge Planning

1. Instruct parents about long-term management.
  a. Administration of medications and monitoring child's response to them
  b. Protection from infection
  c. Compliance with treatment
2. Refer child and parents to appropriate community resources.
  a. Parent, child, sibling groups
  b. Financial supports
  c. Pediatrician

BIBLIOGRAPHY

deBernardi B et al: Localized neuroblastoma, surgical and pathologic staging, *Cancer* 60(5):1066, 1987.

Evans A et al: Prognostic factors in neuroblastoma, *Cancer* 59(11):1853, 1987.

Hockenberry M, Coody D, Bennett B: Childhood cancers: incidence, etiology, diagnosis, and treatment, *Pediatr Nurs* 16(3):239, 1990.

Kelly J: The use of an investigational radio pharmaceutical in neuroblastoma: a nursing perspective ... 1311 — metaiodoben-zylquanidine, *J Pediatr Oncol Nurs* 6(4):133, 1989.

McWilliams N: Screening infants for neuroblastoma in North America, *Pediatrics* 79(6):1048, 1987.

Moshang T, Lee M: Late effects: disorders of growth and sexual maturation associated with the treatment of childhood cancers, *J Assoc Pediatr Oncol Nurs* 5(4):14, 1988.

49 ❖ Non-Hodgkin's Lymphoma

PATHOPHYSIOLOGY

Non-Hodgkin's lymphoma is a malignant neoplasm that can arise in any site in the lymphatic system and lymphoid tissue. No definite cause has been identified. Viruses, immunologic defect, chromosomal aberration, and chronic immunostimulation have been identified as cofactors in precipitating malignant lymphomas. High-risk groups (incidence is 100 to 10,000 times greater than for normal population) include those individuals with an acquired or inherited immunodeficiency syndrome and children receiving immunosuppressive agents. Common sites include the lymph nodes, Peyer's patches of the gastrointestinal (GI) tract, the thymus, and Waldeyer's ring. Extralymphatic sites include the bones and the skin. Abdominal lymphomas are the most rapidly proliferating, most often involving the terminal ileum, the cecum, and the appendix. Abdominal involvement can cause intussusception, and metabolic abnormalities are associated with abdominal involvement. Mediastinal sites rapidly disseminate to the bone marrow and the meninges (sites that are associated with an unfavorable prognosis). Three basic types of lymphomas are classified according to cytomorphologic features: (1) large cell (primarily a B cell tumor); (2) lymphoblastic (primarily a T cell tumor); and (3) undifferentiated lymphomas (Burkitt and non-Burkitt tumors).

Signs and symptoms are related to site of involvement. Staging procedure is performed for diagnostic and treatment purposes.

Staging Procedure

Staging refers to the exact determination of the extent of the disease at the time of diagnosis. Two major types of staging systems are currently used in pediatric practice: (1) the TNM method of classification, which is based on the anatomic factors present, and (2) stage grouping, which uses both anatomic and biologic variables.

Staging can be achieved by the following three methods:

1. Clinical diagnostic staging, which is noninvasive and relies on physical examination and diagnostic studies
2. Surgical evaluation staging, which uses biopsy results
3. Postsurgical (pathologic) treatment staging, which relies on the histologic examination of cancer tissue after its surgical removal

INCIDENCE

1. Non-Hodgkin's lymphoma accounts for approximately 4% of the cancer in children.
2. It accounts for 10% of all cancer in children <15 years of age.
3. It is the third most common malignant neoplasm.
4. Non-Hodgkin's lymphoma occurs 1.5 times more frequently than Hodgkin's disease.
5. Male to female ratio is 3:1.
6. The abdomen is the primary site of involvement in 30% to 40% of children.
7. Ten percent to 15% of cases involve Waldeyer's ring, the nasopharynx, and the sinuses.
8. The 3-year survival rate for all children with non-Hodgkin's lymphoma is 50% to 80%.
9. Central nervous system (CNS) involvement occurs in 30% of children with this disease.
10. Forty percent to 50% are T cell tumors.
11. Forty percent to 50% are B cell tumors.
12. Less than 10% are non–T cell and non–B cell tumors.

CLINICAL MANIFESTATIONS

Initial

1. Cough
2. Sore throat
3. Shortness of breath (with masses in anterior mediastinum)
4. Vomiting
5. Enlarged cervical lymph nodes

Gastrointestinal Involvement

1. Distended abdomen
2. Intussusception associated with ileal involvement

Respiratory Involvement Caused by Pleural Effusion or Tracheal Compression

1. Increased respiratory rate
2. Shortness of breath
3. Cough

Long-term

1. Malaise
2. Fatigue
3. Anemia

COMPLICATIONS

1. Respiratory distress
2. Destruction of superior vena cava
3. Intussusception
4. CNS involvement

LABORATORY/DIAGNOSTIC TESTS

1. Serum uric acid (increased because of cellular destruction from chemotherapy)
2. Serum phosphate (increased because of increased tumor load)
3. Serum potassium (increased because of metabolic alterations)
4. Bone marrow aspiration (assess extent of disease)
5. Gallium scan (assess extent of disease)
6. Complete blood count (CBC) (diagnostic for bone marrow dysfunction)

7. Platelet count (diagnostic for bone marrow involvement)
8. Lumbar puncture (assess for CNS invasion)
9. Biopsy of involved site
10. CT scan—to assess extent of disease
11. Serum lactate dehydrogenase (LDH) (increased)
12. Serum creatinine (increased; to assess for kidney involvement and its extent)
13. Serum calcium (increased with bone involvement)
14. Serum phosphorus (increased with bone involvement)
15. Bone scan (to detect bone sites)
16. Lumbar puncture—used to evaluate CSF
17. Abdominal ultrasound to assess extent of disease

MEDICATIONS

Combination of drugs used for treatment determined by histologic diagnosis.

Prednisone

Prednisone is used in conjunction with antineoplastics for the treatment of cancer. Its dosage is individualized.

Side Effects

1. Metabolic—sodium and fluid retention, hypokalemia, congestive heart failure (CHF), hypertension
2. Neurologic—increased intracranial pressure (ICP), insomnia, convulsions
3. Dermatologic—impaired wound healing, ecchymoses, hyperpigmentation, hirsutism
4. Musculoskeletal—muscle wasting and weakness, osteoporosis, spontaneous fractures
5. Endocrine—resistance to stress, steroid-induced diabetes, weight gain, obesity, sterility

Vincristine (Oncovin)

Vincristine is an antineoplastic that inhibits cell division during metaphase. It is used with other antineoplastics for the treatment of non-Hodgkin's lymphoma. Dosage is highly variable according to protocol.

Side Effects

1. Neuromuscular — peripheral neuropathy, paresthesias of hands and feet, loss of deep tendon reflexes, ataxia
2. Gastrointestinal — stomatitis, nausea, vomiting, diarrhea, abdominal cramps
3. Dermatologic — alopecia, cellulitis, phlebitis after extravasation
4. Other — malaise, fever, polyuria, weight loss, uric acid nephropathy, hyperkalemia

Cyclophosphamide (Cytoxan)

Cyclophosphamide is an alkylating agent that blocks synthesis of DNA, RNA, and protein. It is used with other antineoplastic agents for the treatment of non-Hodgkin's lymphoma. Refer to treatment protocol for dosage.

Side Effects

1. Hematologic — leukopenia, thrombocytopenia, anemia
2. Dermatologic — alopecia
3. Gastrointestinal — nausea, vomiting, weight loss, diarrhea
4. Genitourinary — sterile hemorrhagic and nonhemorrhagic cystitis

Methotrexate (Amethopterin)

Methotrexate is an antimetabolite and folic acid antagonist. It interferes with the mitotic process by inhibiting uptake of folinic acid. It is used with other antineoplastic agents in the treatment of non-Hodgkin's lymphoma. Dosage is highly individualized.

Side Effects

1. Gastrointestinal — ulceration, stomatitis, gingivitis, nausea, vomiting, diarrhea
2. Hematologic — suppression of bone marrow, aplastic bone marrow
3. Neurologic — headache, drowsiness, blurred vision
4. Other — malaise, extreme fatigue, systemic toxicity, chills, fever, pneumonitis, diabetes, decreased resistance to infection

Allopurinol (Zyloprim)

Allopurinol is used to increase renal excretion of uric acid, an end product of protein metabolism. It is used prophylactically for hyperuricemia resulting from use of chemotherapeutic agents. Refer to treatment protocol for dosage.

Side Effects

1. Dermatologic — alopecia, maculopapular rash
2. Gastrointestinal — nausea, vomiting, diarrhea
3. Hematologic — aplastic anemia, bone marrow depression, thrombocytopenia, pancytopenia
4. Neurologic — peripheral neuritis, headache, drowsiness
5. Hypersensitivity — fevers, chills, oral mucosal ulceration, eosinophilia

NURSING ASSESSMENT

Nursing assessment is based on the site of involvement (i.e., the gastrointestinal system and the respiratory system); see Appendix A.

NURSING DIAGNOSES

High risk for injury
Activity intolerance
Fluid volume excess
Sensory/perceptual alterations
Pain
Anxiety
Knowledge deficit
Ineffective individual coping
Ineffective family coping: compromised

NURSING INTERVENTIONS

Diagnosis

1. Monitor child's clinical status; observe or prevent signs and symptoms of complications.
   a. Monitor vital signs as ordered.
   b. Observe for signs and symptoms of respiratory distress.
   c. Observe for signs and symptoms of intussusception.

    d. Observe for signs and symptoms of superior vena caval obstruction (facial plethora and venous engorgement).

    e. Observe for CNS involvement.

2. Provide age-appropriate preprocedural explanations to child to alleviate anxiety.

3. Encourage child and parents to express concerns and fears about diagnosis.

4. Prepare child and parents for upcoming staging surgery.

Home Care/Long-Term Care

1. Administer and monitor child's response to chemotherapy (see "Medications").
   a. Prednisone
   b. Vincristine
   c. Cyclophosphamide
   d. Methotrexate
   e. Radiation (nausea and vomiting)
   f. Allopurinol

2. Monitor for complications and signs of relapse.
   a. CNS relapse
   b. Tumor recurrence
   c. Infection
   d. Urate nephropathy
   e. Leukemic conversion

3. Provide child and family with information about community support systems for long-term adaptation.
   a. School reintegration
   b. Parent groups
   c. Children's cancer groups
   d. Sibling groups
   e. Financial information about third-party providers

BIBLIOGRAPHY

Cap J et al: Non-Hodgkin's lymphoma in children, *Neoplasma* 34(6):735, 1987.

Fraser M, Tucker M: Second malignancies following cancer therapy, *Semin Oncol Nurs* 5(1):43, 1989.

Freeman A, Brecher M: Non-Hodgkin's lymphoma in children, *Pediatr Ann* 9(7):71, 1978.

Hockenberry M, Gody D: Childhood cancer: incidence, etiology, diagnosis, and treatment, *Pediatr Nurs* 16(3):239, 1990.

Jenkin R et al: The treatment of localized non-Hodgkin's lymphoma in children, a report from the Children's Cancer Study Group, *J Clin Oncol* 2:88, 1984.

Link M: Non-Hodgkin's lymphoma in children, *Pediatr Clin North Am* 32(3):699, 1985.

Magarth I: Malignant non-Hodgkin's lymphomas in children, *Hematol Oncol Clin North Am* 1(4):577, 1987.

Rahr V, Tucker R: Non-Hodgkin's lymphoma: understanding the disease, *Cancer Nurs* 13(1):56, 1990.

Truog A, Wozmak S: Cyclosporine-A as prevention for graft versus host disease in pediatric patients undergoing bone marrow transplants, *Oncol Nurs Forum* 17(1):39, 1990.

Tucker R, Ruhr V: Nursing care of the patient with non-Hodgkin's lymphoma: a case study, *Cancer Nurs* 13(4):229, 1990.

50 ❖ Osteogenic Sarcoma/ Amputation

PATHOPHYSIOLOGY

Osteogenic sarcoma is a tumor found in the diaphysis of a long bone (femur, radius, ulna, proximal humerus, and ilium). It also can affect the flat bones, which include the head, pelvis, and spine. The order of site of occurrence is the femur, knee joint, tibia, and humerus. The clinical course occurs in the following sequence: (1) the normal bone is destroyed and is replaced by tumor cells, forming osteoid tissue and bone; (2) growth penetrates the cortex and extends beyond it (radiating spindles of bone are characteristic of this process); and (3) the tumor extends through the bone marrow cavity. Metastasis occurs through veins and involves lungs first.

INCIDENCE

1. Osteogenic sarcoma is the most common bone tumor in children.
2. It occurs most commonly during the adolescent growth period.
3. It is uncommon before age 10 years.
4. Peak incidence is 10 to 15 years of age.
5. Its survival rate is 50%.

CLINICAL MANIFESTATIONS

Symptoms are gradual in onset. The child may have symptoms for 6 to 9 months before he or she seeks treatment. The symptoms are as follows:

1. Local pain during activity, and more severe pain with passage of time (most common symptom)
2. Limping or gait variation
3. Limitation of joint motion
4. Joint tenderness

COMPLICATIONS

Pathologic fractures occur with larger lesions and many times are the initially seen symptoms.

LABORATORY/DIAGNOSTIC TESTS

1. Serum alkaline phosphates (elevated because of osteoid production)
2. Tissue biopsy — to confirm diagnosis
3. Anteroposterior lateral x-ray studies — soft-tissue mass associated with destructive bone lesion and calcification are present
4. Skeletal bone scan — to detect presence of metastatic bone lesions

MEDICATIONS

Methotrexate (MTX)

Methotrexate is an antimetabolite that interferes with the production of folic acid and the reproduction of tissue cells. By depriving cells of folic acid it is hoped methotrexate will cause damage to more cancer cells than normal cells. Dosage is 100 to 250 mg/kg intravenously (IV). No more than 15 mg IV or 75 to 100 mg by mouth (po) should be administered in 5 days.

Leucovorin Calcium (Citrovorum Factor)

Leucovorin calcium is folinic acid in an active form of folic acid. It reverses the action of methotrexate and decreases its toxicity. Administer leucovorin calcium 2 hours after the infusion of methotrexate. Dosage is equivalent to the amount of methotrexate that is administered.

Allopurinol

Allopurinol decreases the level of uric acid, which is a byproduct of chemotherapy, and prevents hyperuricemia.

SURGICAL TREATMENT: AMPUTATION

A malignant tumor is the most common nontraumatic cause of amputation in children. Surgery is determined by age of child and tumor size and location; may be either an amputation or limb salvage. Most amputations are performed on the lower extremities. After amputation, the child is usually fitted for a prosthetic device. Children require frequent prosthetic adjustments because of growth. On the average, the child will need a new limb every year up to age 5 years, biennially between 6 and 12 years of age, and every 3 to 4 years up to age 21.

COMPLICATIONS

1. Reactive hyperemia—reddened skin, particularly the pressure points; subsides as keratoma layer forms
2. Contact dermatitis—most often caused by contact with prosthetic materials (e.g., polyester resins, chrome)
3. Infections—including fungal and pyogenic ones (e.g., furuncles)
4. Epidermal cysts—evident at points of friction at or near the brim of the socket; most often caused by an ill-fitted prosthesis
5. Stump edema syndrome—reactive hyperemia worsens, resulting in oozing and capillary rupture
6. Terminal bone overgrowth
7. Bony spurs—develop at the corners or margins of the amputation as a result of periosteal irritation
8. Neuroma
9. "Phantom limb" feelings of pain and sensation in the amputated limb
10. Stump scarring—caused by inguinal weight bearing and increased shearing force at stump-socket interface

NURSING ASSESSMENT

1. Observe for signs of stump infection.
2. Observe for stump swelling.

NURSING DIAGNOSES

Impaired tissue integrity
Impaired physical mobility

High risk for injury
Pain
Body image disturbance
Fluid volume excess
Impaired home maintenance management
Ineffective individual coping
Altered family processes
Altered growth and development

NURSING INTERVENTIONS

Preoperative Care

1. Prepare operative site according to hospital procedure.
2. Encourage use of exercises to strengthen muscles.
3. Provide emotional support to child and parents.
   a. Provide active listening to concerns.
   b. Encourage expression of feelings of loss.
   c. Provide anticipatory information about emotional responses to surgery.
4. Provide preoperative information to decrease anxiety about unknown aspects.
5. Prepare child before laboratory and diagnostic testing.
   a. Complete blood count (CBC)
   b. Urinalysis
   c. Bone scan
   d. X-ray studies
   e. Type and crossmatch for blood

Postoperative Care

1. Monitor for signs of complications, and report immediately; see "Complications."
2. Observe and monitor for signs of hemorrhage q1 hr for 24 hours, then q4 hr.
3. Promote patency and healing of stump.
   a. Apply pressure dressing to stump.
   b. Institute range-of-motion exercises according to physical therapist's orders.
   c. Reinforce exercise program with physical therapist.
   d. Cleanse stump and socket everyday with soap and water; dry thoroughly.
   e. Avoid use of skin lotions (cause maculation and superficial infection).

      f. Pat stump with wet tea bags (tenniten facilitates development of thickened keratin).

4. Position correctly to prevent deformities.
   a. Trendelenburg's position
   b. Pillow beneath knee for 24 hours to decrease edema
   c. After 24 hours, no pillow beneath knee (causes flexion of knee)
   d. Prone position for several hours everyday (to prevent hip flexion and contracture)
   e. No external rotation or abduction of amputated limb

5. Promote use of and adaptation to prosthetic device.
   a. Prosthetic fitting should be performed immediately after surgery because doing so promotes stump maturation, early ambulation, and resumption of normal activities.
   b. Encourage venting of feelings about being disabled.
   c. Explain restrictions on activities.

6. Monitor administration of chemotherapy.
   a. Provide adequate hydration (hydrate 12 hours before infusion).
   b. Record intake and output q1 hr.
   c. Measure specific gravity to assess hydration.
   d. Monitor urine pH and hematest (54% to 88% of medication is excreted in urine in first 24 hr); urine needs to be alkaline, or its precipitates in kidney will cause tubular necrosis.
   e. Blood chemistry, CBC, platelet count
   f. Urinalysis

7. Monitor for child's or adolescent's untoward and therapeutic responses to chemotherapy.
   a. Oral and gastrointestinal ulcerations
      (1) Diarrhea
      (2) Ulcerative stomatitis (hemorrhagic enteritis and death can occur)
   b. Skin reactions—urticaria, rashes
   c. Cystitis—inflammation of urinary tract
   d. Nausea and vomiting

8. Minimize negative consequences of chemotherapy.
   a. Provide good mouth care.
   b. Patient should stop smoking.

    c. Patient should stay out of the sun; methotrexate can cause skin blotches.

    d. Push fluids.

    e. Administer antiemetics.

    f. Provide bland, soft diet.

    g. Elevate head of bed.

    h. Teach self-hypnosis and relaxation techniques.

9. Monitor for complications.

    a. Pneumothorax (symptoms — shortness of breath, dyspnea, chest pain)

    b. Depression of hematologic values 10 days after methotrexate administration

    c. Renal toxicity — dysuria, oliguria (monitor intake and output)

10. Provide emotional support to parents and child.

    a. Encourage ventilation of feelings.

    b. Provide physical comforts (e.g., sleeping arrangements, hygiene).

    c. Encourage use of preexisting support systems.

    d. Refer to social worker, therapist, or group as necessary.

Home Care/Discharge Planning (Chemotherapy Regimen)

1. Instruct parents and adolescents about home management.

    a. Administer leucovorin calcium *on time* (wake up child if necessary).

    b. Administer antiemetic for nausea and vomiting.

    c. Drink increased amount of fluids (two quarts per day); milk tends to increase mucous secretions.

    d. Check urine for pH.

    e. Stay out of the sun.

2. Refer to community resources for follow-up.

    a. Parent, child, sibling groups

    b. Financial assistance

    c. Public health nurse

    d. Outpatient care

Home Care/Discharge Plans (Postoperative)

1. Instruct child and parents about stump care.

2. Provide reinforcement information about physical therapy regimen.

3. Refer to school nurse and clinic and advise them about child's status.
4. Explore compliance potential by asking about the following:
   a. Means of transportation
   b. Resources for child care
   c. Finances
   d. Level of motivation
   e. Understanding of need for long-term follow-up q3-4 months until growth complete

BIBLIOGRAPHY

Edmonson J: High-dose methotrexate in osteosarcoma: Mayo Clinic studies, *NC Monographs* 5:67, 1987.

Ferguson A: *Orthopedic surgery in infancy and childhood,* ed 5, Baltimore, 1981, Williams & Wilkins.

Filston H: *Surgical problems in children: recognition and referral,* St. Louis, 1982, Mosby–Year Book.

Hockenberry M, Lane B: Limb salvage procedures in children with osteogenic sarcoma, *Cancer Nurs* 11(1):2, 1988.

Lovell W, Winter R: *Pediatric orthopaedics,* Philadelphia, 1978, JB Lippincott.

Meyers P: Malignant bone tumors in children: osteosarcoma, *Hematol Oncol Clin North Am* 1(4):655, 1987.

51 ❖ Osteomyelitis

PATHOPHYSIOLOGY

Osteomyelitis is an infection of the bone that can occur in any bone in the body. The most common locations are the femur and the tibia. The humerus and the hip are rarely affected. The skull is a common location in infants. Usually a predisposing condition such as poor nutrition or poor hygiene exists.

Bacterial emboli reach the small arteries in the metaphysis, where circulation is sluggish. An abscess forms and replaces bone, causing increased pressure and secondary necrosis. This abscess eventually can rupture into the subperiosteal space. The infection spreads beneath the periosteum, thrombosing vessels and causing increased necrosis. The cycle of impaired circulation is thus established. A sinus can form and extend the infection to the skin. Extension to a joint results in septic arthritis. The condition can become chronic and thus quite resistant to therapy, often requiring involved surgical intervention. The epiphysis is usually spared because it has a separate circulation.

Any organism is capable of causing osteomyelitis either through the direct *(exogenous)* route or through seeding through the bloodstream from an infection elsewhere *(hematogenous)*. Exogenous sources include penetrating wounds, open fractures, contamination during surgery, or secondary extension through an abscess, burn, or wound.

The hematogenous route is more common; sources include furuncles, skin abrasions, upper respiratory infections, otitis media, abscessed teeth, and pyelonephritis. The hematogenous form is often subacute because the preceding infection is often treated with antibiotics.

INCIDENCE

The greatest frequency of osteomyelitis occurs in 5- to 14-year-olds. It is twice as common in males as in females.

CLINICAL MANIFESTATIONS

1. Abrupt pain — point tenderness above the bone, as well as swelling and warmth over the bone.
2. Fever
3. Possible dehydration
4. Unwillingness to move the limb or bear weight
5. Holding extremity semiflexed (muscle spasm)
6. Irritability
7. Poor appetite

COMPLICATION

Pathologic fractures occur as a complication of osteomyelitis.

LABORATORY/DIAGNOSTIC TESTS

1. Complete blood count (CBC) — marked leukocytosis
2. Sedimentation rate — elevated erythrocyte sedimentation rate (ESR)
3. Blood culture — positive in 50% of cases; common organisms are as follows:
   a. All ages — staphylococci, primarily *Staphylococcus aureus*
   b. Young children — *Haemophilus influenzae*
   c. Neonates — coliforms *(Escherichia coli)*
   d. Sickle cell anemia — *Salmonella*
   e. Foot — *Pseudomonas*
4. X-ray studies — negative first 10 to 12 days until bone destruction occurs (soft-tissue swelling is evident early)
5. Bone scan — often positive early for inflammation
6. Direct needle aspiration — confirms diagnosis as well as provides culture of site

MEDICATIONS

1. Intravenous (IV) antibiotics. IV antibiotics are often administered for a minimum of 3 or more weeks, depending on duration of symptoms, response to treatment, and sensitivity of the organism; the type of antibiotic that is used to treat osteomyelitis is dependent on culture and sensitivity.
2. Closed-tube antibiotic irrigation of the bone. An additional approach is to perform surgical drainage and place polyethylene tubes in the bone — one for instilling the antibiotic solution (usually the upper tube) and another for drainage. A cast is usually used to ensure immobilization and to avoid dislodging the tubes. Sometimes a window is cut to visualize the site, with tubes emerging from the cast.

NURSING ASSESSMENT

1. Refer to "Skeletal Assessment" in Appendix A.
2. Assess pain — location, duration, intensity.
3. Assess nutritional status — usually poor appetite; assess adequacy of caloric intake, as well as intake of protein and fluids.

NURSING DIAGNOSES

Potential for infection
Hypothermia
Pain
Altered tissue perfusion: peripheral
Impaired tissue integrity
Knowledge deficit
Altered nutrition: less than body requirements

NURSING INTERVENTIONS

1. Immobilize extremity to facilitate healing and prevent complications.
   a. Apply splint, bivalved cast, or complete cast with window.
   b. Allow NO WEIGHT BEARING (high risk of pathologic fracture).
      (1) Use gurney or wheelchair; elevate extremity slightly.

(2) Use physical therapy on unaffected extremity after inflammation subsides.
2. Provide pain relief measures.
   a. Allow comfortable position.
   b. Support affected limb on pillows.
   c. Use care in turning and moving.
   d. Monitor child's response to analgesia and sedation as necessary.
3. Use wound and skin precautions if any drainage occurs.
   a. Provide diversional activities.
   b. Provide rooming-in for young children.
   c. Refer to procedures manual for institutional isolation techniques.
4. Monitor child's response to antibiotic irrigation of site (up to 6 weeks).
   a. For first 3 days, expect blood, debris, and pus (have tendency to clog tubes).
      (1) Reversing flow direction of tubes at intervals can prevent blockage; do with physician consultation only.
      (2) Physician may elect to irrigate with heparin and saline solution if blockage occurs.
      (3) Use prescribed suction (usually low suction).
   b. If tubes are functioning properly, wound and dressing should remain dry.
   c. Maintain records of instillation and output (clarity, color, and volume of drainage); often up to 1000 ml per day are instilled.
   d. When tubes are removed, usually the instillation tube (upper) is removed first, leaving the drainage tube until no further drainage occurs.
   e. Sudden pain at the site of irrigation may indicate blockage of the drainage tube.
5. Monitor child's response to medications.
   a. Antibiotics
   b. Analgesics
   c. Sedatives
6. Provide cast care.
   a. Monitor skin temperature; casting creates concern for thermoregulation in the young infant and child.

   b. Monitor color, heat, sweating, tenderness, motion of digital digits.
7. Promote adequate nutritional intake.
   a. Promote high-caloric intake (juices, gelatin, Popsicles).
   b. Appetite usually returns when acute symptoms subside.
8. Monitor for signs of infection and alterations in thermoregulation.
   a. Increased temperature (institute cooling measure)
   b. Signs of inflammation
   c. Drainage or musty odor with cast
9. Provide age-appropriate diversional activities (see Appendix B, *Growth and Development*).
10. Provide emotional support to parents.
   a. Encourage ventilation of feelings of guilt and self-blame.
   b. Provide and reinforce information about child's condition.
   c. Encourage use of preexisting support systems as necessary.
   d. Provide for physical comforts (e.g., sleeping arrangement and bathing).

Home Care

1. Instruct parents about elements of rehabilitation.
   a. Risks of fractures
   b. Necessity for hospitalization
   c. Necessity for operations
2. Instruct parents about administration of antibiotics.
   a. Therapeutic responses
   b. Side effects—given that many of these antibiotics have negative renal, audiologic, and hepatic effects, these systems must be monitored closely during therapy (some may be on IV medications if treatment is longer than 3 weeks).

BIBLIOGRAPHY

Dich VQ, Nelson JD, Hatalin KC: Osteomyelitis in infants and children, *Am J Dis Child* 129:1273, 1975.

Hilt NE, Cogburn SB: *Manual of orthopedics,* St Louis, 1980, Mosby–
Year Book.

Legg M, Murphy M: Human bite wounds, *J Emerg Nurs* 16(3):145,
1990.

Seringer R et al: Acute osteomyelitis in children remains a current
topic, *Ann Pediatr* 34(10):824, 1987.

Unger E et al: Diagnosis of osteomyelitis by MR imaging, *Am J
Radiol* 150(3):605, 1988.

52 ❖ Otitis Media

PATHOPHYSIOLOGY

Otitis media refers to an infection of the middle ear. Young children under the age of 3 years are particularly susceptible to recurrent episodes of otitis media because their eustachian tubes are wide and short, promoting the entry of pathogens. There are three types of otitis media, which are classified according to causative factors, clinical manifestations, and treatment. It is critical that otitis media be diagnosed and treated because of the possibility of hearing involvement. Hearing impairment can significantly affect the child's development, especially in the acquisition of language.

Acute Otitis Media

Acute otitis media is most commonly caused by viral agents. Bacterial pathogens include pneumococcus, *Haemophilus influenzae,* streptococci, and many enteric organisms. Causative bacterial agents in infants less than 6 weeks old include *Escherichia coli,* staphylococcus, and *Klebsiella pneumoniae.*

Chronic Otitis Media

Chronic otitis media refers to recurrent episodes of otitis media. Infectious causative agents include *Staphylococcus aureus, H. influenzae,* and other gram-negative rods. Allergy is present in 25% of cases. Chronic otitis media occurs most frequently in infants and younger children. One fifth of the children have a recurrence within 3 years. One out of seven children have at least six episodes. The potential for permanent hearing loss increases with repeated episodes of otitis media.

Serous Otitis Media

Although allergies, viral infections, and inadequately treated infections have been associated with serous otitis media, no causative agent has been identified. Serous otitis media involves fluid behind the tympanic membrane, resulting in signs and symptoms of infection. Discoloration of the tympanic membrane and chronically decreased retraction (eardrum) occur.

Surgical Treatment: Myringotomy

Myringotomy refers to the surgical procedure that involves insertion of pressure-equalizer tubes into the tympanic membrane. Insertion of the pressure-equalizer tubes facilitates drainage and ventilation from the middle ear, preventing the formation of a vacuum or the retention of fluid in the middle ear. The tubes spontaneously fall out after 6 to 12 months. The pressure-equalizer tubes may have to be replaced if they become blocked or are ejected too soon. Complications that may result include atrophy of the tympanic membrane, tympanosclerosis (scarring of the tympanic membrane), permanent perforation, and cholesteatoma.

INCIDENCE

1. Otitis media accounts for 10% to 25% of visits to pediatricians.
2. Fifty percent of children experience an episode of otitis media by 1 year of age.
3. Peak incidence of acute otitis media is during the first 2 years.
4. Peak incidence of serous otitis media is during the third to fourth year.
5. One million tympanostomy tubes are inserted each year.
6. Seventy-five percent of otitis media patients have transient-to-significant hearing loss.

7. Fifty percent of children with cleft palate have chronic middle ear infection before correction.
8. Boys are twice as likely as girls to have recurrent acute otitis media.

CLINICAL MANIFESTATIONS

1. Red, infected, congested tympanic membrane
2. Complaint of pain
3. Pulling at ear (infant and young child)
4. Febrile (above 104° F [40° C]).
5. Enlarged postauricular and cervical lymph glands
6. Anorexia

Acute Otitis Media

1. Tympanic membrane is bulging.
2. Tympanic membrane may rupture spontaneously.
3. Middle ear effusion may spontaneously resolve in 8 to 10 weeks.

Serous Otitis Media

1. Tympanic membrane retracted and dull
2. Impaired hearing; sense of fullness in ear
3. Thin, serous, mucoid, or gelatinous fluid in middle ear

Chronic Otitis Media

1. Condition is considered chronic if otitis media persists longer than 2 weeks with treatment.
2. Child has recurrent episodes of otitis media.

COMPLICATIONS (UNUSUAL IF TREATED)

1. Chronic otitis media
2. Hearing loss
3. Meningitis
4. Mastoiditis
5. Brain abscess
6. Otorrhea

LABORATORY/DIAGNOSTIC TESTS

Tympanogram is obtained to measure tympanic membrane stiffness and compliance.

MEDICATIONS

1. Decongestants — used to decrease drainage and inflammation within the middle ear; aids in clearing the eustachian tubes
2. Antihistamines — used to decrease drainage and inflammation within the middle ear; aids in clearing the eustachian tubes
3. Antibiotics — choice of antibiotic dependent on culture and sensitivity

NURSING ASSESSMENT

Assess for the symptoms listed under "Clinical Manifestations."

NURSING DIAGNOSIS

High risk for infection
High risk for injury
Sensory-perceptual alteration: auditory
Knowledge deficit

NURSING INTERVENTIONS

1. Monitor child for therapeutic response to and untoward effects of medications.
   a. Temperature
   b. Complaint of pain in ear
   c. Sense of fullness in ear
   d. Decreased hearing
   e. Irritability and restlessness
   f. Decreased appetite
   g. Lymph gland enlargement in cervical region
2. Observe for signs of complications.
   a. Drainage from ear
   b. No improvement in signs and symptoms of otitis media
3. Assist child in complying with treatment regimen.
   a. Schedule Potizer technique, gum chewing, and inflating balloons at specific time.
   b. Observe child's ability to perform procedure alone (if not supervised).
4. Provide age-appropriate explanations to child and parents about surgical procedures.

a. Myringotomy with insertion of tympanostomy tubes
b. Adenoidectomy

Postoperative Care

Monitor child's response to surgical intervention.
1. Vital signs (increased temperature means infection)
2. Otorrhea from ears (tube insertion)
3. Presence of bleeding (adenoidectomy)
4. Provision of pain measures and medications as needed
5. Hearing (tube insertion)

Home Care

1. Instruct child and parents about maintaining patency of tympanostomy tubes (e.g., when child is swimming, plug ears with ear plugs, petroleum jelly).
2. Administer prophylactic antibiotics (to children who have chronic otitis media).
    a. Administer during winter and spring months (long-term).
    b. Administer for 10 to 14 days postoperatively.
3. Limit child's activities until fully recovered.
    a. Avoid rigorous activities.
    b. Provide frequent rest periods.
    c. Child can return to school after he or she receives medical approval.

BIBLIOGRAPHY

Casey R et al: An intervention to improve follow-up of patients with otitis media, *Clin Pediatr* 24(3):149, 1985.

Dyson A et al: Speech characteristics of children after otitis media, *J Pediatr Health Care* 1(5):261, 1987.

Facione N: Otitis media: an overview of acute and chronic disease, *Nurs Pract: Am J Prim Health Care* 15(10):11, 1990.

Ginsburg C: Otitis media, *Pediatrics* 74(suppl):948, 1984.

Hendrickse W et al: Five vs. 10 days of therapy for acute otitis and media, *J Pediatr Infect Dis* 7(1):14, 1988.

Jones S, Jones P, Katz J: A nursing intervention to increase compliance in otitis media patients, *Appl Nurs Res* 2(2):68, 1989.

Schwartz R: Prevention of otitis media: a multitude of yellow brick roads, *Pediatr Infect Dis* 1(1):3, 1982.

Schwartz-Lookinland S, McKeever C, Saputo M: Compliance with antibiotic regimes in Hispanic mothers . . . children suffering from otitis media, *Patient Educ Counsel* 13(2):171, 1989.

Weiss J et al: Cost effectiveness in the choice of antibiotics for the initial treatment of otitis media in children: a decision analysis approach, *J Pediatr Infect Dis* 7(1):23, 1988.

Woolbert L: Do antihistamines and decongestants prevent otitis media? *Pediatr Nurs* 16(3):265, 1990.

Wuest J, Stern P: Childhood otitis media: the family's endless quest for relief, *Issues Comprehens Pediatr Nurs* 13(1):25, 1990.

Wuest J, Stern P: The impact of functioning relationships with the Canadian health care system on family management of otitis media with effusion, *J Advanc Nurs* 15(5):556, 1990.

Zenk K, Ma H: Pharmacologic treatment of otitis media and sinusitis in pediatrics, *J Pediatr Health Care* 4(6):297, 1990.

53 ❖ Patent Ductus Arteriosus

Patent ductus arteriosus (PDA) refers to the persistent patency of the ductus arteriosus after birth, resulting in the shunting of blood directly from the aorta (higher pressure) into the pulmonary artery (lower pressure). This left-to-right shunting causes the recirculation of increased amounts of oxygenated blood in the lungs, producing increased demands on the left side of the heart. The additional effort of the left ventricle to meet this increased demand leads to progressive dilation and left atrial hypertension. The cumulative cardiac effects cause increased pressure in the pulmonary veins and capillaries, resulting in pulmonary edema. The pulmonary edema results in decreased diffusion of oxygen and hypoxia, with progressive constriction of the arterioles in the lungs. Pulmonary hypertension and failure of the right side of the heart ensue if the condition is not corrected through medical or surgical treatment. Closure of the PDA is primarily dependent on the constrictor response of the ductus to the oxygen tension in the blood. Other factors affecting ductus closure include action of prostaglandins, pulmonary and systemic resistances, size of the ductus, and the condition of the infant (premature or full-term). PDA occurs more frequently in premature infants and is less well tolerated because their cardiac compensatory mechanisms are not as well developed and left-to-right shunts tend to be larger.

Surgical Management: Patent Ductus Arteriosus Repair

PDA ligation marked the beginning of heart surgery in children in 1938. Since then, two major categories of children have been identified as requiring this surgery. The first includes infants with congestive heart failure, usually premature neonates who did not respond to indomethacin therapy. Children more than 1 year of age whose ductus did not close spontaneously (and who are at risk for pulmonary hypertension and subacute endocarditis) comprise the second group. Both groups require a left thoracotomy incision, and bypass is unnecessary. Infants are usually at greater risk for complications, so the PDA is doubly ligated in a comparatively quick procedure. For older children, surgery is advised during their preschool years and is performed by dividing the ductus between clamps and suturing the ends closed. A procedure for closing the PDA during cardiac catheterization by depositing a "plug" in the ductus is a recent development being used in the United States.

The hemodynamic results of PDA ligation are truly curative, in contrast to the palliative procedures of many heart surgeries. Closure decreases the pulmonary flow while increasing the systemic flow, creating normal hemodynamics. Unfortunately, if severe pulmonary hypertension existed before surgery, closure will not reverse this process.

INCIDENCE

Precise incidence varies, depending on gestational age.
1. PDA accounts for 10% of cardiac defects, excluding those of premature infants.
2. Incidence in full-term infants is 1 in 2500 to 5000 live births.
3. Overall incidence in premature infants is 20% to 75%.

CLINICAL MANIFESTATIONS

Manifestations of PDA in premature infants are often clouded by other problems associated with prematurity (e.g., respiratory distress syndrome). Signs of ventricular overload are not apparent for 4 to 6 hours after birth. Infants with small PDA may be asymptomatic; infants with large PDA may manifest signs of congestive heart failure (CHF).

1. Persistent murmur (systolic, then continuous)
2. Tachycardia (apical pulse greater than 170)
3. Prominent to bounding pulses
4. Tachypnea (respiratory rate greater than 70)
5. Temperature instability
6. Increased ventilator requirement (associated with pulmonary problems)
7. Metabolic acidosis (may not be present)
8. Anemia (hematocrit [Hct] less than 45 g)

COMPLICATIONS

1. Hepatomegaly (rare in premature infants)
2. Necrotizing enterocolitis
3. Concurrent pulmonary disorder (e.g., respiratory distress syndrome or bronchopulmonary dysplasia)
4. Gastrointestinal (GI) hemorrhage (decreased platelet count)
5. Hyperkalemia (decreased urinary output)
6. Arrhythmias (digitalis toxicity)

LABORATORY/DIAGNOSTIC TESTS

1. Chest x-ray study—prominent or enlarged left atrium and left ventricle (cardiomegaly)
2. Echocardiography—left-atrial–to–aortic-root ratio greater than 1.4:1 (caused by increased left atrial volume as a result of left-to-right shunt)
3. Contrast echogram (findings can be influenced by fluid volume)
4. Electrocardiogram (ECG)—varies with degree of severity; small PDA—no abnormality noted; large PDA—left ventricular hypertrophy
5. Nuclear angiography—to assess extent of cardiac defect
6. Complete blood count (CBC) (anemic; Hct less than 45 g)
7. Cardiac catheterization—performed only in very severe cases because echocardiogram is diagnostic
8. Doppler vascular probe—noninvasive; applied over carotid arteries to evaluate blood flow and its direction
9. Serum electrolytes (increased potassium and decreased sodium concentration with decreased urinary output)—occurs only if renal failure is present.

10. Blood urea nitrogen (BUN), creatinine (BUN greater than 25 mg; creatinine greater than 1.8 mg with decreased urinary output)
11. Platelet count (decreased)

MEDICATIONS

Furosemide (Lasix)

Furosemide is used to promote diuresis and to decrease fluid overload. It is used in the treatment of edema associated with CHF. Dosage is as follows: 2 mg/kg by mouth (po) as a single dose (may be increased to 1 or 2 mg/kg q6-8 hr) or 1 mg/kg intramuscularly (IM) as a single dose (may repeat 2 hours later, increased by 1 mg/kg).

Indomethacin (Indocin)

Indomethacin inhibits prostaglandins and promotes closure of PDA. Its side effects include causing transitory changes (lasting 72 hours) in renal function (decreased output), decreased serum sodium concentration, increased potassium (K^+), and GI hemorrhage.

Contraindications

1. Do not administer if BUN is greater than 25 mg or creatinine is greater than 1.8 mg because it binds with protein.
2. Do not administer if platelet count is less than 80,000 U because prolongs platelet activity.
3. Do not administer if hematologic abnormalities (GI or central nervous system [CNS] bleeding, hyperbilirubinemia) are present.

Dosage

1. Initial dose — 0.2 mg/kg IV or po given in 2 to 3 doses
2. Second and third doses — 0.1 mg/kg if infant less than 48 hours old; 0.2 mg/kg if infant 2 to 7 days old; 0.25 mg/kg if infant more than 8 days old
3. Administer q12 hr for 3 doses unless contraindicated.

Digitalis (controversial and contraindicated in premature infants)

Digitalis increases the force of contraction of the heart, increases the stroke volume and cardiac output, and decreases cardiac venous pressures. It is used to treat CHF and selected cardiac arrhythmias. Digitalizing dose is 0.03 to 0.05 mg/kg or 0.75 mg/m^2 po, IM, or intravenously (IV). Maintenance dose is one tenth to one fifth of the digitalization dose.

NURSING ASSESSMENT

Refer to "Cardiovascular Assessment" in Appendix A.

NURSING DIAGNOSES

Decreased cardiac output
Activity intolerance
Altered tissue perfusion
Fluid volume excess
Ineffective thermoregulation
High risk for infection
High risk for injury
Altered family processes

NURSING INTERVENTIONS

1. Monitor cardiac and respiratory status (may need to monitor as often as q1 hr during acute phase).
2. Observe and report signs of changes in cardiac status (color, vital signs, peripheral perfusion, level of consciousness [LOC], activity level, signs of CHF).
3. Observe and report signs of respiratory distress and changes in respiratory status.
4. Monitor and report responses to ventilator assistance.
5. Assess and maintain hydration status.
    a. Limit intake of fluids (65 to 100 ml/kg/day).
    b. Monitor urinary output.
    c. Observe for signs of fluid overload.
6. Promote conservation of energy demands (anemic); provide periods of quiet and rest.
7. Promote and maintain body temperature.
    a. Use radiant warmer.
    b. Keep covered.
8. Monitor action and side effects of medications.
    a. Diuretics (e.g., furosemide [Lasix]) — decrease fluid overload, increase urinary output. Check K^+, Cl^-.

b. Indomethacin — inhibits prostaglandins, promotes closure of PDA

c. Digitalis — increases contractility of heart (monitor serum levels)

9. Monitor response and side effects of blood transfusions.
10. Promote process of attachment between parents and infant.
11. Provide developmentally appropriate stimulation activities (see Appendix B, *Growth and Development*).

Preoperative Care

1. Allow parents to vent feelings; despite its being a relatively minor heart surgery, PDA repair is still overwhelming to parents.
2. Prepare child for surgery by obtaining assessment data.
   a. CBC, urinalysis, serum glucose, BUN
   b. Baseline electrolytes
   c. Blood coagulation
   d. Type and crossmatch blood
   e. Chest x-ray study, ECG
3. Child is usually preschool age, so prepare accordingly; do not tell the child that surgery will make him or her "feel better" because he or she is usually asymptomatic.

Postoperative Care

1. Monitor child's or infant's cardiac status (see "Cardiovascular Assessment" in Appendix A).
   a. Vital signs (temperature, apical pulse, respiratory rate, blood pressure)
   b. Arterial blood pressure/central venous pressure (CVP) (often not placed)
   c. Peripheral pulses — quality and intensity
   d. Capillary refill time
   e. Presence of ascites (rare)
   f. Arrhythmias
2. Monitor and report signs and symptoms of the following complications.
   a. Atelectasis
   b. Bleeding
   c. Chylothorax
   d. Hemothorax

    e. Pneumothorax
    f. Phrenic nerve damage
    g. Recurrent laryngeal nerve damage
3. Treat chylothorax.
    a. Provide and monitor child's intake of medium-chain triglyceride diet.
    b. Monitor for signs of respiratory distress.
4. Provide intensive pulmonary toilet.
    a. Perform postural drainage and percussion.
    b. Change position q2 hr.
    c. Encourage deep breathing and use of spirometer q1 hr.
    d. Encourage coughing; if child cannot cough, use suction.
5. Provide intensive pain control, since pain with a thoracotomy incision is usually greater than with a median sternotomy.
6. Monitor child's response to medications.
    a. Diuretics
    b. Digitalis
7. Provide emotional support to infant or child during hospitalization.
    a. Use age-appropriate explanations before treatments.
    b. Encourage, through age-appropriate means, child's expression of fears and anxieties (e.g., verbal expression, play, drawings).
    c. Encourage parental expression of feelings.

Home Care

1. Instruct parents to observe and report signs of cardiac or respiratory distress.
2. Instruct parents about the administration of medications.
3. Provide parents with name of physician or nurse to contact for medical or health care follow-up.
4. Instruct parents about principles of infection control and well child care (e.g., use prophylactic medications before dental care).
5. Encourage and instruct parents about providing developmentally appropriate stimulation activities (see Appendix B, *Growth and Development*).

BIBLIOGRAPHY

Cotton R et al: Early prediction of symptomatic patent ductus arteriosus from perinatal risk factors: a discriminant analysis model, *Acta Pediatr Scand* 70:723, 1981.

Dooley I: Management of the premature infant with a patent ductus arteriosus, *Pediatr Clin North Am* 1159, 1984.

Huddleston K: Patent ductus arteriosus ligation: performing surgery outside the operating room, *AORN J* 53(1):69, 1990.

Moynihan P, King R: Caring for patients with lesions increasing pulmonary blood flow, *Crit Care Clin North Am* 1(2):195, 1989.

Neal W, Mullet M: Patent ductus arteriosus in premature infants: a review of current management, *Pediatr Cardiol* 3:59, 1982.

Rashkind W et al: Nonsurgical closure of patent ductus arteriosus: clinical application of the Rashkind PDA occluder system, *Circulation* 75(3):583, 1987.

Roberts P: Caring for patients undergoing therapeutic cardiac catheterization, *Crit Care Clin North Am* 1(2):275, 1989.

Runton N: Congenital cardiac anomalies: a reference guide for nurses, *J Cardiovasc Nurs* 2(3):56, 1988.

Stevenson J: Acyanotic lesions with increased pulmonary blood flow, *Pediatr Clin North Am* 25(4):743, 1978.

54 ❖ Pneumonia

PATHOPHYSIOLOGY

Pneumonia is an inflammation or infection of the pulmonary parenchyma. The cause of pneumonia is attributable to one or more agents: viruses, bacteria, mycoplasmas, and aspiration of foreign substances. The pattern of the illness is dependent on the following: (1) causative agent; (2) age of the child; (3) child's reaction; (4) extent of lesions; and (5) degree of bronchial obstruction. Pneumonia occurs more frequently in infancy and early childhood than in the school-age and adolescent periods. The clinical features of bacterial, viral, and mycoplasmal pneumonia are listed in the box on pp. 348 and 349.

INCIDENCE

1. Viral pneumonia occurs more frequently than bacterial pneumonia.
2. Staphylococcal pneumonia occurs most frequently during the first 2 years of life — in 30% of children with pneumonia who are less than 3 months old and in 70% of children with pneumonia who are less than 1 year old.
3. Pneumococcal pneumonia accounts for 90% of all lobar pneumonia.
4. Mycoplasmal pneumonia rarely causes pneumonia in children less than 5 years old; it is associated with 20% of cases of pneumonia diagnosed between 16 and 19 years of age.

Clinical Features of Bacterial, Viral, and Mycoplasmal Pneumonia

Bacterial Pneumonia

Staphylococcal, streptococcal, and pneumococcal pneumonia occur most frequently

Initial symptoms
Mild rhinitis
Anorexia
Listlessness

Progresses to abrupt onset
Fever
Malaise
Rapid and shallow respiratory rate (50 to 80)
Expiratory grunt
Greater than 5 years old—headache and chills
Less than 2 years old—vomiting and mild diarrhea
Increased white blood count (WBC)
Chest x-ray result—lobar pneumonia

Viral Pneumonia

Causative viruses include influenza virus, adenovirus, rubeola, varicella, and human cytomegalovirus.

Initial symptoms
Cough
Rhinitis

Onset may be abrupt or insidious
Range of symptoms—mild fever, slight cough, and malaise to high fever, severe cough, and prostration
Obstructive emphysema
Scattered rales, rhonchi
Chest x-ray result—bronchopneumonia
Decreased WBC

5. Pneumonia is more severe in younger children.
6. Respiratory syncytial virus accounts for the largest percentage of viral pneumonia.
7. Viral respiratory infection is the second leading cause of death in infants and young children.

Clinical Features of Bacterial, Viral, and Mycoplasmal Pneumonia — cont'd

Mycoplasmal Pneumonia

Initial symptoms
> Fever
> Chills
> Headache
> Anorexia
> Myalgia

Progresses to insidious or abrupt onset
> Rhinitis
> Sore throat
> Dry hacking cough — blood streaked
> Chest x-ray result — areas of consolidation

---

8. Mycoplasmal pneumonia accounts for 10% to 20% of hospital admissions.

CLINICAL MANIFESTATIONS

Major clinical signs include the following (see box for specific clinical manifestations).

1. Cough
2. Dyspnea
3. Tachypnea
4. Cyanosis
5. Decreased breath sounds
6. Retractions of chest wall
7. Nasal flaring
8. Abdominal pain (caused by irritation of the diaphragm by the adjacent infected lung)
9. Paroxysmal cough simulating pertussis (common in smaller children)
10. Older child does not appear as ill

COMPLICATIONS

1. Chronic interstitial pneumonia
2. Chronic segmental or lobar atelectasis
3. Airway damage

4. Pleural effusion
5. Pulmonary calcification
6. Pulmonary fibrosis
7. Obliterative bronchitis and bronchiolitis
8. Persistent atelectasis

LABORATORY/DIAGNOSTIC TESTS

1. Chest x-ray studies—diagnostic; used to visualize the lungs for presence of infection
2. Blood gas values—to evaluate cardiopulmonary status in terms of oxygenation
3. CBC with differential—used to determine presence of anemia, infection, inflammatory process
4. Gram stain—for initial antimicrobial selection
5. Tuberculin skin test—rules out tuberculosis if child does not respond to treatment
6. White blood count (WBC)—leukocytosis with bacterial pneumonia
7. Pulmonary function—used to assess pulmonary function, determine extent and severity of disease, and assist in diagnosis of condition
8. Static spirometry—used to assess amount of inspired air
9. Blood culture—blood specimen obtained to identify causative agents such as viruses and bacteria
10. Culture of pleural fluid—specimen of fluid from pleural space obtained to identify causative agents such as bacteria and viruses
11. Bronchoscopy—used to visualize and manipulate the main branches of the tracheobronchial tree; tissue obtained for diagnostic testing therapeutically used to identify and remove foreign bodies
12. Lung biopsy—during thoracotomy, lung tissue is excised for diagnostic studies

MEDICATIONS

Antibiotics are used to treat pneumonia. Culture and sensitivity testing is performed to determine the medication to be used (see Appendix D, *Commonly Used Antibiotics*).

NURSING ASSESSMENT

Refer to "Respiratory Assessment" in Appendix A.

NURSING DIAGNOSES

Impaired gas exchange
Hypothermia
Ineffective airway clearance
High risk for injury
Knowledge deficit

NURSING INTERVENTIONS

1. Monitor and maintain patent airway.
   a. Suction as needed.
   b. Perform postural drainage and percussion.
2. Monitor and observe for signs of respiratory distress.
3. Observe and monitor child's response to oxygen therapy.
   a. Monitor respiratory status.
   b. Perform care of mist tent.
   c. Change clothing and linens frequently to prevent chilling.
4. Monitor and maintain hydration status.
   a. Monitor administration of intravenous (IV) fluids.
   b. Assess for dehydration.
5. Monitor child's response to medications' (for bacterial pneumonia) therapeutic and side effects: nafcillin, gentamicin, methicillin, oxacillin, penicillin G, erythromycin.
6. Provide for adequate rest (bed rest while febrile).
7. Observe for signs of complications (see "Complications").
8. Provide age-appropriate, quiet diversional activities and toys.
9. Provide emotional support to child and family during hospitalization.
   a. Provide age-appropriate explanations before procedures.
   b. Encourage parents to ventilate feelings.
   c. Encourage age-appropriate methods to express feelings (e.g., drawings, play therapy).
   d. Provide and reinforce information to parents about condition and hospitalization.

e. Provide for parents' physical comforts (e.g., sleeping arrangements, bathing).

Home Care

1. Instruct parents about the administration of medications.
   a. Appropriate dose, route, time
   b. Side effects
   c. Child's response
2. Provide information to parents about measures for infection control and prevention.
   a. Avoid exposure to infectious contacts.
   b. Adhere to immunization schedule.

BIBLIOGRAPHY

Barkin R: Pediatric respiratory emergencies, *Emerg Care Quart* 5(1):71, 1989.

Dennehy P: Respiratory infections in the newborn, *Clin Perinatol* 14(3):667, 1987.

Hagedorn M, Gardner S: Physiologic sequelae of prematurity: the nurse practitioner's role: respiratory issues, part 1, *J Pediatr Health Care* 3(6):288, 1989.

Kendig E, Chernock O: Disorders of the respiratory tract in children, ed 3, Philadelphia, 1977, WB Saunders.

Koenigeknecht S: Pneumonia, *Top Emerg Med* 2:31, 1980.

Laraga-Carasay L: Pulmonary sequelae of acute respiratory viral infections, *Pediatr Ann* 7(42):47, 1978.

LeBlanc K, Forestell F: Assessment of the neonatal respiratory system, *AACN: Clin Issues Crit Care Nurs* 1(2):401, 1990.

Pinney M: Pneumonia, *Am J Nurs* 81(3):517, 1981.

Sheahan S, Seabolt J: *Chlamydia trachomatis* infections: a health problem of infants, *J Pediatr Health Care* 3(3):144, 1989.

Steele R: Drugs for viral respiratory tract infections, *Choices Resp Manag* 20(5):109, 1990.

Timmons O et al: Association of respiratory syncytial virus and streptococcus pneumonia infection in young infants, *J Pediatr Infect Dis* 6(12):1138, 1987.

55 ❖ Poisonings

INCIDENCE

1. The most prevalent injury of children.
2. The most common poisonings are from nonprescription drugs (such as cough and cold preparations, analgesics, and topical agents).
3. Nonpharmaceutical agents ingested are: household cleaners, plants, cosmetics, and beauty aids.
4. Most poisonings take place in the home. The number-one location is the child's own home, and the second is the grandparents' home.
5. Peak times are mealtimes, weekends, and holidays.
6. The peak age is 22 months.

CLINICAL MANIFESTATIONS

The manifestations depend on the agent that is ingested. The following are some examples:
  1. Hyperthermia or hypothermia
  2. Tachycardia or bradycardia
  3. Salivation
  4. Diarrhea
  5. Seizures
  6. Lethargy
  7. Dry mouth
  8. Dilated pupils
  9. Ileus
10. Urinary retention

11. Ataxia
12. Headache, "flulike syndrome"
13. Coma
14. Nausea and vomiting

COMPLICATIONS

1. Cardiac arrest
2. Respiratory arrest

LABORATORY/DIAGNOSTIC TESTS

1. Blood screen
2. Urine screen

MEDICATIONS/TREATMENT

1. Initial stabilization (the "ABCs")
2. Antidote, if appropriate
3. Decontamination (such as orogastric lavage, or emetic agent like ipecac or activated charcoal).

NURSING ASSESSMENT

1. A detailed history is essential (agent ingested, dose, time of ingestion, underlying problems of the child, signs/symptoms produced, treatment rendered).
2. Complete system-by-system assessment.

NURSING DIAGNOSES

Activity intolerance
Knowledge deficit
High risk for injury

NURSING INTERVENTIONS

1. Teaching regarding prevention and home safety.
2. Use of the poison control center.
3. Close monitoring of the patient.

BIBLIOGRAPHY

Woolf AD, Anderson A: The diagnosis and initial management of pediatric poisonings, *Emerg Care Quart* 6(3):7, 1990.

56 ❖ Renal Failure: Acute

PATHOPHYSIOLOGY

Acute renal failure refers to the abrupt deterioration in renal function that impairs regulation of body fluids and composition. The abnormal excretion rate causes a variety of physiologic disturbances in homeostasis. The two predominant signs of renal failure are oliguria (urine output is <300 ml/kg/day) and azotemia (increased plasma concentration of nitrogenous waste productions, especially blood urea nitrogen [BUN], which is 100 mg/dl or higher).

In a patient with acute renal failure, three basic pathophysiologic processes occur: (1) severe reduction in the amount of plasma filtered by glomeruli; (2) increased permeability of the tubules; and (3) severe alteration in hemodynamics. These processes create a uremic clinical state that leads to multiorgan dysfunction. A variety of causes are associated with acute renal failure and are listed in the box on p. 356. Prognosis is determined by a variety of factors, including age, etiology, severity of condition, metabolic state, and type of treatment.

INCIDENCE

Incidence varies according to the following factors: age group, etiology, associated problems, and geographic location (most likely influenced by location of treatment centers).

Causes of Acute Renal Failure

Acute tubular necrosis — refers to syndrome that is a result of tubular degeneration caused by renal ischemia and toxic agents

Sudden injury or illness associated with shock

Severe renal vasoconstriction

Hemorrhage

Hypotension

Specific disease (e.g., progressive glomerulonephritis or hemolytic-uremic syndrome)

Hemolysis and hypotension following extensive burns

Hemolysis resulting from use of mismatched blood

Complication of cardiac surgery

Respiratory distress syndrome (hyaline membrane disease)

Prolonged perinatal hypoxia

Septicemia

Excessive use of diuretics — associated with salt deprivation

Bilateral renal artery thrombosis (occurs in neonates)

Nephrotoxins

Congenital renal anomalies

Urethral obstructions (by calculi, blood clots, sulfoxamide crystals, or uric acid crystals)

Dehydration and decreased perfusion concurrent with or preceding gastroenteritis

CLINICAL MANIFESTATIONS

1. Oliguria lasting from a few days to several weeks (average of 10 to 14 days)
2. Anuria (30–40 mg/day) for 24 hours
3. Lethargy and nausea (caused by acidosis)
4. Urine — scant, bloody, trace glucose
5. Edema and hyponatremia (caused by unrestricted fluid intake)

6. Infection (associated with secondary conditions)
7. Anemia (caused by deficient red blood cell [RBC] production or RBC destruction)
8. Circulatory congestion
9. Increased weight (caused by decreased urine output, unrestricted fluid intake, fluid retention)
10. Altered serum electrolytes (see "Laboratory/Diagnostic Tests")
11. Hypertension
12. Weakness

COMPLICATIONS

1. Potassium intoxication (caused by potassium released from injured or infected muscles, intravascular hemolysis, or hematomas)
2. Severe infections (caused by associated conditions or effects of prolonged immobility, general deterioration, and metabolic status)
3. Neurologic complications
   a. Coma
   b. Seizures
4. Anemia
5. Diuresis
6. Cardiovascular complications
   a. Pulmonary edema
   b. Cardiac failure
   c. Pericarditis
   d. Diastolic hypertension
   e. Arrhythmias
   f. Acute cardiorespiratory failure

LABORATORY/DIAGNOSTIC TESTS

1. Serum sodium (Na)—in anuric infants and children, hyponatremia is common (<130 mEq/L)
2. Serum potassium (K) (increased; >7.5 mEq/L)
3. Serum calcium (hypocalcemia—4 to 8 mg/dl; impaired production of active vitamin D)
4. Serum phosphorus (increased; >5.5 mg/dl)
5. Serum chloride bicarbonate (HCO_3)—decreased
6. Metabolic acidosis (assess acidosis—venous pH of 6.8 to 7.0)

7. BUN (an increase >100 mg/dl)—influenced by degree of tissue necrosis and protein catabolism
8. Serum creatinine (increased)—influenced by degree of tissue necrosis and protein catabolism
9. Urinalysis (RBCs and/or casts in urine; increased or decreased specific gravity, depending on phase of renal failure)
10. Urinary Na, K, and chloride (Cl) (Na >20 mEq/L)
11. Urine osmolality (decreased; <350 mOsm)
12. Dextrostix, blood glucose
13. CBC, platelets
14. Blood cultures
15. Serum uric acid (10 to 25 mg; exceeds 50 mg with burns)
16. ECG—detects changes associated with hyperkalemia, hypocalcemia, and metabolic acidosis
17. Chest and abdominal x-rays

MEDICATIONS

1. Antihypertensives
   a. Hydralazine (Apresoline)—1.7 to 3.5 mg/kg qd into 4 to 6 doses intramuscularly (IM) or intravenously (IV); po dose 0.75 mg/kg QID
   b. Diazoxide (Hyperstat)—5 mg/kg IV; repeat in 30 to 60 minutes as needed
   c. Sodium nitroprusside (Nipride)—0.5-8 μg/kg/min.
   d. Methyldopa (Aldomet)—10 to 50 mg/kg/day q6 h
   e. Propranolol (Inderal)—0.5 to 2 mg/kg/po TID
   f. Minoxidil 0.1 to 0.5 mg/kg/day TID
2. Diuretics
   a. Mannitol (0.5-1 g/kg in IV dose)—use for prerenal condition but not with diagnosis of acute renal failure
   b. Furosemide (Lasix)—1 to 5 mg/kg; use for oliguric and nonoliguric renal failure
3. Antibiotics (see Appendix D, *Commonly Used Antibiotics*)
4. Anticonvulsants
   a. Phenobarbital—5 to 10 mg/kg for seizures; 3 to 5 mg/kg for maintenance
5. For hyperkalemia:
   a. Kayexalate
   b. Sodium bicarbonate

c. Calcium gluconate
d. 50% glucose

NURSING ASSESSMENT

Refer to "Renal Assessment" in Appendix A.

NURSING DIAGNOSES

Fluid volume excess
High risk for injury
High risk for infection
Activity intolerance
Ineffective individual coping
Altered family processes

NURSING INTERVENTIONS

1. Monitor and maintain fluid balance.
   a. Monitor type of fluids and administration rate to avoid fluid overload and cerebral edema.
   b. Record accurate input and output.
   c. Record daily weights (during acute phase record BID).
   d. Monitor blood pressure and pulse pressure to assess hydration.
   e. Replace fluids from urinary loss with isotonic solution (saline or lactated Ringer's) cubic centimeter for cubic centimeter.
   f. Assess hydration status q4-6 hr during acute phase.
   g. Replace fluids lost during hypovolemic shock.
   h. Monitor arterial pressure and central venous pressure (CVP).
2. Monitor and observe for signs of electrolyte imbalances.
   a. Hyperkalemia—muscular irritability; ECG changes (peaked T wave, wide QRS complex, prolonged PR interval); cardiac arrhythmias
   b. Hypocalcemia—coma, convulsions
   c. Hyponatremia—seizures
   d. Hypoglycemia—seizures
3. Observe and report signs and symptoms of impending complications.
   a. Shock
   b. Infection

   c. DIC
   d. Heart failure
   e. Potassium intoxication
   f. Overhydration
   g. Seizures
   h. Neurologic disturbance—lethargy, coma, hyperactivity
   i. Pulmonary edema
   j. Hypertension
4. Monitor for therapeutic and untoward responses to administered medications (refer to "medications" for list).
5. Prevent infection.
   a. Patient must cough and deep breathe.
   b. Perform mouth care.
   c. Perform daily catheter care.
   d. Protect patient from infectious contacts.
6. Prepare child and family for dialysis if indicated. Indications for dialysis follow.
   a. Anuria for 24 to 48 hours
   b. Central nervous system disturbance
   c. Congestive heart failure
   d. Bleeding (gastrointestinal or cutaneous)
   e. BUN results—100 mg/dl
   f. Uncontrollable hyperkalemia
   g. Hyponatremia (Na <130 mEq/L)
   h. Change in neurologic status—lethargy to coma or hyperactivity
   i. Hyperphosphatemia (>8 mg/100 ml)
   j. Severe metabolic acidosis
   k. Hypocalcemia (<8 mg/100 ml)
7. Encourage child and parents to ventilate feelings of concern about child's condition. Child's response will be affected by the following.
   a. Developmental needs
   b. Presence of primary caretakers
   c. Extent of immobilization
   d. Nutritional needs
   e. General malaise
8. Provide preprocedural information, and reinforce data provided to child and parents.

BIBLIOGRAPHY

Chan J: Current problems in end-stage kidney disease, *Clin Pediatr* 14(6):539, 1975.

Edelman C, ed: Pediatric kidney disease, Boston, 1978, Little, Brown and Co.

Ellis D, Gartner J, Galvis A: Acute renal failure in infants and children: diagnosis, complications, and treatment, *Crit Care Med* 9:607, 1981.

Fine R: Peritoneal dialysis. In Gellis S, Kagan B: *Current pediatric therapy 13*, Philadelphia, 1990, WB Saunders.

Lieberman E: Acute renal failure. In Lieberman E, ed: Clinical pediatric nephrology, Philadelphia, 1976, JB Lippincott.

McCormick A et al: Acute renal failure of the neonate, *Dimens Crit Care Nurs* 13(5):257, 1986.

Ruley E, Brock G: Acute renal failure in infants and children. In Shoemaker W et al, eds: *Textbook of critical care,* ed 2, Philadelphia, 1989, WB Saunders.

57 ❖ Renal Failure: Chronic

PATHOPHYSIOLOGY

Chronic renal failure refers to the progressive impairment of renal function that occurs over a prolonged time. Cardinal signs observed in chronic renal failure are (1) a severely impaired glomerular filtration rate (urinary output <80 ml/min) and (2) a serum creatinine level less than 2 mg/dl (not age related). Causes of chronic renal failure are associated with a variety of congenital and acquired factors. These factors can be broadly categorized into five types of diseases: (1) glomerular disease (e.g., focal and segmental polycystic); (2) obstructive uropathies (e.g., reflux); (3) renal hypoplasia (e.g., segmental hypoplasia or dysplasia); (4) hereditary neuropathies (e.g., polycystic kidney); and (5) vascular neuropathies (e.g., hemolytic-uremic syndrome).

Numerous manifestations resulting from multisystem involvement and disturbance in acid-base balance are associated with chronic renal failure, and metabolic acidosis results. Electrolyte imbalances include hyperkalemia, hyperphosphatemia, hypermagnesemia, hyponatremia, hyperuricemia, and hypocalcemia. Anemia (hemoglobin [Hb] <6 g/dl; hematocrit [Hct] <20%) results from impaired production of erythropoietin. Carbohydrate intolerance (hyperinsulinism) results from impaired tissue anabolism caused by insufficient energy intake. Decreased caloric intake results from altered taste perception caused by uremia. Manifestations of calcium-phosphate metabolism include renal osteodystrophy, osteomalacia, osteoporosis, and osteosclerosis. Severe growth retardation may occur secondary to metabolic imbalances.

Cardiac involvement associated with chronic renal failure includes cardiac failure and pericarditis. Neurologic disturbances range from muscular irritability and weakness to alterations in levels of consciousness. The signs and symptoms of chronic renal failure are variable (i.e., the child may exhibit any number of clinical manifestations). The disease is noncurable; medical and nursing care is directed symptomatically. Concurrent illness and death are ever-present threats to the child's clinical status.

INCIDENCE

1. Incidence — 2.5 per million in children 16 years old and younger; 5 per million in children 0 to 21 years old
2. Occurs more often in males than in females
3. Onset variable; dependent on category
4. Increased incidence in children less than 9 years of age because of obstructive and hereditary neuropathies and renal hypoplasia
5. Increased incidence in patients less than 8 years old who have glomerular disease
6. Terminal renal disease in more than 50% of patients whose disease is discovered by 5 years of age
7. Incidence of renal osteodystrophy — 21.2% to 42.1%

CLINICAL MANIFESTATIONS

1. Nocturia with enuresis
2. Marked polyuria
3. Marked polydipsia
4. Recurrent fevers
5. Undue fatigue during exertion
6. Poor appetite
7. Hypertension
8. Edema (first observed as puffy eyes or, in males, swollen scrotum [first sign may be tight underpants])
9. Frequent epistaxis
10. Pallor
11. Neurologic dysfunction (lethargy, coma, twitching, convulsions)

12. Malaise
13. Headaches
14. Growth retardation
15. Muscle cramps
16. Nausea

COMPLICATIONS

1. Anemia
2. Renal rickets
3. Failure to grow
4. Delayed sexual maturation
5. Recurrent infections (e.g., urinary tract infections, upper respiratory infections)
6. Cardiac failure
7. Hypertension
8. Water and electrolyte disturbances

LABORATORY/DIAGNOSTIC TESTS

1. Blood urea nitrogen (increased; reflects progression of renal disease)
2. Serum creatinine (decreased; reflects progression of renal disease)
3. Serum electrolytes (decreased sodium, increased potassium, decreased chloride, increased carbon dioxide)
4. Venous and arterial blood gas values (metabolic acidosis)
5. Hypercalcemia, hypophosphatemia
6. Complete blood count (decreased red blood cells, decreased renal erythropoietin production, decreased white blood cells, increased susceptibility to infection, decreased reticulocyte count)
7. Percutaneous kidney biopsy (diagnostic)
8. Nephrosonogram (diagnostic)
9. Renal scan (diagnostic)
10. Voiding cystourethrogram (identification of organic and functional abnormalities)

MEDICATIONS

1. Diuretics (to treat hypertension)
   a. Furosemide (Lasix) — 1 to 10 mg/kg by mouth (po) or intravenously (IV) BID

    b. Ethacrynic acid — 1 to 10 mg/kg/day po
    c. Hydrochlorothiazide — 1 to 2 mg/kg/day po
    d. Chlorothiazide — 10 to 20 mg/kg BID po
2. Sodium polystyrene sulfonate (Kayexalate) — 1 g/kg/dose
3. Immunosuppressive
    a. Steroids
    b. Cyclophosphamide (Cytoxan)
4. Antihypertensives
5. Calcium
    a. Ergocalciferol (Calciferol) — 2000-25,000 units/day po
    b. Calcium carbonate
    c. Calcium gluconate or calcium lactate — 10 to 20 mg/kg/day po
6. Multivitamins, folic acid 1-2 mg/kg/day
7. Phosphate binders (aluminum hydroxide gel [Amphojel, AlternaGEL] and aluminum carbonate gel [Basaljel])
8. Anticonvulsants
9. Allopurinol — decreases uric acid levels

NURSING ASSESSMENT

Refer to "Renal Assessment" in Appendix A.

NURSING DIAGNOSES

Fluid volume excess
High risk for injury
High risk for infection
Activity intolerance
Ineffective individual coping
Social isolation
Altered family processes

NURSING INTERVENTIONS (CONSERVATIVE TREATMENT)

1. Maintain metabolic balance — work with dietician to offer foods that child likes within limits of diet.
    a. Provide high-calorie, high-protein diet.
    b. Limit intake of salt (no added salt).
    c. Avoid foods rich in potassium (e.g., bananas, 7-Up).
    d. Avoid foods rich in phosphorus (e.g., cow's milk).
    e. Administer supplemental vitamins (e.g., D, C, pyridoxine, folic acid)

2. Monitor child's therapeutic and untoward responses to medications.
   a. Alkylating agents (e.g., sodium bicarbonate)
   b. Antihypertensives
   c. Diuretics
   d. Immunosuppressives
   e. Antibiotics
3. Provide emotional support to child and parents during hospitalization.
   a. Encourage child's and family members' verbalization of feelings.
   b. Provide age-appropriate teaching before procedures.
   c. Provide and reinforce information about condition and hospitalization.
   d. Encourage use of social support network (e.g., neighborhood, friends, relatives).
   e. Refer to social worker as needed.
   f. Provide age-appropriate toys and recreational activities.
   g. Elicit expression of fears concerning body mutilation, death, and separation.

Refer to nursing care plan for renal transplantation and continuous peritoneal dialysis in Chapter 58, *Renal Transplantation*.

BIBLIOGRAPHY

Erlich L: Use of EPOGEN for treatment of anemia associated with chronic renal failure, *Crit Care Nurs Clin North Am* 2(1):101, 1990.

Habib R, Broyer M, Benmaig H: Chronic renal failure in children, *Nephron* 11:290, 1973.

Innerarity S: Electrolyte emergencies in the critically ill renal patients, *Crit Care Nurs Clin North Am* 2(1):89, 1990.

Novis M: Management of acute conditions in chronic renal failure, *DCCN* 2:328, 1983.

Sander V, Murray C, Robertson P: School and the in-center pediatric hemodialysis patient, *ANNA J* 16(2):72, 1989.

Weiss R, Edelman C: End stage renal disease in children, *Pediatr Rev* 5(10):295, 1984.

58 ❖ Renal Transplantation

PATHOPHYSIOLOGY

Renal transplantation is the treatment of choice for children with irreversible renal insufficiency. Primary diseases that can lead to renal transplantation include the glomerular diseases: lupus nephritis, chronic glomerulonephritis, and nephrotic syndrome with focal sclerosis. Children with bilateral Wilms' tumor are candidates, although their prognosis is improved if transplantation is delayed for 1 year after diagnosis. Transplantation is performed for congenital conditions such as polycystic disease and cystinosis. Twenty-five percent of children who have transplants have obstructive uropathy. The mortality rate is higher in children than in adults who have transplants, especially when the kidney was obtained from cadaveric sources. Nevertheless, extended hemodialysis and renal transplantation have increased the survival rate of children with irreversible renal insufficiency. The major problem associated with transplantation is rejection of the kidney. Rejection is the result of one of a variety of causes: cellular and/or humoral immune response, technical failures, severe systemic infection, noncompliance, and renal artery stenosis. Long-term consequences of transplantation include retarded bone growth (short stature) and osteodystrophy. Pubertal development proceeds normally after successful transplantation.

INCIDENCE

1. Occurrence—one in 1 million in children less than 15 years old; one to three in 1 million in children older than 15 years
2. In-hospital or dialysis-center cost—$30,000 per year
3. Home dialysis cost—$14,000 during first year, $7000 in successive years
4. Transplant cost—$14,000 per year
5. Survival rates
   a. Hemodialysis—83% for 2 years and 81% for 3 years
   b. Allograft—60% for 2 years
   c. Living-related transplant—70% for 2 years
   d. Cadaver transplant—55% for 2 years
6. Decreased survival with subsequent grafts

CLINICAL MANIFESTATIONS

Before Transplant

Refer to specific renal condition (e.g., nephrotic syndrome).

Transplant Surgery

1. Kidney is placed in extraperitoneal cavity in iliac fossa; renal artery and vein are anastomosed to external or common iliac artery and hypogastric vein.

COMPLICATIONS AFTER TRANSPLANT

1. Hyperacute, acute, or chronic rejection
   a. Fever
   b. Hypertension
   c. Graft tenderness
   d. Oliguria
   e. Proteinuria
   f. Anuria
   g. Hyperchloremic metabolic acidosis
   h. Increased serum creatinine (0.3 mg/dl)
2. Ureteral obstruction
3. Acute tubular necrosis
4. Bleeding at transplant site
5. Infection (peritonitis, *Candida* infections, cytomegalovirus, viral infections)
6. Corticosteroid toxicity

7. Surgical complications (lymphocele)
8. Transplant nephrectomy for irreversible technical complications or hyperacute rejection

PRETRANSPLANT EVALUATION

1. Extensive serologic studies, including general survey panel, CBC with differential, platelets, viral screening, blood culture
2. Meticulous search for infection, including dental exams, sinus films
3. ECG, chest x-ray, VCUG
4. Urinalysis, urine culture and sensitivity, urine collection for creatinine clearance, and total protein
5. Histocompatibility testing
   a. ABO blood type
   b. Antibody screening
   c. Human leukocyte antigens (HLA) typing (A, B, C, D, Dr)
   d. WBC crossmatch
   e. Mixed lymphocyte culture

POSTOPERATIVE LABORATORY/DIAGNOSTIC TESTS

1. BUN, creatinine, electrolytes, CBC, glucose
2. Renal scan
3. Cyclosporine levels
4. Urine for protein, creatinine, electrolytes
5. Renal biopsy (diagnostic for rejection)

MEDICATIONS

Dosages and scheduling vary with different transplant centers.
1. Cyclosporine — immunosuppressant
2. Azathioprine — immunosuppressant
3. Prednisone — corticosteroid, immunosuppressant
4. Antacids — to buffer acid in stomach
5. Nystatin — prophylactic for *Candida* in mouth
6. Diuretics — indicated for hypertension and edema
7. Antihypertensives
8. Antibiotics — used prophylactically or for specifically identified infections

NURSING ASSESSMENT

Refer to "Renal Assessment" in Appendix A.

NURSING DIAGNOSES

Fluid volume excess
High risk for injury
High risk for infection
Body image disturbance
Fear
Ineffective individual coping
Altered family processes

NURSING INTERVENTIONS

Preoperative Care

Prepare donor, recipient, and family for transplantation.
1. Provide information about presurgical routine.
2. Reinforce information given about surgery.
3. Provide age-appropriate preprocedural or preoperative preparation.

Postoperative Care

1. Monitor and report signs of kidney rejection.
2. Monitor vital signs, and report significant changes because may be indicators of rejection, bleeding, infection, hypovolemic shock.
   a. Check vital signs q1 hr for 24 hours; if stable, then check vital signs q4 hr.
   b. Check shunt or fistula for patency.
3. Monitor urinary output; report any significant changes.
   a. Monitor hourly urinary output for 24 hours, then q2 hr for 48 hours.
   b. Check for increased bleeding or clot formation.
   c. Check for decreased urinary output; then assess the following:
      (1) Check for catheter kinking.
      (2) Check for dehydration or hypovolemia.
      (3) Irrigate to remove clots.
4. Observe for drainage on dressing.
   a. Circle extent of drainage.
   b. Notify physician if drainage increases significantly.

5. Observe for child's therapeutic response to or untoward effects of medications.
6. Observe and report signs and symptoms of possible complications.

Home Care

1. Instruct child and family about the therapeutic and untoward reactions of medications.
2. Reinforce the necessity of being compliant with medical regimen.
3. Reinforce information provided about nutritional needs.
   a. High calorie and high protein
   b. Limited sugar
   c. Limited salt
4. Instruct about proper dental care (brushing and flossing).
5. Refer to appropriate community, clinic, agencies, or personnel for psychosocial needs.

BIBLIOGRAPHY

Baxter J: Criteria for selection in renal transplantation, *J Urol Nurs* 9(3):943, 1990.

Chan J: End-stage kidney failure in children, *Clin Pediatr* 15(11):991, 1976.

Fedric T: Immunosuppressive therapy in renal transplantation, *Crit Care Nurs Clin North Am* 2(1):123, 1990.

Fennell R et al: Renal transplantation in children and adolescents, *Clin Pediatr* 18(9):518, 1979.

Fine R et al: Long-term results of renal transplantation in children, *Pediatrics* 61(4):641, 1978.

Hetrick A, Frauman A, Gilman C: Nutrition in renal disease: when the patient is a child, *Am J Nurs* 79(12):2152, 1979.

Hudson K et al: Coping with pediatric renal transplantation, *J Am Nephrol Nurses Assoc* 13(5):261, 1986.

Laquire R: Crossword puzzle: renal transplantation, *ANNA J* 16(6):416, 1989.

Morris P, ed: *Kidney transplantation; principles in practice,* ed 2, Orlando, 1984, Grune & Stratton.

59 ❖ Respiratory Distress Syndrome

PATHOPHYSIOLOGY

The pathogenesis of respiratory distress syndrome, or hyaline membrane disease, is probably attributed to inadequate synthesis, secretion, and/or storage of surfactant (surface-active material) by type II cells. Surfactant is needed to maintain the stability of the alveoli and to allow their adequate perfusion. A decrease in surfactant causes alveolar collapse, resulting in altered oxygen–carbon dioxide exchange (hypoxia), which leads to pulmonary vascular constriction and decreased pulmonary perfusion. Decreased pulmonary perfusion results in capillary damage and alveolar necrosis, contributing to the accumulation of exudate in the alveolar space and the formation of hyaline membrane. An alternative explanation for respiratory distress syndrome suggests that ischemic insult to the lung causes the death of type II cells and alters the enzymatic pathways associated with surfactant production.

INCIDENCE

1. Respiratory distress syndrome is the respiratory disorder most frequently seen in neonatal intensive care units (NICU).
2. It occurs in 0.5% to 2% of all live births.

3. It occurs in 10% of all preterm births.
4. It affects 25% to 30% of infants born early.
5. It affects 60% of infants weighing less than 1000 g.
6. Males are affected twice as often as females.
7. Respiratory distress syndrome occurs five times more often in infants of diabetic mothers.
8. It accounts for 9000 deaths per year.
9. The survival rate is 80% to 90% when respiratory distress syndrome is the only pathologic condition.
10. Mortality during first 72 hours is as follows: first 24 hours—50%; 48 hours—70%; 72 hours—90%; if infants survive longer than 72 hours, recovery is the rule.

CLINICAL MANIFESTATIONS
Symptoms Observed in First 6 to 8 Hours of Life
1. Tachypnea (70 to 120 breaths/min)
2. Diaphragmatic breathing leading to paradoxical breathing
3. Retractions
4. Grunting
5. Rales
6. Systemic hypotension (peripheral pallor, slow capillary filling, hypothermia)
7. Cyanosis when breathing room air
8. Peripheral edema
9. Decreased renal output
10. Ileus
11. Jaundice
12. Muscle flaccidity
13. Acidosis

Long-Term Effects
Prognosis is dependent on development of chronic lung disease and neurologic impairment.
1. Chest x-ray study—interstitial fibrosis or hyperaeration and localized atelectasis for 2 to 5 years
2. Increased small airway resistance for up to 6 years
3. Decreased arterial oxygen tension with or without bronchopulmonary dysplasia from 1 to 5 years
4. Increased pulmonary vascular resistance and right hypertrophy for 1 to 5 years

COMPLICATIONS

1. Acid-base imbalance resulting from hyperventilation or hypoventilation
2. Atrophy of respiratory muscles
3. Retrolental fibroplasia (increased incidence in infants with gestational age less than 8 months because of increased oxygen concentrations)
4. Nasal deformities, corneal lacerations, and necrosis of skin of cheeks and neck caused by pressure from oxygen mask or prongs
5. Pneumothorax, pneumomediastinum, subcutaneous emphysema caused by air leak
6. Tracheal ulceration or stenosis and subglottic stenosis (ET tube)
7. Accidental extubation
8. Lung collapse (tube slips into contralateral mainstem bronchus)
9. Airway occlusion or secretions (endotracheal tube placement)

LABORATORY/DIAGNOSTIC TESTS

1. Chest x-ray studies—evidence of decreased expansion of lungs, radiopacity, and presence of air on bronchograms
2. Pulmonary function tests—decreased tidal volume, decreased crying volume capacity, decreased functional residual capacity, ventilation-perfusion imbalance, decreased lung compliance
3. Complete blood count (CBC)—decreased oxygen saturation
4. Arterial blood gas values (ABGs)—respiratory or metabolic acidosis
5. Serum electrolytes—decreased sodium (Na^+), decreased potassium (K^+), decreased calcium (Ca^+)
6. Serum glucose—decreased glucose
7. Urinary output—decreased osmolarity, increased specific gravity
8. Arterial blood pressure/central venous pressure (CVP)—decreased because of hypotension

MEDICATIONS

1. Theophylline—relaxes the smooth muscle of the bronchi and pulmonary vessels; also stimulates the respiratory

center, causing an increase in vital capacity; dosage — 10 mg/kg/24 hr or 0.3 g/m^2/24 hr BID or TID by mouth (po)
2. Indomethacin (Indocin) — used to constrict patent ductus arteriosus (PDA); alleviates necessity for surgical management of PDA
3. Prostaglandin E — used to dilate closed ductus arteriosus
4. Artificial surfactant via ET tube

NURSING ASSESSMENT

Refer to "Respiratory Assessment," Appendix A.

NURSING DIAGNOSES

Impaired gas exchange
High risk for injury
Altered nutrition: less than body requirements
Hypothermia
Fluid volume excess
Altered tissue perfusion: gastrointestinal
Knowledge deficit
Altered parenting
Altered growth and development
Sensory-perceptual alterations

NURSING INTERVENTIONS

1. Monitor and observe for changes in respiratory status.
2. Monitor and observe infant's response to mechanical ventilation.
3. Monitor infant's response and side effects of prescribed medications.
   a. Theophylline
   b. Indomethacin
   c. Prostaglandin E
   d. Vitamin E_1 — controversial; to prevent or modify bronchopulmonary dysplasia or retrolental fibroplasia
   e. Tolazoline/acetylcholine — controversial; to decrease pulmonary vascular resistance
   f. Metocurine (Metubine) and pancuronium (Pavulon) — skeletal muscle relaxant for mechanical ventilation
4. Promote and maintain caloric intake through intravenous (IV) or gavage feedings.

5. Monitor IV or gavage feedings for hypoglycemia (use Dextrostix — range 45 to 90 mg/dl).
6. Maintain infant in neutral thermal environment (use overhead radiant heating and incubators with heat shield).
7. Record daily weights.
8. Monitor output (2 ml/kg/hr; specific gravity — 1.005 to 1.010).
9. Limit unnecessary handling of infants.
10. Monitor transfusion of blood products.
    a. Whole blood or fresh frozen plasma for rapid expansion of intravascular volume
    b. Packed red blood cells (RBCs)
11. Encourage parental-infant attachment.
12. Provide developmentally appropriate auditory, tactile, and visceral stimulation (see Appendix B, *Growth and Development*).

Home Care

1. Instruct parents about infant cardiopulmonary resuscitation (CPR).
2. Instruct parents about monitoring and observation of signs of respiratory distress.
3. Instruct parents about preventive infection control measures.
   a. Limit and screen visitors to the home.
   b. Use hygienic practices.
4. Instruct parents about strategies to optimize infant's developmental needs (see Appendix B, *Growth and Development*).
5. Refer parents to appropriate community agencies (Visiting Nurse Association, parent support group, infant stimulation programs).

BIBLIOGRAPHY

Blair G, Sharpe L: Nutrition support in respiratory disorders, *Nutr Clin Pract* 4(5):173, 1989.

Cheng M, Williams P: Oxygenation during chest physiotherapy of very low-birth-weight infants: relations among fraction of inspired oxygen levels, number of hand ventilations, and transcutaneous oxygen pressure, *J Pediatr Nurs* 4(6):411, 1990.

Clancy G: Blood gas monitoring and management of neonates with respiratory distress, *J Perinat Neonat Nurs* 1(1):72, 1987.

Engel N: Update on pulmonary surfactant replacement for neonates, *MCN: Am J Matern Child Nurs* 15(3):189, 1990.

Few B: Corticosteroids and respiratory distress syndrome, *MCN* 13(1):17, 1988.

Fox M, Molesky M: The effects of prone and supine positioning on arterial oxygen pressure, *Neonat Network: J Neonat Nurs* 8(4):25, 1990.

Gorden P: High frequency jet ventilation for severe respiratory failure, *Pediatr Nurs* 15(6):625, 1989.

Inselman L: Respiratory distress syndrome, *Pediatr Ann* 7(4):243, 1978.

Ioli J, Richardson M: Giving surfactant to premature infants, *Am J Nurs* 90(3):59, 1990.

Lapido M: Respiratory distress revisited, *Neonat Network* 8(3):9, 1989.

LeBlanc K, Forestell F: Assessment of the neonatal respiratory system, *AACN: Clin Issues Crit Care Nurs* 1(2):401, 1990.

Lynam L: Surfactant replacement therapy: a second look, *Neonat Network* 9(3):79, 1990.

Phelan P, Sandau L, Olinsky A: *Respiratory illness in children,* Oxford, 1982, Blackwell Scientific Publications.

Reynolds M, Wallander K: Surfactant for neonatal respiratory distress syndrome, *J Pediatr Health Care* 4(4):209, 1990.

Simmons M: Supportive care in RDS, *Pediatr Ann* 2:42, 1977.

Toper-Hunter D: Respiratory distress syndrome, *Neonat Network* 2:9, 1982.

60 ❖ Respiratory Syncytial Virus (RSV)

PATHOPHYSIOLOGY

Respiratory syncytial virus (RSV) is a highly contagious pathogen. Its primary effect is on the lower respiratory tract. RSV has an incubation period of 5-8 days, after which it usually causes "upper respiratory tract infection symptoms." The primary mode of transmission (similar to other respiratory pathogens) is contact with respiratory secretions by direct handling of patients or objects contaminated with the virus.

INCIDENCE

1. Annual epidemics occur during winter and early spring.
2. It affects any age group, but most often small children and infants under age 1 to 2 years.
3. Incidence decreases with age.
4. By age 2 years nearly 100% of all children will have acquired RSV.
5. RSV tends to cause more severe illness in very young and debilitated children. Infants age 6 weeks to 3 months and those with cardiac problems, pulmonary problems, or immune diseases are generally the most ill.

CLINICAL MANIFESTATIONS

1. The first symptoms are usually rhinorrhea and pharyngitis.
2. Progresses to coughing and wheezing.
3. Associated otitis media.
4. Lower respiratory tract symptoms: bronchitis, pneumonia, and apnea.
5. Air hunger, retractions, increased respiratory rate, and cyanosis.
6. Hypoxemia.

COMPLICATIONS

1. Respiratory distress, respiratory arrest.
2. Apnea.

LABORATORY/DIAGNOSTIC TESTS

1. CBC with differential.
2. Chest x-ray.
3. Nasal washing (EIA or enzyme immune assay).

MEDICATIONS/TREATMENT

1. Humidified oxygen.
2. Intravenous fluids.
3. Intubation/mechanical ventilation as needed.
4. Ribavirin aerosol.
5. Antipyretics.

NURSING ASSESSMENT

Refer to "Respiratory Assessment" in Appendix A.

NURSING DIAGNOSES

High risk for injury
High risk for infection
Ineffective tissue perfusion
Knowledge deficit

NURSING INTERVENTIONS

1. Monitor respiratory status and hydration status.
2. Use suction as needed; implement pulmonary hygiene.
3. Position with the head of the bed elevated; allow position of comfort.

4. Administer oxygen.
5. Provide adequate fluid intake (IV and oral).
6. Strictly monitor intake and output.
7. Weigh daily.
8. Administer medications as ordered.
9. Take infection control measures.
10. Encourage parental education.

BIBLIOGRAPHY

Nederhand KC et al: Respiratory syncytial virus: a nursing perspective, *Pediatr Nurs* 15(4):342, 1989.

61 ❖ Reye's Syndrome

PATHOPHYSIOLOGY

Reye's syndrome is a nonrecurring encephalopathy associated with the fatty infiltration of the viscera, typically evolving in the wake of a viral illness and for which no other chemical or clinical explanation has been found. Epidemic forms of the syndrome occur following an increased incidence of influenza A or B, and sporadic cases are associated with varicella. Reye's syndrome has been reported in association with bacterial pharyngitis and *Haemophilus influenzae* infection. In addition, recent research proposes that administration of salicylates contributes to the syndrome. The American Academy of Pediatrics (1982) recommends that aspirin be avoided for treatment of the symptoms of chicken pox or influenza.

Although the mechanism of mitochondrial damage is currently unknown, drugs, viruses, metabolic defects, and environmental toxins have all been implicated as causative agents.

Speculation has been advanced that the syndrome is a response to a universal mitochondrial insult. The following changes occur:

1. Cerebral edema and neuronal necrosis
2. Hypoglycemia
3. Altered hepatic function as a result of enlargement and fatty infiltration of the liver and, to a lesser extent, organs such as the kidneys, myocardium, and

other viscera (liver biopsy reveals small droplets of fat within the parenchymal cells and no inflammation)

4. Tissue glycogen depletion
5. Peripheral lipolysis
6. Impairment of biosynthetic processes (specifically, decreased pre-β-lipoproteins, several clotting factors, and components of the complement system)

The survival rate currently is greater than 80%, and there is rapid and complete recovery in most patients. Improved treatment is the most significant factor contributing to increased survival. In addition, early recognition is vital. Neurologic, intellectual, and emotional sequelae may result in survivors. Voice and speech disorders are the predominant disability in survivors.

The severity of the illness at the time of admission apparently is correlated with the likelihood of recovery. A variety of staging systems have been developed with criteria to assess the severity of the condition (see Table 8 for National Institutes of Health's staging).

INCIDENCE

1. Reye's syndrome is the major cause of noninfectious neurologic death following a viral illness in the pediatric age group.
2. Age range of children with this disorder is from neonates to age 19 years; typically the patient is 6 to 11 years of age.
3. There is no gender preference.

CLINICAL MANIFESTATIONS

The prodromal illness has the following signs and symptoms.

1. Upper respiratory tract infection
2. Rapid onset of vomiting
3. Tachypnea
4. Fever
5. Altered mental status
6. Pupillary dilation
7. Marked lethargy
8. Irritability

Table 8. Staging of Reye's Syndrome

Stage	I	II	III	IV	V
Level of consciousness	Lethargy; follows verbal commands, vomiting, sleepiness	Combative or stuporous; verbalizes inappropriately, disoriented	Coma	Coma; seizures	Coma; no respirations, flaccid paralysis
Posture	Normal	Normal	Decorticate	Decerebrate	Flaccid
Response to pain	Purposeful	Purposeful or nonpurposeful	Decorticate	Decerebrate	None
Pupillary reaction	Brisk	Sluggish	Sluggish	Sluggish	None
Oculocephalic reflex ("doll's eyes")	Normal	Conjugate deviation	Conjugate deviation	Inconsistent or absent	None

Modified from National Institutes of Health Consensus Development Conference, March 1981, and Lovejoy FH et al: *Am J Dis Child* 128:136, 1974.

9. Coma
10. Seizures

COMPLICATIONS

1. Varying degrees of decorticate or decerebrate posturing
2. Encephalopathy (usually for 24 to 96 hours)
3. Gastrointestinal hemorrhage (10% of patients)
4. Pancreatitis (severe complication with poor prognosis)

LABORATORY/DIAGNOSTIC TESTS

1. Serum transaminases — elevated serum glutamic-oxaloacetic transaminase (SGOT) and serum glutamic-pyruvic transaminase (SGPT) to at least 1.5 to 2 times normal
2. Prothrombin and partial thromboplastin times — prolonged
3. Serum glucose — decreased
4. Serum amylase — elevated
5. Serum lactic dehydrogenase — elevated
6. Serum ammonia (hyperammonemia) — elevated at least two times normal levels
7. Serum uric acid level — increased
8. Serum creatinine phosphokinase — elevated
9. Serum lipase — elevated
10. Serum cholesterol level — decreased
11. Serum bilirubin — usually normal
12. Liver biopsy — to define histopathologic features (usually with infants and atypical cases only)
13. Lumbar puncture — to rule out bacterial meningitis or viral encephalitis (controversial)

MEDICATIONS

1. Anticonvulsants — prophylactic use of anticonvulsants may be indicated; used for treatment of seizures
2. Antibiotics — culture and sensitivity performed to determine type of antibiotic to use
3. Stool softeners
4. Analgesia — acetaminophen, aspirin (bleeding tendency), and other narcotics (mask neurologic status) are not used

5. Vitamin K — used for prothrombin deficiencies; dose — 5 to 10 mg by mouth (po)/intramuscularly (IM)/intravenously (IV)/subcutaneously (SC)
6. Pancuronium (Pavulon) — used to induce skeletal muscle relaxation; used to sedate children who are on mechanical ventilation; dosage — 0.04 to 0.1 mg/kg q30-60 min IV

NURSING ASSESSMENT

Refer to "Neuromuscular Assessment" in Appendix A.

NURSING DIAGNOSES

Altered tissue perfusion, cerebral
Fluid volume deficit
Sensory-perceptual alteration
Altered nutrition: less than body requirements
High risk for injury
Altered patterns of urinary elimination
Altered growth and development
Altered family processes
Knowledge deficit

NURSING INTERVENTIONS

1. Monitor neurologic status with serial measures.
   a. Report any deterioration or questionable findings; intervention may be required on an emergency basis.
   b. Monitor level of consciousness.
      (1) General appearance
      (2) Arousability
      (3) Orientation
      (4) Restlessness
   c. Monitor vital signs.
      (1) Respiratory pattern
      (2) Blood pressure
      (3) Heart rate
      (4) Temperature
   d. Check pupils: pupils equal, react to light, accommodate (PERLA).
   e. Monitor reaction to pain.
   f. Check head circumference (check fontanels).

g. Use Glasgow Coma Scale (see "Neuromuscular Assessment" in Appendix A).
2. Provide calm, quiet environment.
   a. Provide rooming-in for parents of children.
   b. Do not restrain.
3. Avoid increase in intracranial pressure.
   a. Keep head in midline.
   b. Elevate head of bed 30 to 45 degrees.
   c. Avoid flexed knees.
   d. Avoid using restraints.
   e. Avoid patient's crying.
4. Maintain adequate nutrition and fluid balance.
   a. Monitor nasogastric (NG) tube and use of antacids.
   b. Monitor for residuals before feedings.
   c. Irrigate q4 hr with normal saline solution.
   d. Monitor infusion of hypertonic glucose and electrolytes.
   e. Monitor central venous pressure (CVP) and arterial pressure.
   f. Monitor input and output as often as q1 hr.
5. Maintain patency of airway.
   a. Monitor respiratory status.
   b. Check patency of endotracheal tube and airway.
   c. Check ventilator settings q1 hr.
   d. Irrigate and suction as needed.
6. Administer and monitor child's response to medications.
   a. Therapeutic response
   b. Side effects
7. Monitor for complications.
   a. Atelectasis
   b. Hypoxia
   c. Respiratory disorders
   d. Coma
   e. Seizures
   f. Increased secretion of antidiuretic hormone (ADH)
8. Maintain bowel and bladder function.
   a. Provide Foley catheter care q8 hr.
   b. Administer stool softeners as needed.
9. Prevent skin breakdown by using frequent skin care, change of position, and pressure mattress or sheepskin.

10. Provide lubrication to eyes to prevent drying and ulceration.
11. Provide environmental stimulation (e.g., auditory and tactile) because child may be able to hear and feel even though unresponsive.
12. Provide for child's developmental needs during hospitalization (when condition permits).
    a. Provide age-appropriate toys (see Appendix B, *Growth and Development*).
    b. Incorporate home routines into hospitalization (e.g., feeding practices, bedtime rituals).
    c. Encourage ventilation of feelings through age-appropriate means.
    d. Use age-appropriate explanations before procedures.
13. Provide emotional support to family.
    a. Encourage ventilation of concerns.
    b. Refer to social service as needed.
    c. Provide for physical comforts (e.g., place to sleep, bathing).
    d. Encourage use of preexisting support systems.

Home Care/Discharge Planning

1. Instruct parents about long-term management.
    a. Administration of medications
    b. Level of exercise
    c. Infection control
2. Anticipatory guidance related to recovery includes the following:
    a. Abnormalities present in the early phase of recovery often improve or disappear completely in 6 to 12 months; the most common sequelae are motor and intellectual deficits.
    b. Hearing impairments have been reported and may require individual evaluation if indicated.
    c. Voice and speech disorders such as aphonia, slurred speech, and dysfluency may occur. Severely impaired voice function does not necessarily imply that child is intellectually impaired. When voice and speech problems persist for more than 2 months, it is recommended that nonvocal communication aids such as computers and communication boards be used.

3. Emotional support of the child and family referral for follow-up rehabilitation services are important aspects of the nursing care.

BIBLIOGRAPHY

Aspirin dosage and Reye's syndrome, *Nurses' Drug Alert* 12(10):80, 1988.

Baker GA: The role of decompressive craniectomy in Reye's syndrome, *J Natl Reye's Syndrome Found* 1:73, 1980.

Belkengren RP, Sapala S: Reye's syndrome, clinical guidelines for practitioners in ambulatory care, *Pediatr Nurs* 7(2):26, March/April 1981.

Committee on Infectious Disease of the American Academy of Pediatrics: Aspirin and Reye's syndrome, *Am Acad Pediatr*, June, 1982.

Danis D: Reye's syndrome, *J Emerg Nurs* 14(2):110, 1988.

Davidson PN et al: Neurological and intellectual sequelae of Reye's syndrome, *Am J Ment Defic* 82:535, 1978.

DeVivo DC: Reye's syndrome: a metabolic response to an acute mitochondrial insult, *Neurology* 28:105, 1978.

Diliberti JH, Laxer KD: Brain stem auditory evoked potentials in a case of Reye's syndrome, *Clin Pediatr* 23(4):238, 1984.

Frewen JC et al: Outcome in severe Reye's syndrome with early phenobarbital coma and hypothermia, *J Pediatr* 100:663, 1982.

Haller J: Intracranial pressure monitoring in Reye's syndrome, *Hosp Pract* 15:101, 1980.

Kaufman R et al: Aspirin use and Reye's syndrome, *Pediatrics* 79(6):1049, 1987.

Lovejoy FH et al: Clinical staging in Reye's syndrome, *Am J Dis Child* 128:136, 1974.

Maheady D: Reye's syndrome: review and update, *J Pediatr Health Care* 3(5):246, 1989.

Partin JS et al: Serum salicylate concentrations in Reye's syndrome: a study of 130 biopsy-proven cases, *Lancet* 1:191, 1982.

Reitman MA et al: Motor disorders of voice and speech in Reye's syndrome survivors, *Am J Dis Child* 138:1129, 1984.

Robinson R: Differential diagnosis of Reye's syndrome, *Dev Med Child Neurol* 29(1):110, 1987.

Rodgers GC, Weiner LB, McMillan JA: Salicylate and Reye's syndrome, *Lancet* 1:616, 1982.

Shaywitz BA, Rothstein P, Venes JL: Monitoring and management of increased intracranial pressure in Reye's syndrome: results of 29 children, *Pediatrics* 66:198, 1980.

Sundwall DA, Bergeson ME, Ortiz A: Reye's syndrome associated with *Haemophilus influenzae* infection, *Clin Pediatrics* 19(5):351, 1980.

Travner DA: Diagnosis of Reye's syndrome, *J Natl Reye's Syndrome Found* 2(1):20, 1981.

Volk D: Reye's syndrome: an update, *Clin Pediatr* 10(8):505, 1981.

62 ❖ Rheumatic Fever: Acute

PATHOPHYSIOLOGY

Acute rheumatic fever refers to the inflammatory disease that follows an infection with a group A beta-hemolytic streptococcus. This disease causes pathologic lesions in the heart, blood vessels, joints, and subcutaneous tissue. The symptoms of rheumatic fever are manifested approximately 1 to 5 weeks after the infection occurs. The initial symptoms, as well as severity of the disease, are widely varied. Arthritis, in the form of migratory polyarthritis, is the most common (75%) symptom that is initially seen. Symptoms can be classified as cardiac and noncardiac and may develop gradually. Diagnosis is based on the Revised Jones Criteria from the American Heart Association (see box on facing page). Two major criteria or one major and two minor criteria indicate an increased possibility of rheumatic fever. Prognosis depends on the severity of cardiac involvement.

INCIDENCE

1. One out of 2000 children between the ages of 5 and 15 years is affected.
2. There is an increased incidence among children whose socioeconomic status is low.
3. There is an increased frequency in males.
4. There is an increased incidence among children who have had a previous attack.

Revised Jones Criteria

Major Criteria

Arthritis
Carditis
Erythema marginatum
Subcutaneous nodules
Sydenham's chorea

Minor Criteria

Previous history of rheumatic fever
Arthralgia
Elevated acute phase reactants
Prolonged PR interval visible on ECG
Fever

Evidence of Streptococcal Infection

Positive culture
Scarlatiniform rash
Elevated streptococcal antibodies

From Stollerman G et al: Jones criteria (revised) for guidance in the diagnosis of rheumatic fever, *Circulation* 32:664, 1965. By permission of the American Heart Association, Inc.

5. A 30% to 67% incidence of heart disease occurs 10 years after an individual has had rheumatic fever.
6. There is a decreased incidence in the United States and Europe (seen in the United States in the late winter and early spring).

CLINICAL MANIFESTATIONS

1. Arthritis—painful, warm, red, and swollen; knee, elbow, wrist, ankle most often affected
2. Arthralgia
3. Low-grade fever that usually spikes in late afternoon
4. Chest pain (symptom of carditis)
5. Shortness of breath (symptom of carditis)
6. Tachycardia—especially during rest or sleep
7. Bradycardia

8. Complains of sore throat
9. Chorea
10. Subcutaneous nodules
11. Abdominal pain (symptom of carditis)
12. Cough (symptom of carditis)

LABORATORY/DIAGNOSTIC TESTS

1. Echocardiography — to diagnose pericarditis
2. Pericardiocentesis — to diagnose pericarditis
3. Chest x-ray examination — to detect cardiomegaly
4. ECG (atrioventricular [A-V] block and prolonged PR are present in carditis)
5. Antistreptolysin O (ASO) titer (increased)
6. Antihyaluronidase antibody titers (increased) — to detect streptococcal antibodies
7. Nicotinamide adenine dinucleotidase (NADase), anti-NADase, and antideoxyribonuclease (antiDNAse) B (increased) — to detect streptococcal antibodies
8. Streptozyme — a streptococcal antibody test can be performed in lieu of ASO titer
9. Increased erythrocyte sedimentation rate (ESR) (increased with inflammation)
10. C-reactive protein (increased with inflammation)
11. Throat culture — to diagnose streptococcus
12. Hemoglobin (Hb)
13. White blood count (WBC) (increased with infections)

MEDICATIONS

1. Antibiotics — to treat infections
   a. Penicillin (buffered penicillin G, penicillin V, phenethicillin) — 200,000 to 250,000 units TID or QID by mouth (po) for 10 days
   b. Penicillin G benzathine — 0.6 million units if < 60 pounds; 1.2 million units if > 60 pounds
   c. Erythromycin (used if allergic to penicillin) — 20 mg per pound daily in divided doses for 10 days
   d. Sulfonamides — used for secondary infections
   e. Tetracycline — used for secondary infections
2. Corticosteroids (e.g., prednisone) (2 mg/kg q24 hr po) — used if patient has carditis

3. Aspirin (1.5 g/m^2 q24 hr QID po)—to decrease inflammation

NURSING ASSESSMENT

Refer to "Cardiac Assessment" in Appendix A.

NURSING DIAGNOSES

Activity intolerance
High risk for injury
Pain
Hyperthermia
Decreased cardiac output
Altered family processes
Anxiety
Altered nutrition: less than body requirements
Knowledge deficit

NURSING INTERVENTIONS

1. Conserve energy needs during acute phase of disease.
   a. Maintain bed rest until laboratory results and clinical status improve.
   b. As condition improves, monitor gradual increase in level of activity.
   c. Monitor vital signs q4 hr as needed.
2. Monitor child's response to and possible untoward effects of prescribed medications.
   a. Assess for signs of clinical improvement.
   b. Monitor for side effects of the following medications: aspirin—bleeding tendencies, tinnitus; corticosteroids—cushingoid symptoms, increased weight gain, mood swings, psychotic behavior; antibiotics (penicillin)—allergic rash, anaphylaxis.
3. Provide pain relief measures (for arthralgia).
   a. Minimize handling.
   b. Use bed cradle for sheets.
   c. Maintain proper body alignment.
   d. Administer aspirin.
   e. Change position q2 hr.
4. Implement safety precautions (for chorea and muscle weakness).

       a. Provide bed rest as needed.
       b. Pad siderails.
       c. Assist with ambulation as needed.
       d. Restrain in chair when sitting as needed.
    5. Provide emotional support to child and family.
       a. Encourage parents to ventilate feelings of guilt (may
          have labeled child as "behavior problem"; may feel
          helpless and angry).
       b. Encourage child to share feelings of helplessness,
          shame, and fear regarding manifestations of disease
          (e.g., chorea, carditis, and muscle weakness).
       c. Act as child and family advocate and liaison with
          other members of the team and with hospital organi-
          zation.
       d. Encourage to maintain contact with peers.
       e. Encourage maintenance and involvement in age-
          appropriate recreational and diversional activities.
    6. Support and maintain nutritional status (child may be
       anorexic during acute phase).
       a. Offer small, frequent meals (include fluids).
       b. Incorporate child's food preferences.
       c. Encourage independence in eating when possible
          (muscle weakness may impose limits); choose items
          from menu; arrange foods attractively on tray; ar-
          range meal schedule.
       d. Offer high-quality, nutritious foods.

Home Care

Instruct parents about methods of secondary prevention.
1. Observe for signs and symptoms of recurrence.
2. Administer prophylactic antibiotics (oral administered
   on continuous basis; IM administered once per month)
   and explain rationale for use.
3. Obtain follow-up throat culture 4 or 5 days after oral
   penicillin is discontinued, 3 weeks after IM benzathine
   penicillin is discontinued, and 3 weeks after IM benzathine penicillin G is discontinued.
4. Assist in planning activities if child is to remain in bed
   after hospitalization.
5. Alert dentist about child's condition before any dental care.

BIBLIOGRAPHY

Bernhard R: The mysterious return of acute rheumatic fever, *Emerg Med* 19(20):3, 1987.

DiSciasio G, Taranta M: Rheumatic fever in children, *Am Heart J* 99:635, 1980.

Ferrieri P: Acute rheumatic fever: the comeback of a disappearing disease, *Am J Dis Child* 141(7):725, 1987.

Grimes D, Woolbert L: Facts and fallacies about streptococcal infection and rheumatic fever, *J Pediatr Health Care* 4(4):186, 1990.

Kaplan E: Acute rheumatic fever, *Pediatr Clin North Am* 25(4):817, 1978.

Rultenberg H: Acute rheumatic fever in the 1980's, *Pediatrician* 13(4):180, 1986.

Schulman S, Ayoub E: The control of rheumatic fever, *Clin Pediatr* 14(4):319, 1975.

Schwartz R, Hepner S, Zias M: Incidence of acute rheumatic fever, *Clin Pediatr* 22(12):798, 1983.

63 ❖ Scoliosis

PATHOPHYSIOLOGY

Scoliosis, a frequently occurring orthopedic problem, is the lateral curvature of the spine, which can occur anywhere along the spine. Curvatures in the thoracic area are the most common, although curves of the cervical and lumbar areas are the most deforming. There are two basic types of scoliosis: functional and structural. Functional scoliosis is secondary to a preexisting problem such as poor posture or unequal leg length. This form of scoliosis can be corrected through exercises or the use of shoe lifts. Structural scoliosis results from the congenital deformity of the spinal column. This condition often occurs in children with myelomeningocele and muscular dystrophy. The structural form of scoliosis can be classified into three basic types: (1) infantile, which occurs during the first year of life (more than 20% of patients resolve spontaneously); (2) juvenile, which occurs between 5 and 6 years of age (bracing is used for management); and (3) adolescent, which is not evident until 11 years of age (when skeletal maturation occurs). Management of scoliosis may include nonsurgical and/or surgical methods. Most curvatures do not progress more than 20%. The curvature is flexible initially and becomes rigid with age.

INCIDENCE

1. Familial tendency is noted in one third of diagnosed clients.

2. Male to female occurrence is 1:6.
3. Adolescent scoliosis is the most common form.

CLINICAL MANIFESTATIONS

Localized lordosis, axial rotation, and lateral curvature of the spine are the major clinical manifestations of scoliosis.

1. Shortened trunk
2. Associated skin and soft-tissue changes
3. Patches of hair in sacral area
4. Unequal leg lengths
5. Asymmetrical scapulae
6. Malalignment of trunk and pelvis
7. Asymmetry of shoulders
8. Asymmetry of hips
9. Asymmetry of flanks
10. Asymmetry of breasts

COMPLICATIONS

1. Urinary problems (most common)
2. Neurologic problems
3. Cardiopulmonary impairment

LABORATORY/DIAGNOSTIC TESTS

1. Cobb diagnostic method — to assess angle of curvature
2. Anteroposterior/lateral x-ray studies of spine — to evaluate curvature of spine
3. Intravenous pyelogram (IVP) — to assess presence of urinary problems
4. Myelogram — to assess for neurologic complications
5. Forward bending test — to assess inequality of flank and ribs

MEDICATIONS

Use of pain medications postoperatively depends on the intensity of the pain experience as assessed by the physician, the nurse, and the patient.

NURSING ASSESSMENT

1. Refer to "Skeletal Assessment" in Appendix A.
2. Assess for asymmetry of flank, ribs, scapulae, and hips.
3. Assess for malalignment of trunk and pelvis.

NURSING DIAGNOSES

Impaired physical mobility
High risk for injury
Impaired skin integrity
Fluid volume deficit
Pain
Impaired home maintenance management
Noncompliance
Knowledge deficit
Impaired adjustment
Ineffective individual coping

NONSURGICAL MANAGEMENT TECHNIQUES

1. Milwaukee brace is used for treatment of lateral curvature of 20 to 40 degrees. Brace consists of neck ring and pelvic girdle. It must be worn 23 hours a day until curvature is corrected.
2. Orthoplast jacket is a molded plastic jacket that is used for the same purpose as the Milwaukee brace.

SURGICAL MANAGEMENT

A posterior spinal fusion is the treatment of choice for a spinal curve greater than 40% or for progressive worsening of a curve in spite of nonsurgical treatment. Spinal fusion provides a permanent method of halting the progressive worsening of the spine. Several different types of instrumentation are used to stabilize the spine internally, including the Harrington rod, Luque rod (segmental spinal instrumentation), and Dwyer cables. The Luque rod instrumentation is a more recent and more preferred technique used in the surgical correction of scoliosis. During the surgery bone chips from the posterior iliac crest are positioned on top of the spine. External immobilization with the use of a body cast is then not needed because greater internal immobilization is achieved with this position.

NURSING INTERVENTIONS

Preoperative Care

1. Prepare child and family before procedures for the sequence of events and sensations that will be experienced.

a. Complete blood count (CBC) — to assess for anemia
b. Blood chemistry — to assess for electrolyte imbalances
c. Coagulation studies (prothrombin)
d. X-ray skull study
e. Pulmonary function — to assess for pulmonary complications
f. Arterial blood gas values — to assess for pulmonary complications
g. Myelography — to rule out genitourinary and neurologic abnormalities
h. Spinal x-ray studies — to assess curvature of the spine

2. Provide preoperative preparation to prepare child for surgery.
3. Provide emotional support to parents during hospitalization.
4. Orient child to intensive care unit and treatment procedures used postoperatively (e.g., blow gloves and spirometer).

Postoperative Care

1. Monitor vital signs; report deviations to physician.
   a. Monitor arterial lines.
   b. Monitor temperature, respirations, blood pressure, and pulse q1-2 hr until stable, then q4 hr.
   c. Auscultate breath sounds; report changes in respiratory status (increased respirations, increased congestion, or color change).
2. Monitor for signs and symptoms of potential complications.
   a. Spinal nerve trauma — observe lower extremities for warmth, sensation, movement, pulses, and pain
   b. Pulmonary complications — infections, atelectasis (chest pain, pallor, dyspnea, cyanosis, increased temperature)
   c. Shock caused by bleeding — skin temperature and color, vital signs (increased respirations, increased apical pulse, decreased blood pressure)
   d. Paralytic ileus
3. Monitor dressing for intactness and signs of complications.

   a. Note bleeding along incision.
   b. Monitor for signs of infection.
4. Promote proper body alignment.
   a. Turn q2 hr (log roll only).
   b. Monitor for reddened areas and pressure.
   c. Keep flat in bed until doctor orders activity (flat with log rolling only until body jacket arrives).
   d. Institute passive range of motion (PROM) exercises second postoperative day.
5. Promote pulmonary ventilation.
   a. Monitor vital signs as often as q2 hr.
   b. Cough, turn, and deep breathe as often as q2 hr.
   c. Use incentive spirometer q2 hr.
   d. Monitor respiratory status q2 hr until stable, then q4 hr.
6. Monitor fluid and electrolyte balance.
   a. Monitor and record input and output—intravenous (IV) fluids, urine, nasogastric drainage.
   b. Monitor bowel sounds.
   c. Advance diet as tolerated (clear liquid to regular diet).
   d. Monitor for signs and symptoms of dehydration and fluid overload (dehydration—decreased urinary output, increased specific gravity, doughy skin, dry mucous membranes; fluid overload—increased AP, increased respiratory rate, pulmonary congestion, dyspnea, edema [initially of extremities]).
7. Provide pain relief measures as necessary.
   a. Medicate routinely q2-4 hr for first 72 hours.
   b. Medicate before procedures.
   c. Provide diversional activities and relaxation techniques.

Postoperative Home Care

1. Instruct child and family about various aspects of care (vary according to procedure).
   a. Physical restrictions
   b. Use of body cast or jacket
   c. Equipment (e.g., firm mattress), log rolling technique
   d. Signs of infection (increased temperature, odor from cast)

2. Encourage child and family to ventilate fears, concerns and anxieties, and body image concerns.
3. Refer to community resources (public health nurse, home health nurses).
4. Encourage adherence to follow-up care (clinic visits for 6 to 12 months postoperatively).

Home Care with Nonsurgical Interventions

1. Instruct child or adolescent and parent in use of Milwaukee brace or orthoplast jacket.
   a. Application and removal of brace or jacket
   b. Cleaning of brace or jacket
   c. Skin inspection for pressure sores or skin breakdown
   d. Bathing before application
   e. Use of undergarments
2. Instruct and reinforce child or adolescent and parents in use of exercises.
3. Instruct child or adolescent and parents about participation in sports and recreational activities.
4. Encourage child or adolescent to express feelings of concern and inadequacy concerning brace.
   a. Distortion of body image
   b. Feelings of rejection from peers
5. Initiate community referrals.
   a. School nurse to facilitate school adaptation
   b. Financial assistance to cover costs incurred through treatment of condition
6. Instruct child or adolescent and family about cast care.
   a. Skin care (use alcohol only)
   b. Assessing for sensation and movement
   c. Exercise for unaffected extremities
   d. Assessing for signs of infection (musty odor, drainage on cast)
   e. Petal cast edges

BIBLIOGRAPHY

Allard J, Northrup W: Nursing care: segmental spinal instrumentation—Luque rod instrumentation, *AORN J* 38(1):45, 1983.
Allen B, Ferguson R: Topic of interest in pediatric orthopedics, *Pediatr Clin North Am* 32(5):1333, 1985.

Anderson B, D'ambra P: Symposium of orthopedic nursing: the adolescent patient with scoliosis; a nursing care standard, *Nurs Clin North Am* 11(4):699, 1976.

Block C: Scoliosis: school screening specifics, *School Nurse* 4(2):7, 1988.

deToleda C: The patient with scoliosis: the defect: classification and detection, *Am J Nurs* 79(9):1588, 1979.

Dickson JH: Spinal instrumentation and fusion in adolescent idiopathic scoliosis: indications and surgical techniques, *Contemp Orthop* 4:397, April 1982.

Ferguson RL, Allen Jr BL: Segmental spinal instrumentation for routine scoliotic curve, *Contemp Orthop* 2:450, Sept 1980.

Francis E: Lateral electrical surface stimulation treatment for scoliosis, *Pediatr Nurs* 13(3):157, 1987.

Jacobs-Zachy J et al: Nursing care of adolescents having posterior spinal fusing with Cotrel-Dubousset instrumentation, *Orthop Nurs* 7(1):17, 1988.

Johnson J, Killman Y: Adolescence, anxiety and adaptation: preparing for posterior spine fusion with instrumentation, *J Pediatr Nurs* 3(5):348, 1988.

Luque, ER: Segmental spinal instrumentation for correction of scoliosis. In *Clinical orthopaedics and related research*, Philadelphia, 1982, JB Lippincott.

Poussa M, Harkonen H, Mellin G: Spinal mobility in adolescent girls with idiopathic scoliosis and in structurally normal controls, *Spine* 14(2):217, 1989.

Scoloveno M, Yarcheski A, Mahon E: Scoliosis treatment effects on selected variables among adolescents, *Western J Nurs Res* 12(5):616, 1990.

Weisz I et al: Back shape in brace treatment of idiopathic scoliosis, *Clin Orthop Rel Res* 240:157, 1989.

64 ❖ Seizure Disorders

PATHOPHYSIOLOGY

Seizure refers to a sudden, transient alteration in brain function because of excessive and abnormal neuronal and electrical activity. This activity can be partial, involving a specific area of the cerebral cortex, or generalized, involving both hemispheres of the brain. Clinical manifestations vary, depending on the area(s) of brain involvement. The types of seizures affecting children and adolescents are listed in the box on pp. 404 and 405. Generalized seizures are more common in children between birth and 2 years of age because of central nervous system immaturity. Five percent of the children develop chronically recurring seizures. The mortality rate of infants with seizures is low. Up to 10% of all children experience a single episode of seizure activity by adolescence.

The causes of seizures include perinatal hypoxia, congenital malformations, metabolic disturbances, neurologic damage, maternal drug addiction during pregnancy, toxic influences, vascular disorders, neoplasms, febrile conditions, infections, trauma, and genetic alterations. Structural abnormalities such as atrophy have also been reported. In addition, immunizations, allergies, and immune reactions have been proposed as causative factors. After the age of 3 years, the cause of recurrent seizures is not diagnosed in the majority of children. Most children diagnosed with seizures will respond to treatment and become seizure-free.

Types of Seizures

Generalized Seizures

Generalized tonic—clonic
    Loss of consciousness
    Tonic phase—rigid extension of body, apnea, cyanosis, loss of bladder and bowel control
    Clonic phase—rhythmic jerking movements lasting 1 to 2 minutes or longer
    Sleep and confusion in postictal phase
Absence
    Brief loss of awareness
    Minor muscle twitching may be present
    May be several to hundreds of brief episodes daily
    Onset—3 to 8 years of age
Minor motor—atonic
    Brief loss of muscle tone in head and upper portion of total body
    Frequency varies
    Onset—3 to 8 years of age
Minor motor—myoclonic
    Brief muscle flexor spasms
    Involves head, arm, or trunk
    Frequency varies
Infantile spasms
    Considered a symptom and not a type of seizure
    Brief flexion of neck and trunk. "Jackknife" movements of legs
    Clusters of episodes up to hundreds of times daily
    Characteristic EEG pattern of hyperarrhythmia
    Frequently the child will develop psychomotor impairment and have other types of seizures in childhood
    Onset—3 to 9 months of age

Partial Seizures

Partial Simple
    No loss of consciousness
    Often unilateral
    Localized motor or sensory impairment:
        Twitching of face, hand, or entire side of body

Types of Seizures — cont'd

Tingling, numbness, or altered sensation in a body part

Weakness in muscle group lasting hours to days — frequency varies

Partial Complex

Manifestations vary widely and include the following: staring, lip smacking, eye blinking, chewing, hand movements, purposeless behaviors, confused state, muffled speech

Frequency varies — usually lasts 5 to 10 minutes

Postictal sleep and fatigue

Status Epilepticus

Usually generalized tonic-clonic seizures that are repeated

Child does not regain consciousness between seizures

Potential for respiratory depression, hypotension, and hypoxia

Requires immediate emergency medical treatment

INCIDENCE

1. Epilepsy occurs in approximately 4 million Americans.
2. One percent to 1.5% of the population is affected with a seizure disorder.
3. Incidence is highest in the first year of life and after the age of 55 years.

CLINICAL MANIFESTATIONS

See box on pp. 404 and 405.

LABORATORY/DIAGNOSTIC TESTS

1. Electroencephalogram (EEG) — used to locate seizure foci in the brain through the use of electrodes placed on the scalp. The diagnosis of epilepsy does not depend solely on abnormal EEG findings. Natural sleep is preferred. If sedation is used, chloral hydrate is preferred. If this does

not work, then meperidine (Demerol) and promethazine (Phenergan) is given IM.
2. Computed or computerized tomography (CT scan) — uses x-ray studies to detect differences in tissue radio-density. Using a rotating x-ray source, assessment of tissue densities is developed into a composite three-dimensional picture. The scan can take up to ½ hour to complete. CT scans are used to evaluate trauma, tumors, infections, hydrocephalus, and strokelike syndromes.
3. Lumbar puncture — used primarily to rule out meningitis and bleeding into cerebrospinal fluid (CSF).
4. Evoked potentials — used to determine integrity of sensory pathways in the brain. Scalp electrodes are used to record the response to brief sensory stimuli such as a sound, flash of light, or tap. Absent or delayed response may be indicative of pathology.
5. CT scan — used to rule out trauma.
6. Complete blood count (CBC) — used to rule out infectious process as causative agent.
7. Fasting glucose, serum calcium, phosphorus and lead levels, and metabolic screen — used to rule out metabolic causes for seizure activity.

MEDICATIONS

1. Phenobarbital, an anticonvulsant — limits the spread of seizure activity by increasing the threshold for motor cortex stimuli; dosage — 3 to 5 mg/kg q12 to 24 hr po.
2. Phenytoin (Dilantin), an anticonvulsant — acts to decrease the voltage, frequency, and spread of electrical discharges within the motor cortex, resulting in the decrease of seizure activity; used to control generalized tonic-clonic, partial complex seizures, and nonepileptic seizures; 5 mg/kg is administered as a single dose or divided into two dosages (rarely used in children because of side effects).
3. Carbamazepine (Tegretol), an anticonvulsant — acts to decrease the voltage frequency and spread of electrical discharges within the motor cortex, resulting in the decrease of seizure activity; used to control generalized psychomotor and nonepileptic seizures.

   a. Children 6 to 12 years old—100 mg BID increased to TID maintenance dose—400 to 800 mg qd in divided doses.
   b. Children more than 12 years old—200 mg BID increased to TID maintenance dose—800 to 1200 mg/day.
4. Valproic acid (Depakene), an anticonvulsant—used alone or with other anticonvulsants to control absence and mixed seizures.
   a. Initial dose—15 mg/kg/day BID po; increase every week by 5 to 10 mg/kg/day until seizures controlled or side effects evident
   b. Maximal dose—60 mg/kg/day
5. Primidone (Mysoline), an anticonvulsant—used alone or with other anticonvulsants to control focal, partial complex, and generalized seizures
   a. Children less than 8 years old—125 mg q6-12 hr; increase by 125 mg every week until maximal daily dose of 1 g achieved
   b. Children more than 8 years old—initially 250 mg qd q6-12 hr; increase 250 mg every week until maximal daily dose of 2 g achieved
6. Clonazepam (Clonopin), an anticonvulsant—used to control absence seizures; also used to treat infantile spasms and generalized tonic-clonic convulsions; dosage for children up to 10 years old—0.01 to 0.03 mg/kg/day, not to exceed 0.05 mg/kg/day TID; can be increased in increments of 0.25 to 0.5 mg q3 days to achieve maintenance dose of 0.1 to 0.2 mg/kg/day TID
7. Ethosuximide (Zarontin), an anticonvulsant—depresses impulses to motor cortex and elevates central nervous system (CNS) threshold to stimuli; used in the management of absence seizures; may be used alone or with other anticonvulsants

NURSING ASSESSMENT

1. Refer to "Neuromuscular Assessment" in Appendix A.
2. Refer to box on pp. 404 and 405 for specific types of seizure disorders.

NURSING DIAGNOSES

High risk for suffocation
High risk for trauma
High risk for injury
Body image disturbance
Fear
Knowledge deficit
Altered family processes

NURSING INTERVENTIONS

1. Turn child on side.
   a. Suction mouth as needed to remove secretions and clear airway.
   b. Hold head to side to facilitate drainage of secretions.
2. Protect the child from injury.
   a. Loosen clothing.
   b. Pad siderails of bed.
   c. Lay on ground to avoid falls.
   d. If child is in a chair and safe, leave him or her alone.
   e. Do not put anything in mouth.
3. Observe and record seizure activity.
   a. Time and date of seizure
   b. Aura
   c. Type of seizure activity
   d. Use of medications
   e. Suctioning prn
   f. Level of consciousness (LOC) following seizure
   g. Vital signs (record in some instances as often as q15 min)
4. Provide for sleep, rest, quiet place after seizure.
5. Monitor child's therapeutic and untoward responses to medications.
   a. Phenobarbital — nausea, vomiting, hyperactivity, drowsiness, skin rash, and irritability; cognitive and behavioral effects with continued use in young children
   b. Phenytoin — gingival hypertrophy, drowsiness, ataxia, anemia, nystagmus, malaise, rash, vomiting
   c. Carbamazepine — nausea, vomiting, aplastic anemia, liver toxicity, fever, rash, urinary frequency, or retention

    d. Valproic acid — nausea, reversible alopecia, leukopenia, liver toxicity, weight loss or gain

    e. Primidone — drowsiness, irritability, ataxia

    f. Clonazepam — drowsiness, increased salivation, blood dyscrasias

    g. Trimethadione — nausea, photophobia, nephrosis

    h. Ethosuximide — nausea, vomiting, anorexia, dizziness, hiccups, lupus, blood dyscrasia, liver damage

6. Provide for child's developmental needs during hospitalization.

    a. Encourage use of age-appropriate toys and recreational activities.

    b. Provide association with age-appropriate peers in hospital.

    c. Encourage contact with friends.

    d. Provide age-appropriate roommate.

    e. Encourage academic studies in hospital (e.g., hospital teacher, work from school).

7. Provide an outlet for child's emotional expression; alleviate anxiety of hospitalization.

    a. Provide age-appropriate explanations before procedures.

    b. Provide play therapy.

    c. Explore child's feelings of vulnerability and decreased self-worth.

8. Provide emotional support to parents.

    a. Encourage expression of feelings (e.g., self-blame, anxieties about the child's condition).

    b. Provide parents with explanations of child's condition and treatment.

    c. Provide for physical comforts (e.g., sleeping arrangements, bathing).

Status Epilepticus

1. Maintain patency of airway (see number 1 of previous section).

2. Monitor child's response to oxygen if it is needed.

    a. Color

    b. LOC

3. Have resuscitation equipment ready in case of respiratory depression from medications.

4. Monitor infant's or child's response to medications used to control seizures.

Home Care

1. Instruct parents of importance of taking medications regularly and not abruptly discontinuing treatment.
2. Provide information about anticipatory guidance.
   a. Use of Medic-alert bracelet.
   b. Safety measures (i.e., water safety, heights).
3. Provide information to parents and child about seizure disorder.
   a. Clarify child's and family's knowledge about epilepsy, convulsions, and emotional responses.
   b. Determine underlying fears about the disorder.
   c. Discuss how to deal with seizures when they occur.
   d. Review seizure-triggering mechanisms.
   e. Help them understand process by which healthy self-concept is developed.
   f. Discuss age-appropriate developmental tasks.
4. Refer family to National Epilepsy Foundation for long-term follow-up.
5. Refer family and child for support and counseling as indicated.

BIBLIOGRAPHY

Austin J: Childhood epilepsy: child adaptation and family resources, *J Child Adolesc Psych Ment Health Nurs* 1(1):18, 1988.

Austin J: Comparison of child adaptation to epilepsy and asthma, *J Child Adolesc Psych Ment Health Nurs* 2(4):139, 1989.

Austin J: Predicting parental anticonvalescent medication compliance using the theory of reasoned action, *J Pediatr Nurs* 4(2):88, 1989.

Austin JK, McBride AB, Davis HW: Parental attitude and adjustment to childhood epilepsy, *Nurs Res* 33(2):92, March/April 1984.

Boer HR, Gal P: Neonatal seizures: a survey of current practice, *Clin Pediatr* 21(8):453, 1982.

Chee CM: Seizure disorders, *Nurs Clin North Am* 15(1):71, March 1980.

Esposito N et al: Continuous EEG monitoring in the PICU, *J Pediatr Nurs* 2(4):272, 1987.

Frank J: Epilepsy: the school nurse's dilemma, *J School Health* 60(1):34, 1990.

Kennedy C et al: Post traumatic surgeries and post traumatic epilepsy in children, *J Head Trauma Rehab* 1(4):66, 1986.

Leonard B: The adolescent with epilepsy. In Blum RW ed: *Chronic illness and disabilities in childhood and adolescence,* Orlando, Grune & Stratton.

Martin J: Pediatric management problems . . . epilepsy, *Pediatr Nurs* 16(4):394, 1990.

Parrish MA: A comparison of behavioral side effects related to commonly used anticonvulsants, *Pediatr Nurs* 10(2):149, 1984.

Rogers A, Dykstra C: EEGs: a closer look at a familiar diagnostic test, *J Neurosci Nurs* 21(4):27, 1989.

Sagraves R: Antiepileptic drug therapy for pediatric generalized tonic-clonic seizures, *J Pediatr Health Care* 4(6):314, 1990.

Singer H: Computed tomography in pediatric neurologic disorders, *Pediatr Rev* 2(5):139, 1980.

Tse A: Seizures and societal attitudes: a teaching tool for children, siblings, classmates, parents and classroom teachers, *Issues Compr Pediatr Nurs* 9(5):299, 1986.

Willis JK, Oppenheimer E: Children's seizures and their management, *Issues Compr Pediatr Nurs* 2(2):54, 1977.

65 ❖ Short Bowel Syndrome

PATHOPHYSIOLOGY

Short bowel syndrome refers to the signs and symptoms that result after intestinal resection or because of a congenitally malfunctioning bowel. Short bowel syndrome may result from either congenital or acquired causes (Table 9) and is characterized by chronic diarrhea with impaired absorption of nutrients, vitamins, and fats, leading to malnutrition, anemia, and substantial weight loss. The progression of short bowel syndrome occurs as follows:

Stage 1

1. Irretractable diarrhea with massive fluid and electrolyte loss
2. Gastric acid hypersecretion
3. Decreased secretion of pancreatic lipase, resulting in steatorrhea

Stage 2 (few months to years)

1. Improved functioning because of intestinal adaptation
2. Variable nutrient absorption

Stage 3 (many children do not reach this stage)

1. Maximal adaptation of small intestine
2. Increased oral intake

Table 9. Etiology of Short Bowel Syndrome

Prenatal	Postnatal
Vascular accidents— intestinal atresia (multiple)	Necrotizing enterocolitis
Abdominal wall defects— gastroschisis, ompha- locele	Midgut/segmental volvulus
	Inflammatory bowel disease
Midgut volvulus (as- sociated with malro- tation)	Trauma
	Venous thrombosis
Segmental volvulus (associated with intraabdominal bands, omphalomesenteric duct, etc.)	Arterial thrombosis

From Schwartz M, Maeds K: Short bowel syndrome in infants and children, *Pediatr Clin North Am* 32(5):1265, 1985.

Prognosis is dependent on the three following factors:
1. Length of remaining intestinal segment (at least 30%)
2. Amount and condition of remaining ileum
3. Presence of ileocecal valve (increased transit time and decreased bacterial colonization of small intestine).

Most common cause of death is end-stage liver disease resulting from total parenteral administration.

CLINICAL MANIFESTATIONS

1. Intractable diarrhea
2. Substantial weight loss
3. Anemia
4. Pallor
5. Listlessness
6. Malaise

COMPLICATIONS

1. End-stage liver disease
2. Retarded growth

3. Urinary tract infections
4. Pulmonary infections
5. Cardiovascular problems

LABORATORY/DIAGNOSTIC TESTS

1. Complete blood count (CBC) (increased white blood count [WBC])
2. Serum electrolytes (decreased sodium [Na^+], decreased potassium [K^+])
3. Abdominal x-ray study (distention of small bowel)
4. Mean cell hemoglobin (MCH); mean cell volume (MCV); mean cell hemoglobin concentration (MCHC) (increased because of increased fluid loss)
5. Olein absorption (decreased because of impaired absorption)
6. Urinalysis (increased glucose, increased acetone)
7. Laparotomy (diagnostic)
8. Alkaline phosphatase (to assess liver function)
9. Total bilirubin (to assess liver function)
10. 17-hydroxycorticosteroid (increased adrenocorticosteroid production after surgery)
11. Gastric pH (increased after resection)

MEDICATIONS

1. Anticholinergic drugs (e.g., atropine)—decrease the frequency of contractions of the smooth muscles in the stomach and gastrointestinal (GI) tract; cause decrease in the amount of gastric secretions; dosage—0.01 mg/kg q4-6 hr by mouth (po), intramuscularly (IM), or intravenously (IV)
2. Antacids
   a. Aluminum carbonate gel (Basaljel)—acts by neutralizing gastric acids; reacts with gastric acid to form aluminum phosphate, which is then excreted in the feces; dosage—5 to 10 ml q2 hr po
   b. Aluminum hydroxide gel (Amphojel)—acts by neutralizing gastric acids; reacts with gastric acid to form aluminum chloride; dosage—5 to 10 ml q1-3 hr after meals and at bedtime po
3. Vitamin and mineral supplements

NURSING ASSESSMENT

Refer to "Gastrointestinal Assessment" in Appendix A.

NURSING DIAGNOSES

Fluid volume deficit
High risk for infection
High risk for injury
Altered nutrition: less than body requirements
Altered growth and development
Altered parenting
Knowledge deficit
Altered family processes

NURSING INTERVENTIONS

1. Monitor and support adequate nutritional and fluid intake.
   a. Monitor total parenteral nutrition (TPN) infusion.
   b. Maintain accurate input and output.
   c. Monitor specific gravity, glucose, and acetone as often as q2 hr.
   d. Monitor for signs and symptoms of dehydration — doughy skin, decreased urinary output, dry mucous membranes, and increased specific gravity.
   e. Assess response to gastrostomy and oral feedings.
2. Monitor and report signs of complications.
   a. Infection (pulmonary or urinary tract infection)
   b. Cardiovascular problems (caused by fluid overload and electrolyte imbalances)
3. Monitor and report signs of electrolyte imbalances.
   a. Calcium
   b. Magnesium
   c. Phosphate
   d. Sodium
   e. Potassium
4. Monitor child's therapeutic and untoward responses to medications, antacids, and anticholinergics.
5. Provide for child's developmental needs during hospitalization.
   a. Encourage use of age-appropriate toys and recreational activities.

    b. Encourage rooming-in of parents (for infants, toddlers, and preschoolers).
    c. Provide consistent one-to-one nursing care to ensure consistency of care and sense of trust.
    d. Encourage contact with age-appropriate peers in hospital.
    e. Encourage contact with friends.
    f. Encourage pursuit of academic studies in hospital (e.g., hospital teacher, work from school).
    g. Provide age-appropriate roommate.
6. Provide emotional support to parents.
    a. Encourage expression of feelings — self-blame, anxieties over child's condition.
    b. Provide parents with explanations of child's condition and treatment.
    c. Provide for parents' physical comforts (e.g., sleeping arrangements, bathing).

Home Care

1. Instruct parents about administration of TPN.
2. Encourage parents to ventilate feelings about their child's condition and changes in lifestyle.
3. Encourage parents to communicate with child about the following:
    a. Concerns about body image
    b. Focus of mutilation
    c. Feelings of inferiority
    d. Sibling and peer relationships
4. Discuss with parents strategies to normalize child's life.
    a. Peer friendships
    b. Schooling
    c. Social and group activities
    d. Play activities

BIBLIOGRAPHY

Conn J, Chanlz C, Faen W: The short bowel syndrome, *Ann Surg* 175(6):803, 1972.

Rossi R: Endoscopic examination of the colon in infancy and childhood, *Pediatr Clin North Am* 35:331, 1989.

Schwartz M, Maeds K: Short bowel syndrome in infants and children, *Pediatr Clin North Am* 32(5):1265, 1985.

Thompson J: The current status of surgical therapy for the short bowel syndrome, *Contemp Surg* 33(12):27, 1988.

Weser E: Nutritional aspects of malabsorption: short gut adaptation, *Am J Med* 67:1014, 1979.

66 ❖ Sickle Cell Anemia

PATHOPHYSIOLOGY

Sickle cell anemia, or homozygous sickle cell disease (Hb SS), is an inherited autosomal recessive disorder. The basic defect is a mutant autosomal gene that effects a substitution of valine for glutamic acid on the hemoglobin chain. The result is a person with the disease or with sickle cell trait (heterozygous gene Hb AS). Sickled red blood cells are crescent shaped, have decreased oxygen-carrying capacity, and have a greater destruction rate than do normal red blood cells. In addition, the life span of sickled cells is diminished to 30 to 40 days. Sickle cells are extremely rigid because of the gelled hemoglobin, cellular dehydration, and an inflexible membrane. The rigid cells become trapped in the circulatory system, leading to a vicious cycle of infarction and progressive sickling.

Splenic hypofunction and, later, splenic atrophy result in reticuloendothelial failure and a 600-times-greater incidence of infection in children with sickle cell disease than in the normal population. Red blood cells with Hb S increase after the child is 6 months of age, resulting in chronic anemia.

Sickle cell crises result from physiologic changes that result in a decrease in oxygen available to the hemoglobin. Sickling of cells results in clumping of red blood cells in the vessels, decreased oxygen transport, and increased destruction of red blood cells (erythropoiesis). Ischemia, infarcts,

Early Detection: Newborn Screening Programs

Morbidity and mortality can be significantly reduced with newborn screening and early intervention.

Screening should include both prenatal maternal and neonatal screening.

Public education is critical for effective neonatal screening. Target groups include day care centers, schools, and the media.

and tissue necrosis result from the obstruction of vessels and decreased blood flow. Three types of crises occur: (1) vasoocclusive (painful); (2) splenic sequestration; and (3) aplastic. Sickle cell crises occur less frequently with age. Mortality in the first years of life is usually caused by infection and sequestration crisis.

INCIDENCE

1. Incidence of sickle cell disease among blacks is estimated at 1 in 400.
2. Sickle cell trait occurs in one of every 10 black Americans.
3. Twenty-five percent of deaths occur before age 5 years.
4. Approximately 50% of patients survive to the age of 40, and many live into their 50s and 60s.

CLINICAL MANIFESTATIONS

1. Vasoocclusive crisis (painful crisis)
   a. Irritability
   b. Vomiting
   c. Fever
   d. Anorexia
   e. Pain in joints
   f. Dactylitis (hand-and-foot syndrome) — range of motion decreased and extremities inflamed
   g. Leg ulcers
   h. Cerebrovascular accidents (CVA)
   i. Ocular hemorrhages

    j. Proliferative retinopathy
    k. Ischemia in tissues distal to occlusion, resulting in a variety of signs and symptoms such as hemiplegia or stroke
2. Sequestration crisis (usually seen in children less than 5 years old)
    a. Rapid enlargement of spleen (splenomegaly)
    b. Rapid fall in hemoglobin level
    c. Enlargement of liver
    d. Circulatory collapse and shock
    e. Tachycardia, dyspnea, pallor, and weakness (common)
3. Aplastic crisis resulting from rapid destruction of red blood cells
    a. Weakness
    b. Pallor of mucous membranes
    c. Scleral icterus
    d. Anorexia
    e. Increased susceptibility to infection
    f. Tachycardia
    g. Decreased reticulocyte count

COMPLICATIONS

1. Sleep loss
2. Delayed onset of puberty
3. Impaired fertility
4. Priapism
5. Gallstones
6. Leg ulcers
7. Chronic heart, liver, and kidney disease
8. Osteomyelitis
9. Depression, isolation, and low self-esteem
10. Enuresis
11. High risk for drug addiction
12. Strained parent-child relationships

LABORATORY/DIAGNOSTIC TESTS

1. Cellulose acetate followed by citrate agar electrophoresis
2. Isoelectric focusing
3. High-pressure liquid chromatography on cord blood or dried heel-stick blood spot

MEDICATIONS

Analgesics are used to control pain during a crisis period.

NURSING ASSESSMENT

Refer to "Cardiovascular Assessment" and "Respiratory Assessment" in Appendix A.

NURSING DIAGNOSES

Impaired gas exchange
Activity intolerance
Altered tissue perfusion: renal, cerebral, and peripheral
Pain
High risk for infection
High risk for injury
Altered growth and development
Ineffective family coping: compromised
Knowledge deficit

NURSING INTERVENTIONS

1. Prevent or minimize effects of sickle cell crisis.
   a. Early assessment and intervention of crisis episode are *keys* to prevention of morbidity and mortality.
   b. Avoid cold and vasoconstriction during pain episode; cold promotes sickling.
   c. Keep well-hydrated; dehydration increases risk of sickling.
2. Provide and promote hydration and fluid and electrolyte balance.
   a. Maintain strict input and output.
   b. Assess for signs of dehydration.
      (1) Elevated temperature
      (2) Poor skin turgor
      (3) Dry mucous membrane
      (4) Decreased urine output
      (5) Increased specific gravity
      (6) Tachycardia
   c. Provide fluids one-and-one-half to two times normal maintenance rate; calculate as follows:
      (1) 0 to 10 kg at 100 ml/kg
      (2) 11 to 20 kg at 50 ml/kg
      (3) 21 kg and up at 20 ml/kg

3. Prevent infection.
   a. Assess for signs of infection.
      (1) Fever
      (2) Malaise or irritability
      (3) Inflamed and swollen soft tissue and lymph nodes
   b. Patients are particularly susceptible to pneumococcal sepsis and pneumonia, and salmonella osteomyelitis.
4. Promote oxygenation of tissues.
   a. Monitor for signs of hypoxia.
      (1) Cyanosis
      (2) Hyperventilation
      (3) Increased apical pulse, increased respiratory rate, and increased blood pressure
      (4) Cyanosis
      (5) Mental confusion
   b. Provide frequent rest periods to decrease oxygen expenditure.
   c. Monitor use of oxygen equipment.
      (1) Flow rate
      (2) Humidification of oxygen
      (3) Tubing, masks, and nasal cannula
5. Monitor for signs of complications.
   a. Vascular collapse and shock
   b. Splenomegaly
   c. Bone and joint infarction
   d. Leg ulcers
   e. Strokes
   f. Blindness
   g. Chest pain or dyspnea
   h. Delay in growth and development
6. Administer and monitor use of blood products.
   a. Assess for signs of transfusion reactions.
      (1) Fever
      (2) Restlessness
      (3) Cardiac dysrhythmias
      (4) Chills and shaking
      (5) Nausea and vomiting
      (6) Chest pain
      (7) Red or black urine
      (8) Headache
      (9) Flank pain
      (10) Signs of shock or renal failure

    b. Monitor for signs of circulatory overload.
      (1) Dyspnea
      (2) Increased respiratory rate
      (3) Cyanosis
      (4) Chest pain
      (5) Dry cough
7. Provide age-appropriate explanation to the child about hospitalization and procedures.
8. Provide emotional support to child and family.
    a. Encourage ventilation of feelings.
    b. Encourage performance of normal activities.
    c. Encourage use of preexisting support systems.
    d. Encourage networking with other children and families who have sickle cell anemia.
9. Instruct parents to screen their family members.
    a. Newborn screening for hemoglobinopathies
      (1) Identification at birth makes possible early prophylaxis against infections.
      (2) Use of prophylactic penicillin is recommended beginning in the newborn period (4 months).
    b. Screening of siblings for disease and trait

Home Care/Discharge Planning

1. Counsel child to prevent hypoxia resulting from strenuous physical exertion.
2. Provide genetic counseling.
3. Provide parent teaching and anticipatory guidance to ensure that the child is seen by a physician at the first signs of illness.
4. Provide parent teaching and anticipatory guidance about the prevention of infections and excessive life stress.
5. Provide parents with information about routine immunization as well as *Haemophilus influenzae* B vaccine (18 months) and *Streptococcus pneumoniae* vaccine at 2 years of age.

BIBLIOGRAPHY

Consensus Conference: Newborn screening for sickle cell disease and other hemoglobinopathies, *JAMA* 258(9):1205, 1989.

Feance E, Dawson J: Sickle cell disease: implications for nursing care, *J Adv Nurs* 11(6):729, 1986.

Gaston M et al: Prophylaxis with oral penicillin in children with sickle cell anemia, *N Engl J Med* 25(314):1593, 1986.

Goldberg MA et al: Treatment of sickle cell anemia with hydroxyurea and erythropoietin, *N Engl J Med* 323(6):366, 1990.

Gradolf B: Sickle cell anemia in children, *Iss Compr Pediatr Nurs* 6(5/6):295, 1983.

Ives T et al: Constant morphine infusion for severe sickle cell crisis pain, *Drug Intell Clin Pharm* 21(7/8):625, 1987.

Leikin SL et al: Mortality in children and adolescents with sickle cell disease, *Pediatrics* 84(3):500, 1989.

Savitt TL, Goldberg MF: Herrick's 1910 case report of sickle cell anemia: the rest of the story, *JAMA* 261(2):266, 1989.

Schecter NL, Berrien FB, Katz SM: PCA for adolescents in sickle cell crisis, *Am J Nurs* 719, 1988.

Thomas R et al: Sickle cell disease, ways to reduce morbidity and mortality, *Postgrad Med* 81(5):265, 1987.

67 ❖ Spina Bifida

PATHOPHYSIOLOGY

There are two distinct types of failure of fusion of the vertebral laminae of the spinal column: spina bifida occulta and spina bifida cystica.

Spina bifida occulta is a defect in closure in which the meninges are not exposed on the surface of the skin. The vertebral defect is small, usually involving the lumbosacral region. External abnormalities (present in 50% of cases) may include a hair tuft, nevus, or hemangioma. A pilonidal sinus may require surgical closure if it becomes infected.

Spina bifida cystica is a defect in closure that results in protrusion of the spinal cord and/or its coverings. *Meningocele* is a protrusion that includes the meninges and a sac containing cerebrospinal fluid (CSF); it is covered by normal skin. No neurologic abnormalities are present, and the spinal cord is not involved. Hydrocephalus occurs in 20% of cases. A meningocele usually is in the lumbosacral or sacral area.

Myelomeningocele is a protrusion of the meninges and a portion of the spinal cord, as well as a sac containing CSF. Eighty percent occur in the lumbar or lumbosacral area. Infants with a myelomeningocele are prone to injury during the birth process. Hydrocephalus occurs in most children (85% to 90%), and 60% to 70% have a normal intelligence quotient.

The specific cause of spina bifida is unknown. Multiple factors such as heredity and environment are thought to interact to produce these defects. The neural tube is normally complete 4 weeks after conception. The proposal that vitamin deficiency in the mother is a causative factor remains theoretical.

Advances in the use of medications and neurosurgery have resulted in increasing numbers of children with spina bifida surviving to adolescence and young adulthood. Diminished self-esteem is characteristically common to children and adolescents with this condition. Adolescents express concerns about sexual adequacy, social mastery, peer relationships, and physical maturity and attractiveness. The severity of disability is more directly related to *self-perception* of the disability rather than to the actual disability of the adolescent.

Surgical Management: Myelomeningocele or Meningocele

Surgical repair is performed in the neonatal period to prevent rupture. Surgical repair of the spinal lesion and shunting of CSF in infants with hydrocephalus is performed at birth. Skin grafting is necessary if the lesion is large. Prophylactic antibiotics are administered to prevent meningitis. Nursing interventions will depend on the presence and extent of dysfunction of various body systems.

INCIDENCE

1. The highest number of cases is in Great Britain.
2. In the United States, the incidence of spina bifida cystica is estimated at 1 in 1000 live births.
3. Spina bifida occulta is detectable with x-ray studies in almost 50% of normal children.
4. The risk of having a second child with this disorder increases to one in 20 to 50.

CLINICAL MANIFESTATIONS

Varying degrees of dysfunction result from spina bifida, depending on the portion of the spinal cord involved.

1. Motor, sensory, reflex, and sphincter abnormalities— may result in varying degrees
2. Flaccid paralysis of legs; loss of sensation and reflexes

3. Spasticity
4. Lower-limb deformities because of muscle imbalance
5. Dislocation of hip
6. Scoliosis
7. Loss of sensation in the extremities
8. Bladder and bowel functions — vary from normal to ineffective
9. Vasoconstriction of lower limbs — caused by depression of sympathetic activity
10. A variety of related congenital malformations — skeletal anomalies and hydrocephalus

COMPLICATIONS

Birth-related complications of spina bifida include the following:

1. Cerebral palsy
2. Mental retardation
3. Optic atrophy
4. Epilepsy
5. Osteoporosis
6. Fractures (caused by decreased muscle mass)
7. Painless ulcerations, injuries, decubiti

LABORATORY/DIAGNOSTIC TESTS

1. Complete blood count (CBC) — routine preoperative testing
2. Urinalysis — routine preoperative testing
3. Culture and sensitivity (C and S) — to detect presence of microorganisms (i.e., in throat/pharynx, urine, stool)
4. Blood chemistry — to assess serum electrolytes
5. Type and cross match — for blood typing in case blood is needed during surgery
6. Chest x-ray examination — routine preoperative testing

MEDICATIONS

1. Antibiotics — used prophylactically to prevent urinary tract infections (selection depends on C and S)
2. Cholinergics — used to increase bladder tone
3. Antispasmodics — used to decrease hypertonic bladder
4. Stool softeners and laxatives — used for bowel training and evacuation of stool

NURSING ASSESSMENT

Refer to "Neuromuscular Assessment" in Appendix A.

NURSING DIAGNOSES

Impaired physical mobility
High risk for infection
High risk for injury
Urinary incontinence and reflex
Altered bowel elimination
Impaired skin integrity
Body image disturbance
Altered sexuality patterns
Altered family processes
Altered growth and development
Altered nutrition: more than body requirements

NURSING INTERVENTIONS

Preoperative Care

1. Encourage parental expression of grief over loss of "perfect" child.
   a. Feelings related to guilt, self-blame
   b. Feelings of anger about child's condition
   c. Feelings of inadequacy for procreating the infant
   d. Feelings of being overwhelmed with the situation and the unknown
2. Provide emotional support to parents.
   a. Encourage expression of feelings.
   b. Provide and reinforce information given to parents.
   c. Encourage use of preexisting supports.
   d. Provide for physical comforts (e.g., sleeping arrangements and bathing).
3. Monitor infant's vital signs and neurologic status.
   a. Temperature, apical pulse, respiratory rate, and blood pressure as often as q2 hr
   b. Neurologic assessment (see "Neuromuscular Assessment" in Appendix A)
4. Promote preoperative fluid and nutritional status.
   a. Monitor for dehydration or fluid overload.
   b. Monitor administration of maintenance fluids (by mouth [po] or intravenously [IV]).

   c. Monitor and record input and output.

   d. Record daily weight.

5. Maintain integrity of defect; prevent further injury.

   a. Monitor for signs and symptoms of infection—fever, drainage, odor, swelling, and redness.

   b. Maintain child in prone position.

   c. Maintain sterility of dressing.

6. Prepare parents and infant for surgery.

   a. Infant

     (1) Obtain laboratory specimens before surgery.

     (2) Allow nothing by mouth (NPO) after midnight before surgery.

     (3) Refer to institutional manual for specific guidelines.

   b. Parents

     (1) Provide and reinforce information about surgery and procedures.

     (2) Encourage parents to room-in.

     (3) Encourage incorporation of some home routines into hospital experience.

Postoperative Care

1. Maintain nutritional and fluid intake.

   a. Assess for signs of dehydration or fluid overload.

   b. Monitor for bowel sounds.

   c. Monitor administration of IV fluids.

   d. Monitor and record input and output.

   e. Record daily weight.

2. Monitor for signs and symptoms of infections.

   a. Fever (obtain C and S when infant is febrile)

   b. Drainage from surgical site

   c. Redness and inflammation

3. Promote healing of surgical site; use sterile technique when changing and reinforcing dressing.

4. Monitor vital signs and neurologic status.

   a. Monitor temperature, pulse, respirations, and blood pressure.

   b. Perform neurologic assessment (see "Neuromuscular Assessment" in Appendix A.)

   c. Monitor head circumference.

5. Provide emotional support to parents.
   a. Provide teaching to parent to decrease anxiety about holding child and to clarify misconceptions.
   b. Provide explanations to parents before treatments and tests.

Home Care

1. Instruct parents about long-term management of bowel and bladder training.
   a. Bladder training
      (1) Use of Credé's method
      (2) Self-catheterization of child
      (3) Ileal conduit as last resort
   b. Bowel training
      (1) Regular intervals on the toilet after meals
      (2) Dietary adjustment
      (3) Use of enemas, laxatives, suppositories, and daily digital evacuation.
2. Provide teaching to parent and child about the following:
   a. Prevention of decubiti, increasing range of motion (ROM) and mobility, and importance of skin care
   b. Prevention of bladder infections
   c. Modification of diet for bladder control
3. Provide information to parent and child about techniques to facilitate mobility and independence.
   a. Use of braces, specific devices, and weight bearing (encouraged not only to provide mobility and independence but also to prevent osteoporosis and contractures)
   b. Use of wheelchairs
   c. Physical therapy and ROM exercises
4. Provide education to parents about normal growth and development and deviations from the norm.
   a. Call attention to the special problems and needs of the handicapped child.
   b. Act as liaison with parents, teachers, and school to establish developmentally and intellectually appropriate expectations.
5. Instruct adolescents and provide information about the following areas of concern:

   a. Sexual counseling (based on evaluation of genital re-
      sponsiveness)
   b. Vocational counseling and weight control mea-
      sures prn

BIBLIOGRAPHY

Alexander M, Steg N: Myelomeningocele: comprehensive treat-
    ment, *Archiv Phys Med Rehabil* 70(8):637, 1989.
Blum R: The adolescent with spina bifida, *Clin Pediatr* 22(5):331,
    1983.
Brown J: A practical approach to teaching self-catheterization to
    children with myelomeningocele, *J Enterost Ther* 17(2):54, 1990.
DiConden M: Pediatric rehabilitation: special patients, special
    needs, *J Rehabil* 56(3):13, 1990.
Dimmock W: An approach to bladder and bowel management in
    children with spina bifida, *Am Urolog Assoc Allied J* 8(4):9, 1987.
Erickson D: Mental functioning of infants with spina bifida in the
    Bayley scales of infant development, *Canad J Rehabil* 3(3):159,
    1990.
Feldman WS, Varni JW: Conceptualizations of health and illness by
    children with spina bifida, *Child Health Care* 13(3):102, 1985.
Hambley J et al: Assessing the need for management of the neuro-
    genic bowel in a pediatric population, *Canad J Rehabil* 3(1):17,
    1989.
Macedo A et al: Nursing the family after the birth of a child with
    spina bifida, *Issues Compr Pediatr Nurs* 10(1):55, 1987.
McAndres I: Adolescents and young people with spina bifida, *Dev
    Med Child Neurol* 21:619, 1979.
Rauen K: Documentation of the nursing process in an outpatient
    clinic, *J Nurs Qual Assur* 4(4):55, 1990.
Shaw N: Common surgical problems in the newborn, *J Perinat
    Neonat Nurs* 3(3):50, 1990.
Smith K: Bowel and bladder management of the child with my-
    elomeningocele in the school setting, *J Pediatr Health Care*
    4(4):175, 1990.
Ziviani J, Hayes A, Chant D: Handwriting: a perceptual-motor
    disturbance in children with myelomeningocele, *Occup Ther J Res*
    10(1):12, 1990.

68 ❖ Sudden Infant Death Syndrome

PATHOPHYSIOLOGY

Sudden infant death syndrome (SIDS) refers to the sudden and unexpected death of an infant for unexplained reasons as demonstrated by autopsy. The following autopsy findings have been reported: (1) pulmonary edema and congestion; (2) petechiae on the pleura, pericardium, and thymus (85% of cases); (3) delayed myelinization of several tracts; (4) absence of lethal trauma and malformation; (5) normal to near-normal nutritional status; and (6) symptoms of chronic hypoxemia—retained brown fat, bone marrow hyperplasia, cor pulmonale, brainstem changes, hepatic erythropoiesis, and increased muscle in small pulmonary arteries. One third of infants do not exhibit abnormalities on autopsy. Risk factors associated with the incidence of SIDS are listed in the box on p. 433.

Many explanations have been offered to account for SIDS (none are conclusive):

1. Airway obstruction caused by anatomic and developmental factors
2. Abnormality in cardiorespiratory control
3. Abnormal oropharyngeal neuromuscular control, causing airway obstruction
4. Hyperactive airway reflexes
5. Posterior displacement of tongue
6. Abnormality in autonomic nervous system

Risk Factors Associated with SIDS

Infant

Prematurity
Low birth weight for gestational age
History of apnea
Nonwhite
Neonatal intensive care unit (NICU) graduate
More males than females
Mild respiratory tract infection in 40% to 75% of infants during week preceding SIDS

Familial

Lower socioeconomic status
History of sibling with SIDS (20 in 1000)
Twin or triplet birth

Maternal

Young, unmarried mother <20 years old
History of smoking
History of narcotic ingestion
Anemia
Second or third pregnancy
Unexpected drop of 20 to 60 mm Hg in diastolic blood pressure during third trimester
Methadone addiction (10 times greater risk for SIDS)
Short intergestational interval

---

7. Possible increase in sympathetic nervous activity
8. Muscle tone abnormality (shoulder hypotonia)
9. Physiologic handicaps before birth

INCIDENCE

1. Most common manner of death during the first year after the neonatal period
2. Peak incidence—2 to 3 months; rarely occurs before 2 weeks of age or after 6 months of age
3. Seasonal occurrence—winter

4. Most frequent occurrence of death—between midnight and 9 AM
5. Ethnic distribution (according to incidence rates per live birth)—1.3 in 1000 whites; 1.7 in 1000 Hispanics; 0.5 in 1000 Asians; 2.9 in 1000 blacks
6. Worldwide incidence (varies)—0.3 to 3.0 per 1000 live births
7. Accounts for an estimated 7000 to 10,000 infant deaths per year
8. Apparent life-threatening event (ALTE)—the child is found limp, blue, and unresponsive and needs resuscitation. The link to SIDS is unknown and not well-defined; the child experiencing ALTE is thought to be at slightly greater risk for SIDS, but this needs to be empirically validated.

Parental Response After SIDS

1. Acute grief—acute somatic distress, shortness of breath, choking sensation, sighing, depression, crying, and social isolation
2. Chronic grief—constellation of bereavement behaviors
3. Placing guilt and blame (may feel responsible for death)

LABORATORY/DIAGNOSTIC TESTS (ALTE)

Preventive Care

1. Blood chemistries (electrolytes, serum glucose, phosphorus [P], magnesium [Mg], and blood urea nitrogen [BUN]—assess for metabolic abnormalities)
2. Arterial blood gas (ABG) values—to assess respiratory status and determine abnormal ventilatory drive
3. Chest x-ray study—to assess presence of upper respiratory infection (present in 40% to 75% of SIDS victims)
4. 12-lead electrocardiogram (ECG)—to detect presence of arrhythmias (e.g., bradycardia caused by apnea)
5. Upper gastrointestinal study—to detect reflex apnea
6. Apnea monitor—to detect periods of apnea
7. 12- to 24-hour ECG monitoring (rhythm analysis)

After Death

An autopsy is performed to confirm the diagnosis of SIDS.

NURSING INTERVENTIONS

Refer to "Respiratory Assessment" in Appendix A.

NURSING DIAGNOSES

Dysfunctional grieving
Altered family processes

NURSING INTERVENTIONS

Prevention

1. Assess ability of family members to participate in in-home apnea monitoring program (a controversial practice—American Academy of Pediatrics does not support this practice). Monitoring does not prevent SIDS.
2. Provide psychosocial referral, when appropriate, to strengthen family's adaptive responses.
3. Refer family to appropriate community-based support group.

After SIDS

1. Support family during acute grieving period.
   a. Encourage parents to provide permission for autopsy to confirm SIDS diagnosis as a means to alleviate guilt because they may feel "responsible" for death.
   b. Counsel and reassure parents that they are not responsible for the infant's death.
   c. Encourage parents to express feelings of guilt and remorse.
2. During bereavement period, refer family to appropriate resources to deal with issues such as infertility during first year after SIDS, miscarriage during first year after SIDS, and chronic grief.
   a. National Sudden Infant Death Syndrome Foundation
      10500 Little Patuxent Parkway
      Suite 420
      Columbia, MD 21044
      1-800-638-7437
   b. Council of Guilds for Infant Survival (has 12 guilds in seven states)
      PO Box 3586
      Davenport, IA 52808
      (319)322-4870

BIBLIOGRAPHY

Andrews M et al: Home apnea monitoring in the intermountain west, *J Pediatr Health Care* 1(5):255, 1987.

Bultreys M: High incidence of sudden infant death syndrome among Northern Indians and Alaska natives compared to Southwestern Indians: possible role of smoking, *J Commun Health* 15(3):185, 1990.

Chan M: Sudden infant death syndrome and families at risk, *Pediatr Nurs* 13(3):166, 1987.

Davis N, Sweeney L: Infantile apnea monitoring and SIDS, *J Pediatr Health Care* 3(2): 67, 1989.

Deal J, Bordeaux S: The phenomenon of SIDS, *Pediatr Nurs* 6(1):48, 1980.

Grether J, Schulman J, Croen L: Sudden infant death syndrome among Asians in California, *J Pediatr* 116(4):525, 1990.

Guntheroth W, Lohmann R, Spiers S: Risk of sudden infant death syndrome in subsequent siblings, *J Pediatr* 116(4):520, 1990.

Haglund B, Crattingius S: Cigarette smoking as a risk factor for sudden infant death syndrome: a population based study, *Am J Publ Health* 80(1):29, 1990.

Herbst J et al: When sudden infant death strikes, *Patient Care* 18:18, 1984.

Paige P: Noninvasive monitoring of the neonatal respiratory system, *AACN: Clinic Issues in Critic Care Nurs* 1(2):409, 1990.

Swoiskin S: Sudden infant death: nursing care for the survivors, *J Pediatr Nurs* 1(1):33, 1986.

Valdes-Depana M: Sudden infant death syndrome: a review of the medical literature 1974-1979, *Pediatrics* 66:597, 1980.

69 ❖ Tetralogy of Fallot

PATHOPHYSIOLOGY

Tetralogy of Fallot is a cyanotic congenital heart defect comprising four structural defects, resulting in decreased pulmonary blood flow (approximately one fourth to one third less systemic circulation) and hypertrophy of the right ventricle. This defect includes (1) a ventricular septal defect; (2) pulmonic stenosis, which may be infundibular, valvular, supravalvular, or a combination of them, causing obstruction of the blood flow into the pulmonary arteries; (3) right-ventricular hypertrophy; and (4) varying degrees of overriding of the aorta. The ventricular septal defect is invariably large. In patients with tetralogy of Fallot, the diameter of the aorta is larger than normal, whereas the pulmonary artery is smaller than normal. Congestive heart failure (CHF) rarely occurs because the chamber pressures of the right and left ventricles are equal because of the septal defect. Hypoxia is the primary problem. The degree of cyanosis is related to the severity of the anatomic obstruction to the blood flow from the right ventricle into the pulmonary artery, as well as to the physiologic status of the patient.

Most children with tetralogy of Fallot are candidates for surgical repair, which can be performed at any age but is usually performed when the child is 1 to 4 years old. Shunt procedures may be performed before total correction as palliative measures to correct hypoxia secondary to inadequate pulmonary flow. Blalock-Taussig and Waterston-Cooley are examples of preliminary shunt procedures. Surgical correction is indicated for children with severe hypoxia and polycythemia (hematocrit [Hct] greater than 60%). Surgical risk is associated with the size of the diameter of the pulmonary arteries; risk is less than 10% if the diameter of the pulmonary arteries is at least one third of the size of the aortic diameter.

SURGICAL MANAGEMENT

Palliative Measures

Blalock-Taussig anastomosis. A Blalock-Taussig subclavian-pulmonary anastomosis is the palliative intervention generally recommended for children who are unsuitable for corrective surgery with tetralogy of Fallot, pulmonary atresia with an intact ventricular septum, or transposition of the great arteries and tricuspid atresia. The subclavian artery opposite the side of the aortic arch is ligated, divided, and anastomosed to the contralateral pulmonary artery. The advantage of this shunt is the ability to construct very small shunts, which grow with the child, and it is easy to remove during definitive repair. The modified Blalock-Taussig anastomosis is essentially the same, but using a prosthetic material, usually polytetrafluoroethylene. In this shunt, the size can be better controlled, and it is easier to remove since most complete repairs are performed at a young age.

The hemodynamic consequence of the Blalock-Taussig shunt is to allow systemic blood to enter the pulmonary circulation through the subclavian artery, increasing pulmonary blood flow under low pressure, thus avoiding pulmonary congestion. This blood flow allows stabilization of the cardiac and respiratory status until the child grows enough for corrective surgery to be safe. Collateral circulation will develop to ensure adequate arterial flow to the arm, although a blood pressure will not be obtainable in that arm.

Waterston-Cooley anastomosis. Waterston-Cooley anastomosis is a palliative procedure used for infants with defects associated with decreased pulmonary blood flow, such as tetralogy of Fallot, pulmonary atresia with intact ventricular septum, or transposition of the great arteries when their anatomy is unsuitable for a Blalock-Taussig anastomosis. It is a closed-heart surgery in which the posterior ascending aorta is sewn directly to the anterior of the right pulmonary artery, creating a fistula. Although this shunt is difficult to remove during definitive repair, it has generally replaced the Potts-Smith-Gibson, or Potts, anastomosis, which is a side-to-side shunt between the descending aorta and left pulmonary artery, because it is technically the easiest to create.

The desired hemodynamic response is for the blood from the aorta to flow into the pulmonary artery and thus increase the pulmonary blood flow. This procedure should relieve anoxia, cyanosis, and clubbing. A machine-type murmur is produced.

Definitive Repair

Complete repair of tetralogy of Fallot used to be postponed until the preschool years but now can be safely accomplished when the child is 1 to 2 years old. Indications for surgery at a young age include severe polycythemia (hematocrit greater than 60%), hypercyanotic ("tet") spells, hypoxia, and decreased quality of life. A median sternotomy incision is performed, and bypass is used, with deep hypothermia added for some infants. If a previous shunt is in place, it is removed. Unless the repair cannot be completed through the right atrium, a right ventriculotomy is avoided because of the importance of the ventricles as a pumping chamber. Any right-ventricular outflow obstruction is resected and widened, using Dacron with pericardial backing, being careful to avoid pulmonary insufficiency. The pulmonary valve is incised. The ventricular septal defect is closed with a Dacron patch to complete the operation. Performing a Rastelli procedure might be necessary in cases of severe right-ventricular outflow tract obstruction. The desired response to surgery should be a heart with normal hemodynamics that depend on the correction.

INCIDENCE

1. Tetralogy of Fallot affects males and females equally.
2. There is a higher prevalence with older maternal age.

3. Few patients survive beyond 20 years without surgery.
4. Tetralogy of Fallot accounts for 10% of all congenital defects.
5. It accounts for 50% of individuals with an inoperative congenital heart defect with decreased pulmonary blood flow beyond infancy.
6. It accounts for three of four children with heart disease with decreased pulmonary blood flow after age 4.
7. There is a 5% mortality rate (slightly higher in infants) for patients who undergo cardiac repair.
8. Ten percent of survivors have unsatisfactory results.
9. The mortality rate for patients with shunts is 10%.

CLINICAL MANIFESTATIONS

1. Cyanosis—appears after several months of age; rarely seen at birth; becomes progressively more severe; varies from deep-purple to undetectable desaturation
2. Paroxysmal hyperpnea (hypercyanotic spells)
   a. Increased rate and depth of respiration
   b. Increased cyanosis, which can progress to limpness and syncope and ultimately result in seizures, cardiovascular accident (CVA), and death (occurs in 35% of cases)
3. Clubbing evident (subtle to pronounced)
4. Initially normal blood pressure—can increase after several years of marked cyanosis and polycythemia
5. Assumes squatting position—decreases venous return from lower extremities and increases pulmonary blood flow and systemic arterial oxygenation
6. Undernourished and underweight
7. Anemia—contributes to worsening of symptoms
   a. Decreased exercise tolerance
   b. Increased dyspnea
   c. Increased frequency of paroxysmal hyperpnea
8. Acidosis
9. Murmur (systolic and continuous)
10. Ejection click after first heart sound
11. Prefer knee or head-to-chest position during spells or after exercise

COMPLICATIONS

1. Pulmonary vascular disease
2. Deformity of the right pulmonary artery

After Blalock-Taussig Anastomosis

1. Bleeding—especially prominent in children with heart disease with decreased pulmonary blood flow postoperatively
2. Cerebral embolism or thrombosis occurs due to increased Hct and increased viscosity, especially if anemic, septic
3. Congestive heart failure if the shunt is too large
4. Early occlusion of the shunt
5. Hemothorax
6. Persistent right-to-left shunt at the atrial level, especially in infants
7. Persistent cyanosis
8. Phrenic nerve damage
9. Pleural effusion

LABORATORY/DIAGNOSTIC TESTS

1. Chest x-ray study—indicates increase or decrease in pulmonary flow; no heart enlargement evident
2. Electrocardiogram (ECG)—indicates right-ventricular hypertrophy, left-ventricular hypertrophy, or both
3. Arterial blood gas values (ABGs)—reflect obstructive pulmonary blood flow (increased partial pressure of carbon dioxide [P_{CO_2}], decreased partial pressure of oxygen [P_{O_2}], and decreased pH)
4. Hematocrit (Hct)/hemoglobin (Hgb)—detects iron deficiency anemia; hypovolemia results from increased viscosity caused by polycythemia
5. Echocardiogram—reveals aortic enlargement
6. Cardiac catheterization—increased systemic pressures in right ventricle; decreased pulmonary artery pressures with decreased aortic hemoglobin saturation
7. Platelet count—decreased
8. Barium swallow—demonstrates displacement of trachea to left of midline
9. Radiogram of abdomen—detects existence of congenital anomalies
10. Complete blood count (CBC)—hypochromic and microcytic red blood cells (RBC) caused by iron deficiency anemia or polycythemia

MEDICATIONS

1. Antibiotics—selection dependent on the results of the culture and sensitivity (C and S)

2. Diuretics (e.g., furosemide [Lasix]—used to promote diuresis; decreases fluid overload; used in the treatment of edema associated with CHF; dosage—2 mg/kg by mouth [po] as single dose [may be increased by 0.5 mg/kg q6-8 hr] or 1 mg/kg intramuscularly [IM] as single dose [may repeat 2 hours later, increased by 1 mg/kg])

3. Digitalis—increases the force of contraction of the heart, the stroke volume, and cardiac output and decreases cardiac venous pressures; used to treat CHF and selected cardiac arrhythmias (rarely given before correction unless shunt too large)
   a. Digitalizing dose—0.03 to 0.05 mg/kg or 0.75 mg/m^2 po, IM, or intravenously (IV)
   b. Maintenance dose—one tenth to one fifth of digitalization dose

4. Iron (Fe)—6 mg/kg/24 hr (elemental Fe) or 7 mg/0.6 ml po (ferrous sulfate [Fer-in-Sol] drops)

5. Propranolol (Inderal), a beta blocker—reduces heart rate and decreases force of contraction and myocardial irritability; used to prevent/treat hypercyanotic spells
   a. Doses have been established for adults only—0.5 mg/kg/day, not to exceed 1 mg/min, TID, or QID/24 hr po.
   b. Dose can be repeated after 2 minutes and not again for 4 hr IV.

6. Morphine, an analgesic—increases pain threshold; also used to treat hypercyanotic spells by depressing the respiratory center and cough reflex; children's dose—0.1 to 0.2 mg/kg IM or subcutaneously (SQ); single dose not to exceed 15 mg

7. Sodium bicarbonate (NaHCO$_3$), a potent systemic alkalizer—used to treat acidosis by replacing bicarbonate ions and restoring buffering capacity of body

NURSING ASSESSMENT

Refer to "Cardiovascular Assessment" in Appendix A.

NURSING DIAGNOSES

Activity intolerance
Decreased cardiac output
Altered tissue perfusion
Fluid volume excess

High risk for infection
High risk for injury
Altered family processes
Ineffective individual coping
Altered nutrition: less than body requirements

NURSING INTERVENTIONS

Maintenance Care

1. Monitor for changes in cardiopulmonary status.
2. Monitor and maintain hydration status.
   a. Input and output; specific gravity
   b. Signs of dehydration
3. Monitor child's response to medications (see "Medications").
   a. Iron—for iron deficiency anemia and polycythemia
   b. Antibiotics—administered before, during, and after surgery as prophylaxis against subacute bacterial endocarditis
   c. Diuretics (furosemide)—for CHF before or after surgery
   d. Digitalis—for CHF before or after surgery
   e. Morphine—to alleviate hypercyanotic spells
   f. Propranolol—to alleviate hypercyanotic spells (long-term management)
   g. Sodium bicarbonate—if documented acidosis develops
4. Provide foods high in iron (to treat iron deficiency anemia) and protein (to promote healing).
   a. Cereals, egg yolk, and meat
   b. Supplemental iron
5. Monitor and observe child's response and need for oxygen supplementation.
   a. Respiratory status
   b. Color
   c. Use and maintenance of respiratory equipment (oxygen mask, ventilator, or tent)
6. Protect from potential infectious contacts, and promote preventive practices (to prevent subacute bacterial endocarditis).
   a. Screen visitors for infections.
   b. Instruct child and family about good dental care.

      (1) Brushing and flossing of teeth
      (2) Frequent dental checkups for detection of caries and gingival infections
      (3) Importance of antibiotic prophylaxis for dental extractions
   c. Close surveillance and timely reporting of fever and abrasions for antibiotic prophylaxis
7. Observe and monitor for signs of complications and child's response to treatment regimen.
   a. Acidosis
   b. Anemia
   c. Brain abscess
8. Observe for phrenic nerve damage and diaphragmatic paralysis.
9. Observe for respiratory complications.
10. Observe for shunt occlusion requiring reoperation or for shunt that is too small.

Preoperative Care

1. Allow parents to vent feelings.
   a. Feelings of being overwhelmed
   b. Feelings of guilt
   c. Fears concerning child's well-being
2. Prepare child for surgery by obtaining assessment data.
   a. CBC, urinalysis, serum glucose, and blood urea nitrogen (BUN)
   b. Baseline electrolytes
   c. Blood coagulation
   d. Type and crossmatch for blood
   e. Chest x-ray study and ECG
3. Provide age-appropriate explanations when child is old enough to understand.

Postoperative Care

Blalock-Taussig or Waterston-Cooley anastomosis

1. Assess child's clinical status.
   a. Immediately postoperatively, expect arm with involved subclavian artery to be cool and without blood pressure.
      (1) Flush blood pressure should equal mean arterial blood pressure.

     (2) Note pulse pressure; wide pulse pressure indicates a large shunt.
- b. Note pulses; bounding pulses indicate large shunt.
- c. Note cyanosis; hypoxemia or signs of acidosis indicate early occlusion of shunt.
- d. Assess for Horner's syndrome.
2. Monitor the child for any postoperative complications (Waterston-Cooley anastomosis).
   - a. Bleeding
   - b. CHF if the shunt is too large
   - c. Increased pulmonary blood flow and pulmonary hypertension
3. Monitor child's response to administered medications — digitalis and diuretics are administered if needed.
4. Monitor and maintain fluid and electrolyte balance.
   - a. Monitor for signs of dehydration — lack of tearing, doughy skin, specific gravity >1.020, and decrease in weight and urine output.
   - b. Monitor fluids at 50% to 75% of maintenance volume during first 24 hours (1000 ml/m^2, then 1500 ml/m^2).
5. Promote and maintain optimal respiratory status.
   - a. Perform percussion and postural drainage q2-4 hr.
   - b. Use suction as needed.
   - c. Use spirometer q1-2 hr for 24 hours, then q4 hr.

Tetralogy of Fallot

1. Monitor child's clinical status, and monitor for postoperative complications.
   - a. Arrhythmias
     - (1) Right bundle branch block caused by right ventriculotomy or ventricular septal defect repair
     - (2) Complete heart blocks
     - (3) Supraventricular arrhythmias
     - (4) Ventricular tachycardia
   - b. Congestive heart failure caused by incision of the right ventricle, which decreases the pumping ability of the heart (more common if pulmonary hypertension is present)
   - c. Hemorrhage caused by low platelet count in children with heart disease with decreased pulmonary blood flow

    d. Low cardiac output (most common cause of death)
    e. Neurologic complications caused by thromboembolic problems
    f. Persistent pulmonary regurgitation
    g. Residual ventricular septal defect affects 10% of patients

2. Monitor child's response to medications.
    a. Pressors for low cardiac output
    b. Digitalis and diuretics several weeks to months after surgery for CHF

3. Assess child's cardiac function q1 hr for 24 to 48 hours, then q4 hr.
    a. Vital signs, including rectal temperature
    b. Color
    c. Peripheral pulses and capillary refill time
    d. Arterial blood pressure and central venous pressure (CVP)
    e. Hepatomegaly
    f. Periorbital edema
    g. Pleural effusion
    h. Pulsus paradoxus
    i. Heart sounds
    j. Ascites (rare)

4. Monitor for cardiac arrhythmias.

5. Monitor for signs and symptoms of hemorrhage.
    a. Assess child's tube output q1 hr.
    b. Assess for bleeding from other sites.
    c. Maintain strict input and output.
    d. Assess for ecchymotic lesions and petechiae.

6. Monitor and maintain child's fluid and electrolyte balance.
    a. IV fluids infused at 50% to 75% of maintenance volume for first 24 hours (1000 ml/m^2, then 1500 ml/m^2)
    b. Signs and symptoms of dehydration

7. Monitor and maintain child's respiratory status.
    a. Perform chest physiotherapy.
    b. Place in semi-Fowler's position.
    c. Humidify air.
    d. Monitor for chylothorax.
    e. Provide adequate pain medications.

8. Provide for child's and family's emotional needs (see "Preoperative Care").

Home Care

1. No air can be allowed to enter IV lines since systemic venous blood shunts to aorta.
2. Family should be aware that antibiotic prophylaxis for dental work and surgery is required.
3. Exercise limitations may continue.
4. Instruct parents about the administration of medications and child's response to them.
5. Instruct parents about the use of cardiopulmonary resuscitation (CPR).
6. Instruct parents about parenting skills.
   a. Need to maintain usual expectations for behavior and misbehavior
   b. Continuing with disciplinary measures
   c. Methods and strategies to assist child in living normally and dealing with concerns
7. Instruct parents about infection control measures.

BIBLIOGRAPHY

Adams F, Emmanouilides G, Riemenschneider T: *Heart disease in infants, children, and adolescents,* ed 4, Baltimore, 1989, Williams & Wilkins.

Byrd L, Bruton-Maree N: Tetralogy of Fallot, *AANA J* 57(2):169, 1989.

Kawabori I: Cyanotic congenital heart defects with increased pulmonary blood flow, *Pediatr Clin North Am* 25(4):759, 1978.

Krovetz L, Gessner J, Schiebler G: *Handbook of pediatric cardiology,* Baltimore, 1979, University Park Press.

Maloney S: Tetralogy of Fallot: using pulmonary allograft conduits to reconstruct the right ventricular outflow tract, *JORN* 50(3):554, 1989.

McAnear S: Parental reaction to chronically ill child, *Home Healthcare Nurse* 8(3):85, 1990.

70 ❖ Thalassemia

PATHOPHYSIOLOGY

Thalassemia is a group of hereditary hemolytic anemias caused by deficiency of the synthesis of hemoglobin polypeptide chains. Subcategories of the disorder are named according to the polypeptide chain affected. The two major types of the disorder are thalassemia major (Cooley's anemia) and thalassemia minor (an asymptomatic disorder). Within each type of classification, there are varying degrees of severity.

Thalassemia major is an autosomal recessive disorder (the individual inherits two thalassemia genes). This disorder is especially prevalent among the following groups: Italians, Greeks (and individuals from other Mediterranean countries), and Asians. In individuals with thalassemia major, the synthesis of the beta-globulin molecule is insufficient, resulting in anemia with several secondary effects. The biochemical and physiologic responses to the anemia include the following: (1) increased production of erythropoietin; (2) erythroid hyperplasia; (3) extramedullary erythropoiesis; (4) expanded marrow space; (5) hepatosplenomegaly; and (6) severe hypochromic anemia.

As a result of their thalassemia major, cardiac, hepatic, and infectious complications of hemochromatosis after hypertransfusions invariably prove fatal before patients reach 20 years of age. *Hemosiderosis* and *hemochromatosis* refer to the excessive amount of iron stored in the body tissues.

INCIDENCE

1. Most common form of thalassemia is thalassemia major.
2. Highest prevalence is among individuals of Mediterranean descent.

CLINICAL MANIFESTATIONS

1. Increased risk of fractures
2. Bone deformities
3. Short stature
4. No growth spurt during adolescence
5. Sexual infantilism—growth retardation in the second decade of life; delayed puberty in girls and delayed development of secondary sex characteristics; the majority of males do not undergo puberty
6. Jaundice
7. Diabetes
8. Thickened cranial bones
9. Flat nose
10. Malocclusions of teeth
11. Severe progressive hemolytic anemia beginning at 6 months of age
12. Splenomegaly
13. Skeletal changes resulting from hyperplastic bone marrow

COMPLICATIONS

1. Congestive heart failure resulting from fibrosis and hypertrophy of cardiac muscle, which occur because of excessive iron deposits (hemochromatosis) from blood transfusions
2. Cirrhosis and gallbladder dysfunctions resulting from progressive hemochromatosis
3. Cardiac arrhythmias
4. Folic acid deficiency

LABORATORY/DIAGNOSTIC TESTS

1. Complete blood count (CBC)—to determine presence of abnormal red blood cells (RBCs); RBCs show marked variation in size and shape, many target cells, severe microcytosis, and hypochromia; hemoglobin (Hb) less than 5 g/dl indicates severe anemia

2. Reticulocyte count—increased because of microcytic anemia
3. Free erythrocyte protoporphyrin (FEP)—normal in patients with thalassemia minor
4. Hgb electrophoresis—high percentage of fetal hemoglobin
5. Serum iron—elevated because of increased hemolysis
6. Serum bilirubin—elevated in patients with thalassemia major only
7. Blood smear—indicates severe hypochromic, microcytic anemia
8. Skeletal x-ray studies—indicate skeletal changes

MEDICATIONS

1. Deferoxamine mesylate (Desferal), a chelating agent that binds to ferric ions to form ferrioxamine complex, a chelate easily excreted by the kidneys—used in the management of hemochromatosis and hemosiderosis, which are secondary to an increase in the stores of iron resulting from multiple transfusions; for the treatment of thalassemia major; dosage—1 to 2 g (20 to 40 mg/kg/day) administered continuously over 8 to 24 hr, using an infusion pump
2. Folic acid (vitamin B_9), a vitamin B complex necessary for nucleoprotein synthesis and normal erythropoiesis—stimulates the production of RBCs, white blood cells (WBCs), and platelets in patients with megaloblastic anemia; used in the treatment of thalassemia major; dosage—infants: up to 0.1 mg qd; children up to 4 years: up to 0.3 mg qd; children more than 4 years: up to 0.1 mg qd.

NURSING ASSESSMENT

Refer to "Cardiovascular Assessment" in Appendix A.

NURSING DIAGNOSES

High risk for injury
Activity intolerance
Decreased cardiac output
Fatigue
Knowledge deficit

Altered growth and development
Altered family processes
Ineffective individual coping
Anxiety

NURSING INTERVENTIONS

1. Monitor child's clinical status during transfusions.
   a. Transfusion reactions
      (1) Fever
      (2) Restlessness
      (3) Cardiac arrhythmias
      (4) Chills and shaking
      (5) Nausea and vomiting
      (6) Chest pain
      (7) Red or black urine
      (8) Headache
      (9) Flank pain
      (10) Signs of shock or renal failure
   b. Signs of circulatory overload
      (1) Dyspnea
      (2) Increased pulse
      (3) Cyanosis
      (4) Chest pain
      (5) Dry cough
2. Monitor for signs and symptoms of complications (see "Complications").

Home Care/Discharge Planning

1. Provide anticipatory guidance and parent teaching to prevent spontaneous fractures.
2. Provide supportive care to child who requires blood transfusions; goal is maintenance of hemoglobin above 10 g/dl.
3. Encourage child to express feelings related to chronic disorder and altered physical appearance.
4. Refer parents to genetic counseling; individuals with thalassemia minor can transmit thalassemia major to their children if their partner has either the disorder or the trait. The trait can be transmitted even when the partner displays neither the trait nor the disorder.
5. Instruct parents to monitor side effects of the following:

a. Deferoxamine mesylate administered through slow subcutaneous infusion pump for iron chelation after the age of 3 to 4 years (side effects are allergic reactions and cataracts)
b. Prophylactic antibiotics after splenectomy
c. Recommended pneumococcal and meningococcal vaccines

BIBLIOGRAPHY

Cohen A, Mezanin J, Scherartz E: Rapid removal of excessive beta with daily high-dose intravenous chelation therapy, *J Pediatr* 115(1):151, 1989.

Hall F et al: Screening for alpha-thalassemia in routine erythrocyte measurements, *Am J Clin Pathol* 87(3):389, 1987.

Lucarelli G et al: Marrow transplantation in patients with advanced thalassemia, *N Engl J Med* 316(17):1050, 1987.

Maurer H et al: A prospective evaluation of iron chelation therapy in children with severe beta-thalassemia: a six-year study, *Am J Dis Child* 142(3):287, 1988.

Propper R, Burton L, Nathan D: New approaches to the transfusion management of thalassemia, *Blood* 55:55, 1980.

Rudolph A, Hoffman J: *Pediatrics,* ed 14, Norwalk, Conn, 1987, Appleton and Lange.

Weatherall D, Clegg J: Thalassemia revisited, *Clin Pediatr* 29:7, 1982.

71 ❖ Urinary Diversions

PATHOPHYSIOLOGY

A urinary diversion is performed as treatment for the following conditions: exstrophy of the bladder, uremia, tumors of the lower urinary tract, severe dilation of the urinary tract, neurogenic bladder dysfunction, nonretractable incontinence, outlet obstruction, and nonresponse to reconstructive surgical procedures. There are basically two types of urinary diversions: cutaneous and internal. Cutaneous types include end-cutaneous ureterostomy, ileal conduit, and sigmoid conduit. Ureterosigmoidostomy is the internal form of urinary diversion. These types are described below.

Cutaneous Urinary Diversions

End-cutaneous ureterostomy. At least one dilated ureter is necessary for this procedure. The ureter or ureters are directly anastomosed to the skin.

Ileal conduit. The ureter is anastomosed to the ileum. The end of ileum is brought to the surface of the abdomen as an enterostomy stoma. Revision has been necessary in 40% of children. Increased incidence of late complications has been demonstrated.

Sigmoid conduit. Ureters are anastomosed to a portion of the sigmoid colon. Sigmoid colon is used because its muscular wall is thicker than that of the small bowel. The ureters can be anastomosed in an antireflux fashion to the sigmoid colon. Fewer long-term problems are associated with the sigmoid conduit. This procedure is performed when an ileal conduit and ureterosigmoidostomy have failed.

Internal Urinary Diversion

An internal urinary diversion (ureterosigmoidostomy) is performed on children with exstrophy of the bladder, lower urinary tract malignancies, and epispadias. The urinary tract is diverted into the intestinal tract in a two-stage procedure. During the first stage, a nonrefluxing sigmoid conduit is formed. At approximately 18 months of age, in the second stage, the conduit is anastomosed to the intact sigmoid colon.

CLINICAL MANIFESTATIONS

A permanent urinary diversion provides the child with the means to attain urinary control. The child derives psychologic benefit from attaining this control. Long-term management is dependent on the type of procedure performed. A urinary diversion preserves and maintains renal functioning and prevents further renal injury.

COMPLICATIONS

1. Urinary tract deterioration
2. Chronic bacilluria
3. Bilateral ureterectasis (ureterosigmoidostomy)
4. Increased incidence of carcinoma of colon (at site of ureterosigmoidostomy)
5. Infection ascending through colon
6. Watery stools (ureterosigmoidostomy)
7. Hyperchloremic stools (ureterosigmoidostomy)
8. Intestinal obstruction (ureterosigmoidostomy)
9. Stomal stenosis (cutaneous ureterostomy, ureterosigmoidostomy)
10. Stomatitis with bleeding and encrustation (ureterosigmoidostomy)
11. Pyelonephritis
12. Calculus formation
13. Distal ureteral fibrosis (cutaneous diversions)
14. Ischemic ureteral stricture (cutaneous diversions)
15. Electrolyte imbalance (ureterosigmoidostomy)

LABORATORY/DIAGNOSTIC TESTS

1. Complete blood count (CBC) — preoperative assessment
2. Urinalysis — preoperative assessment
3. Prothrombin time (PT), partial thromboplastin time (PTT) — to assess bleeding time
4. Diagnostic urography
5. Diagnostic pyelography
6. Chest x-ray examination — routine preoperative assessment

MEDICATIONS

Analgesics are used, with their type and amount dependent on child's level of pain intensity and weight/m^2/age.

NURSING ASSESSMENT

Refer to "Renal Assessment" in Appendix A.

NURSING DIAGNOSES

Altered pattern of urinary elimination
Impaired skin integrity
High risk for infection
High risk for injury
Anxiety
Body image disturbance
Pain
Ineffective individual coping

NURSING INTERVENTIONS

Preoperative Care

1. Prepare infant and parents for surgery.
    a. Provide understandable explanations in lay terms.
    b. Encourage ventilation of feelings (anxiety and guilt).
    c. Encourage parents to room-in and participate in the child's care as a means of promoting the child's security.
2. Monitor the child's condition before surgery.
    a. Check vital signs q4 hr.
    b. Monitor fluid and electrolyte balance and input and output.
    c. Monitor for bowel complications (distention).

3. Promote nutritional status before surgery.
   a. Offer diet high in calories and low in residue.
   b. Use alternate route of intake if child cannot take oral fluids.
   c. Assess intake and output accurately q8 hr.
   d. Weigh every day.
4. Prepare the infant physically for surgery.
   a. Monitor the infant's response to laxatives and enemas (to evacuate bowel).
   b. Decompress stomach (insert nasogastric [NG] tube).
   c. Provide nothing by mouth after midnight before surgery.

Postoperative Care

1. Monitor child's response to surgery.
   a. Vital signs
   b. Input and output—urine, stool, NG tube, urethral stent or stoma (restrain prn to ensure safety of stent)
   c. Dressing—amount of drainage, intactness, need for reinforcement
2. Monitor child's urinary output.
   a. Record output per site (stent, stoma, cystostomy).
   b. Monitor appearance of urine (presence of blood, color).
   c. Monitor serum electrolytes.
3. Monitor for signs and symptoms of complications.
   a. Bleeding
   b. Obstruction
   c. Electrolyte imbalance; hypokalemia or hypochloremic acidosis
   d. Stomal bleeding, prolapse, or retraction
   e. Frequency of stools
4. Provide skin care to prevent skin irritation.
   a. Keep site clean and dry.
   b. Maintain an appliance seal that is intact and flush with stoma.
   c. Avoid use of powders or lubricant to decrease skin irritation.
5. Monitor child's response to medications such as sodium bicarbonate (2 to 4 mEq/kg is administered if bicarbonate level is <20 mEq/L).

Home Care/Discharge Planning

1. Instruct parents about long-term management of urinary diversion.
   a. Use of appliance
   b. Complications
   c. Adequate nutritional and fluid intake (push fluids in ureterosigmoidostomy)
   d. Signs of infection
   e. Skin care techniques
   f. Stoma care
2. Discuss and emphasize parental responsibility in preventing complications.
   a. Intravenous pyelogram (IVP) 4 to 6 weeks after surgery (to rule out urinary obstruction)
   b. Periodic renal function studies
   c. Periodic serum electrolyte studies
   d. Proctoscopic examination every year until 5 to 10 years postoperatively (to detect malignancy)

BIBLIOGRAPHY

Althausen A, Hagen-Cook K, Hendren W: Non-refluxing colon conduit: experience with 70 cases, *J Urol* 120:35, 1978.

Cass A: Urinary diversion for neurogenic bladder in children, *J Urol* 118:46, 1976.

Holiday M, Barrett T, Vernmier R, eds: *Pediatric nephrology,* Baltimore, 1987, Williams & Wilkins.

Jeterik P, Bloom S: Management of stomal complications following ileal or colonic conduit operations in children, *J Urol* 106:425, 1971.

Schmidt J et al: Complications, results, and problems of ileal conduit diversions, *J Urol* 109:210, 1973.

Sidi A et al: Enterocystoplasty in the management and reconstruction of the pediatric neurogenic bladder, *J Pediatr Surg* 22(2):153, 1987.

72 ❖ Urinary Tract Infections

PATHOPHYSIOLOGY

Urinary tract infection (UTI) refers to the bacterial colonization of any segment of the urinary tract. The number of organisms in the urine is greater than can be accounted for by the method of collection. More than 100,000 organisms per milliliter obtained on two consecutive cultures is considered diagnostic. The presence of urine and stool surrounding the urinary meatus allows the bacteria to proliferate and ascend upward to the urethra. Children at risk are those with underlying defects of the urinary system, chronic disease, and neurologic disorders. UTI occurs second in frequency to upper respiratory infections.

INCIDENCE

1. The female to male ratio is 9:1.
2. Fifty-seven percent of males and 37% of females with UTI have an underlying abnormality.
3. Peak incidence in girls is 7 to 11 years.
4. Incidence in males less than 16 years old is 1.1%.
5. UTI rarely leads to permanent damage, end-stage renal disease, or chronic pyelonephritis.
6. Prevalence of symptomatic UTI is less than asymptomatic UTI.
7. Thirty percent to 80% of people with UTI experience reinfection within 1 year.
8. Seventy-five percent of reinfections are caused by *Escherichia coli*.

9. The incidence among preschoolers is 1.5% to 2.5%.
10. Peak incidence occurs at 2 to 6 years of age (males).
11. Uncircumcised boys experience 2 to 3 UTIs in child-hood.

CLINICAL MANIFESTATIONS
Infant (Initially Seen with Vague Symptoms)
1. Colic
2. Jaundice
3. Poor eating
4. Vomiting
5. Fever
6. Lethargy
7. Irritability
8. Increased number of wet diapers

Preschool Child
1. Fever (most common)
2. Weak urinary stream or dribbling
3. Foul-smelling urine
4. Hematuria
5. Enuresis
6. Abdominal pain

School-age Child
1. Dysuria
2. Frequency
3. Urgency

All Ages
1. Abdominal distention
2. Dehydration
3. Flank pain
4. Costovertebral angle tenderness
5. Chills and fever
6. Constipation

COMPLICATIONS
1. End-stage renal disease
2. Chronic pyelonephritis
3. Reinfection

LABORATORY/DIAGNOSTIC TESTS

1. Intravenous pyelogram (IVP) — to visualize kidney and bladder
2. Cystourethrogram (CUG) — to establish presence of vesicoureteral reflux and abnormalities
3. Cystoscopy — to visualize interior of bladder and urethra (not routinely performed)
4. Retrograde pyelography — to visualize contour and size of ureters and kidneys
5. Cystometry — to assess filling capacity of bladder and effectiveness of detrusor reflux
6. Suprapubic aspiration — to obtain sterile urine
7. Urine culture — to determine presence and amount of microorganisms (obtain midstream urine)

MEDICATIONS

Use of antibiotics is dependent on results of culture and sensitivity.

NURSING ASSESSMENT

Refer to "Renal Assessment" in Appendix A.

NURSING DIAGNOSES

Altered patterns of urinary elimination
Pain
Knowledge deficit
High risk for injury

NURSING INTERVENTIONS

1. Monitor child's therapeutic response to and untoward effects of medication.
   a. Obtain urinalysis before administration of drugs.
   b. Repeat urinalysis 48 to 72 hours after antibiotics are initiated and 1 week after therapy has ended.
   c. Encourage intake of fluids; norms are as follows:
      (1) First 10 kg — 100 ml/kg/24 hr
      (2) Second 10 kg — no. 1 + 50 ml/kg/24 hr
      (3) Greater than 20 kg — no. 1 + no. 2 + 20 ml/kg/24 hr
2. Prevent reinfection.
   a. Instruct family and child about importance of completing 10 to 14 days of antibiotic treatment.

b. Instruct child to void frequently (retention of urine serves to maintain infection).
c. Instruct about proper hygiene (e.g., anterior-to-posterior wiping).
d. Avoid giving bubble baths.

BIBLIOGRAPHY

Circumcision and urinary tract infections, *Harvard Medical School Health Letter* 14(6):3, 1989.

Herzog L: Urinary tract infections and circumcision: a case-control study, *Am J Dis Child* 143(3):348, 1989.

Lohr A: The foreskin and urinary tract infections, *J Pediatr* 114(3):502, 1989.

Lund M: Perspectives on newborn male circumcision, *Neonat Network* 9(3):7, 1990.

Moffatt M et al: Short-course antibiotic therapy for urinary tract infections in children, *Am J Dis Child* 142(1):57, 1988.

Reid B et al: Radiographic evaluation of children with urinary tract infections, *Radiol Clin North Am* 26(2):393, 1988.

Report of the Task Force on Circumcision, *Pediatrics* 84(2):388, 1989.

Roberts J: Is routine circumcision indicated in the newborn? An affirmative view, *J Fam Pract* 31(2):185, 1990.

Schlayer T et al: Bacterial contamination rate of urine collected in a urine bag from healthy non–toilet-trained male infants, *J Pediatr* 116(5):738, 1990.

Stapleton F, Tinshaw M: Urinary tract infections in children: diagnosis and management, *Iss Compr Pediatr Nurs* 2(6):1, 1978.

Thomas C: Childhood urinary tract infection, *Pediatr Nurs* 8:114, March/April 1982.

Thompson R: Is routine circumcision indicated in the newborn? An opposing view, *J Fam Pract* 31(2):189, 1990.

Wilson D, Killion D: Urinary tract infections in the pediatric patient, *Nurs Practit* 14(7):38, 1989.

73 ❖ Ventricular Septal Defect and Repair

PATHOPHYSIOLOGY

Ventricular septal defect (VSD) is a heart defect with increased pulmonary blood flow that is characterized by a ventricular septal communication that allows direct blood flow between the ventricles, usually from left to right. The defects may vary from 0.5 to 3.0 cm in diameter. Approximately 20% of the ventricular septal defects seen in children are simple (i.e., small). Many of them close spontaneously. Approximately 50% to 60% have a moderate-sized defect and show symptoms in late childhood. This defect is frequently associated with other cardiac defects. The altered physiology can be described as follows:

1. Pressure is greater in the left ventricle and promotes the flow of oxygenated blood through the defect to the right ventricle.
2. Increased blood volume is pumped into the lungs, which eventually may become congested with blood, and may result in increased pulmonary vascular resistance.
3. If the pulmonary resistance is great, right-ventricular pressure may increase, causing a reversal of the shunt, with the unoxygenated blood flowing from the right ventricle to the left one, producing cyanosis (termed Eisenmenger's syndrome).

In a patient with a simple ventricular septal defect, the clinical picture may only be the presence of a murmur. Mild exercise intolerance, fatigue, dyspnea during exertion, and severe repeated respiratory infections may be present. The seriousness of the condition depends on the size of the shunt. If the child is asymptomatic, no treatment is required; however, if he or she has episodes of congestive heart failure (CHF), risk of pulmonary vascular change or extreme shunting, surgical closure of the defect is indicated. The surgical risk is approximately 3%, and the ideal age for surgery is 3 to 5 years old.

For a larger defect the patient will show the same symptoms, but they will be more severe and may appear within the first month or so of life.

INCIDENCE

1. The ratio of males to females with the defect is 1:1.
2. An increase in ventricular septal defects is seen in patients with Down syndrome and Holt-Oram syndrome.
3. The surgical risk is from 10% to 25%, depending on the types of complications involved and the age of the patient.

CLINICAL MANIFESTATIONS

1. Characteristic sign is a loud, harsh, pansystolic murmur that is generally heard best at the left lower sternal border.
2. Severe overloading of the right ventricle causes hypertrophy and obvious cardiac enlargement.
3. With increased pulmonary vascular resistance, dyspnea and frequent respiratory infections are common.
4. Signs of cyanosis are possible, including assuming a squatting position to decrease venous return.

COMPLICATIONS

1. CHF
2. Infective endocarditis
3. Development of aortic insufficiency or pulmonary stenosis
4. Progressive pulmonary vascular disease
5. Damage to the ventricular conduction system

LABORATORY/DIAGNOSTIC TESTS

1. Cardiac catheterization demonstrates an abnormal communication between the ventricles.
2. An electrocardiogram (ECG) and x-ray examination reveal left ventricular hypertrophy.
3. Complete blood count (CBC) is part of routine preoperative testing.
4. Routine prothrombin time (PT) and partial thromboplastin time (PTT) preoperative testing may reveal bleeding tendencies (usually normal; standard tests).

MEDICATIONS

Vasopressors or vasodilators are the medications used for patients with a ventricular septal defect and severe CHF.

1. Dopamine (Intropin)—has a positive inotropic effect on the myocardium, resulting in increased cardiac output and increased systolic and pulse pressures; has minimal or no effect on diastolic pressure; used to treat hemodynamic imbalance caused by open heart surgery; dosage—5 ml in 250 ml D_5W (800 mcg/ml) up to 5 mcg/kg/min to maintain blood pressure and renal perfusion
2. Isoproterenol (Isuprel)—has a positive inotropic effect on myocardium, resulting in increased cardiac output and work; decreases both diastolic and mean pressures while increasing systolic pressure; dosage—0.05 to 1.0 mcg/kg/min IV

SURGICAL MANAGEMENT: VENTRICULAR SEPTAL DEFECT REPAIR

Early repair is preferable if the defect is large. Infants with CHF may require complete or palliative surgery in the form of pulmonary artery banding if they cannot be stabilized medically. Because of the irreversible damage secondary to pulmonary vascular disease, surgery should not be postponed past the preschool years or if progressive pulmonary vascular resistance is present. A median sternotomy is made for this bypass surgery, with the use of hypothermia necessary for some infants. For a membranous defect high in the septum, a right-atrial incision allows the surgeon to repair the defect by working through the tricuspid valve. Otherwise, a right ventriculotomy, or a left ventriculotomy for lesions in the muscular region, is necessary. Generally, a Dacron or pericardial patch is placed over the lesion, although direct suturing may be used if the defect is minimal. Previous banding is removed, and any deformities caused by it are repaired.

Response to Surgery

Surgical response should include a hemodynamically normal heart, although any damage caused by pulmonary hypertension is irreversible. Complications include the following:

1. Potential aortic insufficiency (particularly if present preoperatively)
2. Arrhythmias
   a. Right bundle-branch block for right ventriculotomy
   b. Heart block
3. CHF, especially in patients with pulmonary hypertension and left ventriculotomy
4. Hemorrhage
5. Left-ventricular dysfunction
6. Low cardiac output
7. Myocardial damage
8. Pulmonary edema
9. Residual intraventricular septal defects if repair not complete because of multiple ventricular septal defects

NURSING ASSESSMENT

1. Refer to "Cardiovascular Assessment" in Appendix A.
2. Assess for the following:
   a. Diastolic murmur—indicates aortic insufficiency
   b. Widening pulse pressure—indicates aortic insufficiency
   c. Arrhythmias
   d. CHF
   e. Bleeding
   f. Low cardiac output, especially during first 24 hours after surgery

NURSING DIAGNOSES

Activity intolerance
Decreased cardiac output
Altered tissue perfusion

Fluid volume excess
High risk for infection
High risk for injury
Altered family processes

NURSING INTERVENTIONS

Preoperative Care

1. Prepare child with age-appropriate explanations before surgery.
2. Provide and reinforce information given to parents.
3. Monitor child's baseline status.
   a. Vital signs
   b. Color of mucous membranes
   c. Quality and intensity of peripheral pulses
   d. Capillary refill time
   e. Temperature of extremities
4. Assist and support child during preoperative laboratory and diagnostic tests.
   a. CBC, urinalysis, serum glucose, and blood urea nitrogen (BUN)
   b. Serum electrolytes — sodium, potassium, and chlorine
   c. PT, PTT, and platelet count
   d. Type and crossmatch blood
   e. Chest x-ray examination
   f. ECG

Postoperative Care

1. Monitor child's postoperative status as often as q15 min for first 24 to 48 hours.
   a. Vital signs
   b. Color of mucous membranes
   c. Quality and intensity of peripheral pulses
   d. Capillary refill time
   e. Periorbital edema
   f. Pleural effusion
   g. Pulsus paradoxus if tamponade
   h. Arterial pressures
   i. Cardiac rhythms
2. Monitor for hemorrhage.
   a. Measure chest tube output q1 hr.
   b. Assess for clot formation in chest tube.

    c. Assess for ecchymotic lesions and petechiae.
    d. Assess for bleeding from other sites.
    e. Record blood output for diagnostic studies.
    f. Monitor strict input and output.
    g. Administer fluids at 50% to 75% of maintenance volume during first 24 hours.
    h. Administer blood products as indicated.
3. Monitor child's hydration status.
    a. Skin turgor
    b. Moistness of mucous membranes
    c. Specific gravity
    d. Daily weights
    e. Urine output
4. Monitor for signs and symptoms of CHF.
5. Maintain skin temperature at 36° to 36.5° C and rectal temperature at 37° C.
6. Monitor and promote child's respiratory status.
    a. Turn, cough, and deep breathe.
    b. Perform chest physiotherapy.
    c. Humidify air.
    d. Monitor for chylothorax.
    e. Provide pain medications as needed.
7. Monitor for complications (see "Complications").
8. Provide opportunities for child to express feelings through age-appropriate means (see Appendix B, *Growth and Development*).
9. Provide emotional support to parents.
    a. Encourage verbalization of feelings.
    b. Provide and reinforce information given to parents.
    c. Encourage use of preexisting supports.
    d. Provide for physical comforts (e.g., sleeping arrangements, hygiene).

Home Care

Provide instruction to parents about the following:
1. Medications
2. Time intervals for follow-up care
3. Indications for contacting physician
4. Procedures for treatments
5. Referral to social service
6. Referral to Visiting Nurses Association

BIBLIOGRAPHY

Adams F, Emmanouilides G, Riemenschneider T: *Moss' heart disease in infants, children and adolescents,* ed 4, Baltimore, 1989, Williams & Wilkins.

Foldy S et al: Perioperative nursing care for congenital cardiac defects, *Critic Care Nurs Clin North Am* 1(2):289, 1989.

Moynihan J et al: Caring for patients with lesions increasing pulmonary blood flow, *Critic Care Nurs Clin North Am* 1(2):195, 1989.

Schellinger D et al: Ventricular septa in the neonatal age group: diagnosis and considerations of etiology, *ARN J* 7(6):1065, 1986.

74 ❖ Wilms' Tumor

PATHOPHYSIOLOGY

Wilms' tumor is usually a single tumor that arises from the renal parenchyma. It is separated from the kidney by a membranous capsule. The tumor originates from renoblast cells located in the kidney's parenchyma. A larger tumor will extend across the midline. The tumor may extend to surrounding structures, causing obstruction of the inferior vena cava (from ascites or edema) and/or the intestines (obstruction or constipation). It is associated with congenital anomalies such as hypospadias, cryptorchidism, and aniridia and with hemihypertrophy, cardiac malformations, and neurofibromatosis.

This tumor grows rapidly. Tissue type varies according to "favorable" and "unfavorable" pathology. Favorable histology includes multiocular cysts, nephroblastomatosis, and congenital mesoblastic nephromas. Unfavorable histology includes clear cell sarcoma, anaplasia, and rhabdoid tumor. Metastasis occurs through the bloodstream to the lungs and liver. The tumor may spread through the lymphatics to the retroperitoneal lymph nodes. The most common site for metastasis is in the lungs, followed by the liver, contralateral kidney, and bone (rare). The tumor should not be palpated because doing so can cause seeding of the tumor elsewhere or can cause a pulmonary embolization.

SURGICAL TREATMENT

Staging Procedure

Staging refers to exact determination of the extent of the disease at the time of diagnosis. The NWTS staging system consists of five stages that reflect the extent of the disease. Staging is achieved by surgical evaluation, which uses biopsy results, and postoperative pathologic evaluation, which relies on the holistic examination of cancer tissue after its surgical removal.

Nephrectomy

Nephrectomy is a procedure during which the affected kidney is surgically excised.

MEDICAL TREATMENT

Radiation treatment is initiated immediately after surgery. In some cases, treatment may begin on the day of surgery. Dosage is 1000 rads per week for 3 weeks.

INCIDENCE

1. Wilms' tumor accounts for 5.8% of cancers in white children and 9% in black children.
2. Peak incidence is at 3 to 4 years of age.
3. Prognosis varies according to the stage of the disease at time of diagnosis and the type of cell histology.
4. Overall survival rate is 90%.

CLINICAL MANIFESTATIONS

The first three symptoms are the predominant clinical manifestations.
1. Flank mass
2. Pain
3. Hematuria
4. Hypertension
5. Fever

COMPLICATIONS

1. Metastasis to lungs, bone marrow (anemia), contralateral kidney, and liver
2. Adverse reactions to chemotherapy

LABORATORY/DIAGNOSTIC TESTS

1. Intravenous pyelogram (IVP) and abdominal x-ray studies — used to detect mass
2. Serum glutamic-oxaloacetic transaminase (SGOT), serum glutamic-pyruvic transaminase (SGPT), and lactic dehydrogenase (LDH) — elevated with liver involvement
3. CBC — assess for anemia and potential bleeding problems
4. Urinalysis — to assess for hematuria
5. Urinary catecholamines — to rule out neuroblastoma
6. BUN and creatinine — to assess renal function
7. Chest CT scan: to assess extent of disease
8. Increased erythropoietin levels in urine and serum — indicate presence of metastatic disease
9. Bone marrow aspiration and biopsy — to assess marrow involvement (rare)

MEDICATIONS

Chemotherapy is given with radiation treatment. Its dosage is highly individualized.

1. Dactinomycin (actinomycin D), a cytotoxic antibiotic used for antineoplastic purposes. It is used to inhibit DNA, RNA, and protein synthesis. It potentiates the effect of irradiation and is used in combination with other chemotherapeutic agents and radiation to treat Wilms' tumor.
   a. Side effects
      (1) Toxic renal, hepatic, and bone marrow effects
      (2) Malaise, fever, myalgia, ulcerative stomatitis, and pharyngitis
      (3) Nausea and vomiting
      (4) Bone marrow suppression, excoriation of tissue (at site of intravenous [IV] injection)
2. Vincristine (Oncovin), an antineoplastic that inhibits cell division during metaphase. It is used with other antineoplastics and radiation in the treatment of Wilms' tumor.
   a. Side effects
      (1) Neuromuscular — peripheral neuropathy, paresthesias of hands and feet, loss of deep tendon reflexes, ataxia

      (2) Gastrointestinal — stomatitis, nausea, vomiting, diarrhea, abdominal cramps

      (3) Dermatologic — alopecia, cellulitis, extravasation (at IV site)

      (4) Other — malaise, fever, polyuria, weight loss, uric acid nephropathy, hyperkalemia

   b. Dosage — according to protocol

3. Doxorubicin (Adriamycin), which has antitumor activity and strong immunosuppressive properties.

NURSING ASSESSMENT

1. Refer to "Renal Assessment" in Appendix A.
2. Assess for enlarged abdomen in flank areas.

NURSING DIAGNOSES

Impaired tissue integrity
High risk for injury
Impaired gas exchange
High risk for infection
Anxiety
Pain
Ineffective individual coping
Altered family processes

NURSING INTERVENTIONS

Preoperative Care

1. Avoid palpation of abdomen to prevent seeding of tumor.
2. Monitor child's clinical status; observe and prevent signs and symptoms of complications.
   a. Vital signs
   b. Signs and symptoms of vena caval obstruction (facial plethora and venous engorgement)
   c. Signs and symptoms of renal failure
   d. Bone pain
   e. Anemia and bleeding tendencies
   f. Hypertension
3. Provide age-appropriate preprocedural explanations to child to alleviate anxiety.
4. Encourage child and parents to express concerns and fears about diagnosis.

5. Prepare child and parents for upcoming staging surgery.

POSTOPERATIVE CARE

1. Monitor child's clinical status.
   a. Vital signs monitored as often as q2 hr after surgery
   b. Input and output
   c. Hypertension (caused by removal of kidney)
2. Monitor child's abdominal functioning.
   a. Patency of nasogastric (NG) tube
   b. Bowel sounds
   c. Signs and symptoms of obstruction from vincristine-induced ileus
   d. Postoperative adhesion formation
3. Promote fluid and electrolyte balance.
   a. Monitor infusion of IV solutions.
   b. Monitor for electrolyte imbalances.
   c. Monitor for metabolic alkalosis (results from NG drainage).
4. Maintain and support respiratory status.
   a. Perform pulmonary toilet.
   b. Turn, cough, and deep breathe.
   c. Use suction as needed.
   d. Change position q2 hr.
5. Monitor incisional site for intactness and healing.
   a. Observe for signs and symptoms of drainage.
   b. Monitor for intactness.
   c. Monitor for signs and symptoms of infection (redness, warmth, inflammation).
   d. Change dressing as needed.
6. Provide child's hygienic needs.
   a. Oral and rectal care (especially important because child is immunosuppressed)
   b. Skin care—dry between folds of skin and lubricate
7. Protect child from infection resulting from immunosuppression.
   a. Maintain reverse isolation if white blood count (WBC) decreases (refer to institutional policy).
   b. Limit contacts with public.
   c. Dress child appropriately for weather changes.

8. Monitor side effects of radiotherapy; tumor is remarkably sensitive to radiation.
9. Monitor side effects of chemotherapy.
   a. Dactinomycin
   b. Vincristine

Home Care

1. Instruct parents about the following aspects of medical management.
   a. Therapeutic response to medications
   b. Untoward reactions to medications
   c. Compliance with clinic visits
2. Provide information to parents about the following:
   a. School resources
   b. Financial resources
3. Provide emotional support and referral to support groups for parents, siblings, and affected child.

BIBLIOGRAPHY

D'Angio G et al: The treatment of Wilms' tumor; results of the second national Wilms' tumor study group, *Cancer* 47:2302, 1981.

Ganick D: Wilms's tumor, *Hematol Oncol Clin North Am* 1(4):695, 1987.

Moshang T, Lee M: Late effects: disorders of growth and sexual maturation associated with the treatment of childhood cancer, *J Assoc Pediatr Oncol Nurs* 5(4):14, 1988.

Patore G et al: Epidemiological features of Wilms' tumor: results of studies by the International Society of Pediatric Oncology, *Med Pediatr Oncol* 16(1):7, 1988.

Pilch Y: *Surgical oncology*, New York, 1984, McGraw-Hill Book Co.

PART TWO

Pediatric Diagnostic Tests and Procedures

General Nursing Action

These nursing actions are applicable to all the procedures discussed in this section.

NURSING ASSESSMENT

Assess for the following:
1. Developmental level of cognitive capacity as it relates to ability to understand procedure
2. Previous experience with procedure
3. Acuity level
4. Child's coping abilities
5. Available parental support
6. Parental understanding of procedure
7. Allergies
8. Reaction to medications that may have been taken previously

NURSING INTERVENTIONS

Preprocedural Care

1. Explain the procedure, including sensory information, in age-appropriate language. The younger child may want to practice selected aspects of the procedure (e.g., lying on abdomen).
2. Prepare child for preparatory procedural assessment (e.g., complete blood count [CBC] or urinalysis).

3. Obtain information about usual reaction and sensitivity.
4. Reinforce information given to parents about child's or infant's condition; explain purpose and anticipated outcome of procedure.

Postprocedural Care

1. Provide opportunities for the child to discuss procedure and for clarification of misconceptions.
2. Monitor child's clinical status.
   a. Vital signs
   b. Level of consciousness (LOC)
3. Provide foods and fluids when tolerated.
   a. Discontinue intravenous fluids when alert and awake.
   b. Initially offer small amounts of clear fluids; assess tolerance before progressing to full liquids and solids.

75 ❖ Brain Scan

A brain scan is a noninvasive procedure used to detect intracranial malformations. Accuracy in detection of tumors, malignant gliomas, and meningiomas ranges between 90% and 98%. A brain scan is less accurate in the detection of slow-growing and avascular tumors (e.g., 80% for astrocytoma). It is useful in the detection of blood clots, infections, and other abnormalities that permeate the blood-brain barrier and brain tissue. A radionuclide is injected approximately 15 minutes before scanning. Pathologic tissue absorbs greater concentrations of radionucleotides than does normal brain tissue. The ratio of abnormal-to-normal brain concentration is then measured for diagnostic purposes. A brain scan is used in conjunction with computed tomography (CT) scans.

NURSING ASSESSMENT

Determine the child's sensitivity to dye.

NURSING INTERVENTIONS

Specified observation and postprocedural nursing care are not required.

BIBLIOGRAPHY

Conway-Rutkowski B: *Pediatric neurologic nursing,* St. Louis, 1977, Mosby–Year Book.

Jabbour J et al: *Pediatric neurology handbook,* Flushing, New York, 1976, Medical Examination Publishing Co.

Tilkian S, Conover M, Tilkian A: *Clinical implications of laboratory tests,* St. Louis, 1987, Mosby–Year Book.

76 ❖ Bronchoscopy

Use of bronchoscopy is indicated in the following situations: (1) removal of a foreign body from the bronchus, larynx, or trachea; (2) diagnosis of acquired stenosis of the larynx or trachea after intubation; and (3) diagnosis of the following conditions—laryngeal cysts, papillomas, subglottic hemangiomas, and tracheomalacia. With the patient under general anesthesia in the operating room, an optical telescopic bronchoscope is inserted into the bronchi. The bronchoscopic sheath permits airway control and ventilation, and the bronchoscopic telescope provides clear visualization of the bronchi. One of two methods is used to remove foreign bodies. First, a catheter with a Fogarty balloon is inserted beyond the foreign body. The balloon is then inflated and used to trap the foreign body between it and the lumen. Then the entire bronchoscope is removed. If this procedure is unsuccessful, a Dormia stone basket is used. The foreign body is manipulated into the open wires of the basket, then is clamped within it, and is removed. During the procedure the vital signs (temperature, apical pulse, respiratory rate, and blood pressure) and electrocardiogram (ECG) are monitored.

NURSING ASSESSMENT

Assess the child's respiratory status.
1. Respiratory rate
2. Stridor

3. Aphonia
4. Retraction
5. Cyanosis
6. Hypoxia
7. Wheezing
8. Persistent cough
9. Unexplained fever

NURSING INTERVENTIONS

Preprocedural Care

Provide nothing by mouth 6 hours before surgery (policies vary). If surgery is performed on an outpatient basis, parents should be told to not feed the child breakfast.

Postprocedural Care

1. Monitor the child's clinical status, including respiratory status.
2. Monitor the child's response postoperatively to medications given during the bronchoscopy.
   a. Atropine — decreases secretions; inhibits vagal slowing of heart during airway manipulation
   b. Diazepam — used as sedation

BIBLIOGRAPHY

Fitzpatrick S et al: Indications for flexible fiberoptic bronchoscopy in pediatric patients, *Am J Dis Child* 137:595, 1983.

Johnson D: Bronchoscopy. In Welch K et al: *Pediatric surgery,* ed 4, St. Louis, 1986, Mosby–Year Book.

Wood R, Sherman J: Pediatric flexible bronchoscopy, *Ann Otol Rhinol Laryngol* 89:414, 1980.

Tilkian S, Conover M, Tilkian A: *Clinical implications of laboratory tests,* St. Louis, 1987, Mosby–Year Book.

77 ❖ Cardiac Catheterization

Cardiac catheterization is an invasive procedure that is performed to measure the intracardiac pressures of the heart chambers, as well as oxygen saturation. In addition, contrast dye is injected to outline the anatomic details of the cardiac malformation. A catheter is inserted percutaneously through a large-bore needle into the right femoral artery and vein (if this procedure is not possible, then a cutdown of the saphenous vein and femoral artery is performed). Measurements of chamber pressures, oxygen saturation, cardiac output, and shunt flow, as well as pulmonary vascular resistance, are obtained and recorded (see box on facing page). Cardiac catheterization is used primarily to confirm a diagnosis. It is also performed in neonates and infants who are initially seen with symptoms (e.g., congestive heart failure [CHF], cyanosis, and respiratory difficulty) and preoperatively and postoperatively.

NURSING ASSESSMENT

Assess cardiopulmonary status.
1. Respiratory difficulty
2. Cyanosis
3. Signs of CHF
4. Pedal pulses
5. Skin temperature and color
6. Complete blood count (CBC), bleeding time, and type and crossmatch

Measurements Taken During Cardiac Catheterization

Chamber Pressures

Right-atrial pressure — 3 to 7 mm Hg
Right-ventricular systolic pressure — 25/0 mm Hg
Main pulmonary artery pressure — 25/10 mm Hg
Pulmonary capillary wedge pressure
Left-atrial pressure — 5 to 10 mm Hg
Left-ventricular systolic pressure — 100/70 mm Hg
Left-ventricular end diastolic pressure

Blood Oximetry

Oxygen content measured in chambers
Right atrium — 70 ± 5%
Right ventricle — 70 ± 5%
Left atrium — 97 ± 3%
Left ventricle — 97 ± 3%

Deletion Curves

Presence and location of intracardiac shunt

Pulse Contours

Valvular Gradient

Cardiac Output and Shunt Flow

Pulmonary Vascular Resistance

NURSING INTERVENTIONS

Preprocedural Care

1. Prepare infant or child and parents with explanation of procedure (including anticipation of sensations).
2. Prepare infant or child for procedure.
   a. Provide nothing by mouth before catheterization (from midnight or 4 hours before surgery).
   b. Administer and monitor child's response to pre-medication; infants less than 3 months old are not medicated because doing so can affect pulmonary pressures.

   c. Have the child clothed and chart completed according to institutional policy.
3. Ensure safe transport to catheterization laboratory for clinically symptomatic neonates and infants.
   a. Provide the following equipment:
      (1) Oxygen source
      (2) Suction equipment
      (3) Laryngoscope and blades
      (4) Endotracheal (ET) tubes
      (5) Magill forceps and stylet
      (6) Ambu bag
   b. Keep patient warm to prevent chilling.

Postprocedural Care

1. Monitor clinical status.
   a. Monitor vital signs q15 minutes during first hour; q30 min during second hour; then every hour for 4 hours; then q4 hr.
   b. Monitor extremity for blanching and arterial spasm.
      (1) Locate and palpate pedal pulses.
      (2) Monitor color and temperature of extremity.
2. Monitor patency of insertion site.
   a. Intactness of dressing
   b. Signs of bleeding
   c. Formation of hematoma
3. Provide opportunities for distraction, relaxation, and play.
   a. Provide quiet, passive diversional activities (e.g., read story or watch television).
   b. Hold, cuddle, and comfort.

BIBLIOGRAPHY

King O: *Care of the cardiac surgical patient,* St. Louis, 1975, Mosby–Year Book.

Malinowski M, Doyle J: Cardiac catheterization of the neonate, *Am J Nurs* 85(1):60, 1985.

Tilkian S, Conover M, Tilkian A: *Clinical implications of laboratory tests,* St. Louis, 1987, Mosby–Year Book.

78 ❖ Computed Tomography

Computed tomography (CT) is an invasive (with use of contrast dye) or noninvasive roentgenographic procedure that is performed to detect differences in tissue radiodensity. It is used for the entire body; for example, it provides a 360-degree view of the brain in one-degree angles, providing a view of the intracranial structures and precise location of abnormalities. It is a major diagnostic tool used in the assessment and evaluation of intracranial pathology. Serial evaluations can be performed because the amount of radiation is minimal.

NURSING ASSESSMENT

1. Assess for infant's or child's ability to remain still for 5 to 30 minutes.
2. Assess for allergies.

NURSING INTERVENTIONS

1. Provide explanation of procedure as it is performed (include anticipation of sensations).
2. Monitor infant's or child's reaction to sedation.
   a. Observe for changes in respiratory status.
   b. Monitor untoward allergic reactions.
   c. Secure infant or child safely on scanning table.
3. Monitor infant's or child's pretest reaction to contrast medium; report any signs or symptoms of allergic reaction.

4. If procedure is performed on an outpatient basis, instruct parents about monitoring sedated child after procedure.
   a. Child should rest or sleep until sedation has worn off.
   b. Observe for untoward side effects of medication.

BIBLIOGRAPHY

Conway-Rutkowski B: *Pediatric neurologic nursing,* St. Louis, 1977, Mosby–Year Book.

Gomez M, Reese D: Computed tomography of the head in infants and children, *Pediatr Clin North Am* 23:473, 1976.

Singer H: Computed tomography in pediatric neurologic disorders, *Pediatr Rev* 2(5):139, 1980.

Tilkian S, Conover M, Tilkian A: *Clinical implications of laboratory tests,* St. Louis, 1987, Mosby–Year Book.

79 ❖ Electrocardiography

Electrocardiography is a noninvasive procedure that is used to record the electrical activity of the heart on an electrocardiogram (ECG). It can be used diagnostically to indicate myocardial infarction and ischemia, hypertrophy of the heart chambers, and electrolyte and acid-base imbalances. It is used to detect cardiac arrhythmias and conduction defects, and it can reveal a cardiac rhythm that is typically diagnostic of a specific cardiac disorder. The ECG sinus pattern changes with age. The greatest change occurs during the first year of life, reflecting the alterations in circulation. The ECG tracings of congenital defects (e.g., atrial septal defect and ventricular septal defect) are affected by the size of the defect, the pulmonary vascular resistance, and degree of volume of the left side of the heart and pressure overload of the right side of the heart.

NURSING ASSESSMENT

Determine the child's previous experience with the procedure.

NURSING INTERVENTIONS

1. Explain procedure to child before it is performed.
2. Reassure child and encourage him or her to lie quietly during ECG procedure.

3. Assist in gently holding infant or child (to restrain motion during procedure).
4. Remove conduction gel after procedure is completed.

BIBLIOGRAPHY

Moller J: *Essentials of pediatric cardiology,* ed 2, Philadelphia, 1978, FA Davis.

Perloff J: *The clinical recognition of congenital heart disease,* ed 2, Philadelphia, 1978, WB Saunders.

Tilkian S, Conover M, Tilkian A: *Clinical implications of laboratory tests,* St. Louis, 1987, Mosby–Year Book.

80 ❖ Electromyography

Electromyography is a diagnostic procedure used to measure and record the electrical activity produced by muscular activity. It is used for locating sites of injury, primary muscular disease, and diseases of the anterior horn and peripheral nerves. Needle electrodes are introduced into specific muscles, enabling the electrical potential to be measured. Recordings are made in both the resting and the contracted states.

NURSING ASSESSMENT

Assess the child's need for sedation.

NURSING INTERVENTIONS

1. Explain the procedure to the child in age-appropriate terms.
2. Monitor the child's response to sedation.
   a. Untoward effects
   b. Need for additional amount
3. Allow the child to sleep, with side rails up, until effects of sedation wear off.

BIBLIOGRAPHY

Conway-Rutkowski B: *Pediatric neurologic nursing,* St. Louis, 1977, Mosby–Year Book.

Jabbour J et al: *Pediatric neurology handbook,* Flushing, New York, 1976, Medical Examination Publishing Co.

Tilkian S, Conover M, Tilkian A: *Clinical implications of laboratory tests,* St. Louis, 1987, Mosby–Year Book.

81 ❖ Intracranial Pressure Monitoring

Intracranial pressure (ICP) monitoring is performed to detect intracranial hypertension. It is indicated for the following conditions: intracranial hypertension, tumors, hemorrhage, contusions, edema, and brain injury. It is used for children diagnosed with Reye's syndrome, lead poisoning, hydrocephalus, after neurosurgery, and metabolic disorders. It is an invasive procedure, requiring the drilling of burr holes into the subarachnoid space for the placement of the pressure monitor into the epidural space. One of several techniques may be used. These include ventriculostomy, ventricular taps, shunts, subdural recordings, intraparenchymal recordings, and subarachnoid bolt. Barbiturate coma is induced for monitoring the child.

NURSING ASSESSMENT

Assess the infant's neurologic status.

NURSING INTERVENTIONS

1. Monitor and maintain the functioning of the ICP monitoring.
    a. Report variations greater than the norm.
        (1) ICP—15 mm Hg
        (2) Cerebral perfusion pressure (CCP)— >50 mm Hg
        (3) CCP is calculated as follows: MAP (mean arterial pressure) minus ICP equals CCP.

Pancuronium Bromide (Pavulon)

Pancuronium bromide acts as a neuromuscular blocking agent and has a direct blocking effect on the acetylcholine receptors for heart rate, cardiac output, and arterial pressure: It is used for the management of patients on mechanical ventilation.

Dosage is as follows: initial—0.04 mg to 0.1 mg/kg; additional dosage—0.01 mg/kg administered at 30- to 60-minute intervals.

  b. Note the association between elevations and sleeping and feeding respiratory rate and apical pulse.
2. Monitor for signs and symptoms of complications.
  a. Hemorrhage
  b. Infection
  c. Leakage of cerebrospinal fluid (CSF)
3. Provide explanations to parents about monitoring procedures to alleviate anxiety.
4. Monitor child's response to barbiturate coma (see box above).
  a. Monitor apical pulse, respiratory rate, blood pressure, and arterial pressure q15 min during acute phase, then q1 hr during maintenance phase.
  b. Monitor urinary output q1 hr during acute phase; then q2-4 hr during maintenance phase.
  c. Monitor serum level of drug.

BIBLIOGRAPHY

Levin D, Morriss F: *Essentials of pediatric intensive care,* St. Louis, 1990, Quality Medical Publishing.
Raju T, Vidyasagar D, Papazafiratou C: Intracranial pressure monitoring in the neonatal ICU, *Crit Care Med* 8(10):575, 1980.

82 ❖ Intravenous Pyelogram

The intravenous pyelogram (IVP) makes it possible to identify the presence, absence, size, and configuration of the kidneys, ureters, and bladder through direct intravenous injection of a radiopaque dye at the time of the procedure. Distortions, strictures, scarring, and distention from obstruction can be detected. In addition, masses may be identified by their displacement of the kidneys, ureters, or bladder. First, an x-ray study of the kidneys, ureters, and bladder (KUB) is performed as a "scout" film to ensure the bowel is clear enough to continue with the procedure. After the contrast medium is injected, a sequence of films is taken at 2, 5, 10, 15, 20, 30, and 60 minutes (this time sequence varies). If renal function is normal, the nephrogram fades rapidly and almost disappears within 30 minutes. The contrast medium then moves from the kidneys to the ureters and bladder. The patient (if old enough and cooperative) may be asked to void, and a postmicturition film is taken to estimate residual bladder urine.

Injection of the dye may cause flushing, warm sensations, and a salty taste in the mouth. These are temporary symptoms and are not cause to stop the procedure. Since the dyes contain iodine, there is the potential for mild-to-severe allergic reactions. Antihistamine, epinephrine, a steroid, oxygen, and resuscitation equipment must be available in case they are needed for treating an anaphylactic response.

NURSING ASSESSMENT

1. Obtain a careful allergy history; prior sensitivity to iodinated contrast media is an absolute contraindication for the procedure. A history of allergies other than to iodine requires skin testing.
2. Assess the child's developmental level to plan preparation.
3. Assess the child's previous experience with and reaction to similar procedures.

NURSING INTERVENTIONS

Preprocedural Care

1. Observe for sensitivity to skin test if test is indicated.
2. Administer cathartic the evening before procedure (e.g., citrate of magnesia).
3. Provide nothing by mouth 4 hours before the procedure (policies vary). If procedure is performed on an outpatient basis, parents should be told to not feed the child breakfast.

Postprocedural Care

1. Observe for reactions to the dye; mild reactions include nausea, vomiting, and occasional wheals. Notify the physician if these reactions occur.
2. Give food and fluids to replenish them and to avoid dehydration.

BIBLIOGRAPHY

Kerr DN: Investigation of renal structure and regional function. In Belson PB, McDermott W, Wyngaarden JB, eds: *Cecil: textbook of medicine*, ed 5, Philadelphia, 1979, WB Saunders.

Luckmann J, Sorenson KC: Medical-surgical nursing: a psycho-physiological approach, Philadelphia, 1980, WB Saunders.

Osborn RR, Moline B: Department of radiological sciences procedure manual: diagnostic radiology, nuclear medicine, Los Angeles, Cal, 1984, UCLA Medical Center.

Tilkian S, Conover M, Tilkian A: *Clinical implications of laboratory tests*, St. Louis, 1987, Mosby–Year Book.

83 ❖ Peritoneal Dialysis

Peritoneal dialysis is performed to remove uremic toxins, restore normal biochemical status, and restore fluid depletion. A catheter is inserted through a stab incision into the peritoneal cavity. Gravity pulls the commercially prepared dialysis solution into the abdominal cavity. After equilibration between plasma and dialysis fluid has taken place, the dialysate flows out again. The process is repeated again until amelioration of the symptoms or the condition occurs. The abdominal cavity serves as a semipermeable membrane through which water and small molecular-sized solutes move through osmosis and diffusion. Indications for peritoneal dialysis are listed below.

Acute renal failure

Acute exogenous poisonings

Salt intoxication

Rare inborn errors of metabolism (e.g., maple syrup urine disease)

Severe hyperbilirubinemia

Hydrops fetalis

Reye's syndrome

Hyperuricemia

Deteriorating clinical condition (e.g., gastrointestinal bleeding, hypertension, volume overload, deteriorating neurologic status, congestive heart failure, and hypertensive encephalopathy)

Abnormal laboratory values
   Blood urea nitrogen (BUN) 125 to 150 mg/dl
   Metabolic acidosis
   Metabolic alkalosis
   Serum uric acid > 20 mg/dl
   Serum sodium (Na^+) > 160 mEq/L
   Serum calcium (Ca^+) > 12 mg/dl
   Serum potassium (K^+) ≥ 6.5 mEq/L

NURSING ASSESSMENT

Assess infant's or child's ability to remain still for procedure.

NURSING INTERVENTIONS

1. Prepare infant or child for procedure.
   a. Monitor child's or infant's reaction to sedation.
   b. Use sterile technique with procedure (i.e., use mask and sterile gloves).
   c. Have child empty bladder, and weigh him or her before the procedure.
2. Monitor the child's condition during the procedure.
   a. Respiratory distress
   b. Vital signs
   c. BUN, creatinine, blood chemistry, and blood culture
3. Monitor the child's therapeutic and untoward responses to medications.
   a. Antibiotics
   b. Corticosteroids
   c. Flucytosine (5-Fluorocytosine, 5-FC)
   d. Meperidine (Demerol)
   e. Promethazine (Phenergan)
4. Observe and report signs of complications.

BIBLIOGRAPHY

Arnand D, Northway J, Greshom T: Peritoneal dialysis catheter for small infants, *J Pediatr* 86:985, 1975.

Day R, White H: Peritoneal dialysis in children, *Arch Dis Child* 52:56, 1977.

Tilkian S, Conover M, Tilkian A: *Clinical implications of laboratory tests,* St. Louis, 1987, Mosby–Year Book.

84 ❖ Thoracentesis

Thoracentesis is performed to collect abnormal fluid from the pleural space for diagnostic and therapeutic purposes. Laboratory analysis of the pleural fluid is useful in identifying the cause of pleural effusion. Causes of pleural effusion are transudates (e.g., in children with congestive heart failure or nephrotic syndrome or undergoing peritoneal dialysis) and exudates (e.g., in children with infections, drug reactions, or trauma). A stab incision in the interspace is made through which a large-bore needle is inserted. Fluid that is obtained is sent for laboratory analysis.

NURSING ASSESSMENT

Assess the child's ability to sit upright during the procedure.

NURSING INTERVENTIONS

1. Prepare the child for the procedure.
   a. Position the child (sitting upright is preferable).
   b. Premedicate the child 30 minutes before procedure.
2. Monitor child's response to procedure.
   a. Signs of respiratory distress
   b. Upset or anxious behavior
   c. Extent and duration of immobility
3. Monitor for signs of complications.
   a. Leakage of fluid
   b. Hemorrhage

    c. Tension pneumothorax
    d. Hypotension
    e. Empyema (long-term)
4. Complete postprocedural care.
    a. Send specimen, accurately labeled, to laboratory for analysis (of electrolytes, glucose, protein, cell count, differential, Gram stain, and culture [AFB]).
    b. Obtain chest x-ray film to assess for pneumothorax.

BIBLIOGRAPHY

Funahashi A, Sarkor T, Korg R: Measurements of respiratory gases and pH of pleural fluid, *Am Rev Resp Dis* 108:1266, 1973.

Tilkian S, Conover M, Tilkian A: *Clinical implications of laboratory tests,* St. Louis, 1987, Mosby–Year Book.

Appendixes

❖ Nursing Assessments

CARDIOVASCULAR ASSESSMENT

1. Vital signs
   a. Apical pulse—rate, rhythm, and quality
   b. Peripheral pulse—rate, rhythm, quality, and presence or absence; major differences between upper and lower extremities
   c. Respirations—rate, depth, position of comfort, symmetry, and presence of retractions
   d. Blood pressure
2. General appearance
   a. Activity level
   b. Height, weight, and head circumference
   c. Apprehensive and agitated
3. Chest examination and auscultation
   a. Chest circumference
   b. Presence of chest deformity and abnormal chest sounds
   c. Rales, rhonchi, and wheezing
   d. Pattern of breathing
   e. Prolonged inspiratory and expiratory phases
   f. Tachypnea
   g. Retractions—suprasternal, intercostal, subcostal, and supraclavicular
4. Skin
   a. Pallor

   b. Cyanosis—mucous membranes, extremities, nailbeds
   c. Diaphoresis
   d. Duskiness
5. Eyes—periorbital edema
6. Extremities
   a. Edema
   b. Clubbing of fingers and toes
   c. Peripheral pulses—radial, popliteal, pedal, femoral, and carotid

RESPIRATORY ASSESSMENT

1. General appearance
   a. Activity level
   b. Behavior—apathetic, inactive, restless, irritable, and apprehensive
   c. Height, weight, and head circumference
2. Chest examination
   a. Chest circumference
   b. Presence of chest deformity
   c. Anteroposterior diameter
3. Respiratory status
   a. Respirations—rate, depth, and symmetry
   b. Position of comfort
   c. Presence of retractions—suprasternal, intercostal, subcostal, and supraclavicular
   d. Tachypnea
   e. Pattern of breathing
4. Chest auscultation
   a. Abnormal chest sounds, rales, rhonchi, and wheezing
   b. Prolonged inspiratory and expiratory phases
   c. Presence of hoarseness, coughing, and stridor

NEUROMUSCULAR ASSESSMENT

1. Vital signs
   a. Temperature
   b. Respirations—rate, rhythm, quality, and depth
   c. Pulse—rate and rhythm
   d. Blood pressure
   e. Pulse pressure
2. Pupillary reaction
   a. Size

b. Reaction to light, accommodation
c. Equality of responses
3. Level of consciousness
   a. Alertness — response to name and command
   b. Irritability
   c. Lethargy and drowsiness
4. Orientation
   a. Oriented to self, others, and environment (i.e., identify self and location)
   b. Short-term memory
5. Affect
   a. Mood
   b. Lability
   c. Extremes in affect (depressed or euphoric)
   d. Flat affect
6. Intellectual abilities (dependent on developmental level)
   a. Ability to write or draw
   b. Ability to read
   c. Speech
7. Gross motor function
   a. Size — presence of atrophy or hypertrophy of muscles; symmetry in muscle mass
   b. Tone — spasticity, flaccidity, limited range of motion (ROM)
   c. Strength of upper and lower extremities
   d. Abnormal movements — tremors, dystonia, athetosis, chorea
8. Fine motor function
   a. Playing
   b. Manipulating toys
   c. Drawing
9. Gait and posture control
   a. Maintenance of upright position
   b. Presence of ataxia
   c. Presence of swaying
10. Sensory function
   a. Reaction to pain
   b. Reaction to temperature
11. Reflex function
   a. Superficial and deep tendon reflexes (see Table B-1 in Appendix B for infant reflexes)

b. Presence of pathologic reflexes (e.g., Babinski)
12. In infants
   a. Occipital-frontal circumference
   b. Anterior fontanel — soft and slightly depressed, tense and bulging

RENAL ASSESSMENT

1. Vital signs
   a. Pulse — rate and rhythm
   b. Respirations — rate, rhythm, quality, and depth
   c. Temperature
   d. Blood pressure
   e. Pulse pressure

Glasgow Coma Scale

		Score
Eyes open	Spontaneously	4
	To speech	3
	To pain	2
	None	1
Best verbal response	Oriented to time, place, and person	5
	Verbal response indicates confusion and disorientation	4
	Inappropriate words making little sense	3
	Incomprehensible sounds	2
	None	1
Best motor response	Obeys commands to move body part	5
	Purposefully attempts to stop painful stimuli	4
	Decorticate pain response (arm flexion)	3
	Decerebrate pain response (arm extension and internal rotation)	2
	None	1

2. Kidney function
   a. Flank or suprapubic tenderness
   b. Presence of ascites
   c. Presence of edema — scrotal or periorbital
   d. Voiding pattern — steady or dribbling
   e. Dysuria
   f. Frequency or incontinence
   g. Urgency
3. Diagnostic assessment — urinalysis
   a. Clear or cloudy
   b. Color — amber, pink, red, or reddish-brown
   c. Presence of odor — acetone odor, ammonia odor
   d. Specific gravity — 1.010 to 1.030
4. Behavior
   a. Restlessness
   b. Irritability
   c. Lack of energy
   d. Crying during urination
5. Skin
   a. Pallor
   b. Sallow color
   c. Dehydration
6. Genitalia
   a. Irritation
   b. Discharge

SKELETAL ASSESSMENT

1. Gait — arm and leg swing, heel-to-toe gait
2. Joints
   a. Range of motion (ROM)
   b. Contractures
   c. Redness, edema
   d. Abnormal prominences
3. Spine
   a. Body enlargement
   b. Spinal curvature
   c. Presence of pilonidal dimple
   d. Scoliosis and kyphosis
4. Hips
   a. Abduction
   b. Internal rotation

HEMATOLOGIC ASSESSMENT

1. Vital signs
   a. Temperature
   b. Pulse
   c. Respiration
   d. Tachycardia
   e. Signs of congestive heart failure (CHF)
2. General appearance
   a. Height
   b. Weight
   c. Lethargy
   d. Restlessness
   e. Irritability
3. Skin
   a. Pallor or jaundice
   b. Petechiae
   c. Bruises
   d. Bleeding from mucous membranes or injection and venipuncture sites
   e. Hematomas — injection and venipuncture sites
   f. Hydration status
4. Abdomen
   a. Enlarged liver
   b. Enlarged spleen

GASTROINTESTINAL ASSESSMENT

1. Vital signs
   a. Temperature
   b. Pulse
   c. Respirations
   d. Blood pressure
2. Hydration status
   a. Skin turgor and moistness of mucous membranes
   b. Input and output
   c. Stool output — frequency, volume, and characteristics
   d. Stool testing — pH, blood, and sugar
3. Abdomen
   a. Pain
   b. Rigidity
   c. Presence and type of bowel sounds
   d. Vomiting

    e. Cramping
    f. Tenesmus

ENDOCRINE ASSESSMENT

1. Vital signs
   a. Temperature
   b. Pulse
   c. Respirations — Kussmaul respirations
   d. Blood pressure
2. Hydration status
   a. Polyuria
   b. Polyphagia
   c. Dry skin
   d. Excessive thirst
3. General appearance
   a. Weight and height
   b. Stability of mood
   c. Irritability
   d. Headache
   e. Hunger
   f. Shakiness
   g. Impaired healing
4. Neurologic symptoms
   a. Level of consciousness
   b. Headache
   c. Impaired vision

❖ Growth and Development

INFANCY (0 TO 1 YEAR)

Physical Characteristics

0 to 6 months

1. Weight
   a. Birth weight doubles by 6 months.
   b. Infant gains approximately 1½ pounds per month.
2. Height
   a. Average height at 6 months is 26 inches.
   b. Height increases at the rate of 1 inch per month.
3. Head circumference
   a. Head circumference reaches 17 inches at 6 months.
   b. It increases 1/2 inch per month.

6 to 12 months

1. Weight
   a. Birth weight triples at the end of 1 year.
   b. Approximate weight at 1 year is 22 pounds.
   c. Infant gains 1 pound per month.
2. Height
   a. Most extensive growth occurs in trunk.
   b. Infant grows 1/2 inch per month.
   c. Total height increases by 50% at 1 year.
3. Head circumference
   a. Head circumference increases 1/4 inch per month.
   b. Head circumference at 1 year is 20 inches.

Gross Motor Development

1 to 4 months

Raises head when prone
Can sit for short periods with firm support
Can sit with head erect
Bounces on lap when held in standing position
Attains complete head control
Lifts head while lying in supine position
Rolls from back to side
Arms and legs assume less flexed posture
Precrawling attempts

4 to 8 months

Holds head erect continuously
Bounces forward and backward
Rolls from back to side
Can sit with support for short intervals

8 to 12 months

Sits from standing position without help
Can stand erect with support
Cruises
Stands erect alone momentarily
Pulls self to crawling position
Crawls
Walks with help

Fine Motor Development

1 to 4 months

Purposeful attempts to grab objects
Follows objects from side to side
Attempts to grasp objects but misses
Brings objects to mouth
Watches hands and feet
Grasps objects with both hands
Holds objects momentarily in hands

4 to 8 months

Uses thumb and fingers for grasping
Explores grasped objects
Uses shoulder and hand as single unit

Picks up objects with cupped hands
Able to hold objects in both hands simultaneously
Transfers objects from hand to hand

8 to 12 months

Releases objects with uncurled fingers
Uses pincer grasp
Waves with wrist
Can locate hands for play
Can put objects in containers
Feeds crackers to self
Drinks from cup with help
Uses spoon with help
Eats with fingers
Holds crayons and makes marks on paper

Sensory Development

0 to 1 month

Distinguishes sweet and sour taste
Withdraws from painful stimuli
Distinguishes odors — able to detect mother's scent
Turns head away from aversive odors
Discriminates sounds of different pitch, frequency, and duration
Responds to changes in brightness
Begins to track objects but easily loses location
Prefers human face
Visual acuity 20/400 — able to focus on objects up to 8 inches away
Quiets when hears voices

1 to 4 months

Discriminates mother's face and voice from those of female stranger
Evidences accurate visual tracking
Discriminates between visual patterns
Recognizes familiar and unfamiliar faces

4 to 8 months

Responds to changes in color
Follows object from midline to side

Table B-1. Infant's Reflexes

Reflexes	Description	Appearance	Absent
Babinski	Fanning of toes with upward extension when sole of foot is stroked	Birth	9 months
Galant	Arching of trunk toward stimulated side when stroked along spine	Birth	Neonatal period
Moro (startle)	Sudden outward extension of arms with midline return when infant is startled by loud noise or rapid change in position	Birth	4 months
Palmar (grasp)	Grasping of object with fingers when palm is touched	Birth	4 months
Parachute	Extension forward of arms and legs in protective manner when held in horizontal prone and moving-downward position	8 months	Indefinite
Placing	Attempting to raise and place foot on edge of surface when touched on top	Birth	12 months
Plantar	Inward flexion of toes when balls of feet are stroked	Birth	12 months

Righting	Attempting to maintain head in upright position	Birth	24 months
Rooting	Turning head toward stimulated side of cheek when touched	Birth	6 months
Sucking	Sucking initiated when object is placed in mouth	Birth	Indefinite
Swimming	Mimicking swimming movement when held horizontally in water	Birth	4 months
Walking	Stepping movements elicited when infant is held upright with feet touching a surface	First weeks; reappears at 4 to 5 months	12 months

Follows objects in any direction
Tries to locate sounds
Attempts hand-eye coordination
Has highly developed sense of smell
Reaches adult limits of visual acuity
Responds to unseen voice
Demonstrates taste preference

8 to 12 months

Increases depth perception
Knows own name

Cognitive Development (Sensorimotor Stage)

Child learns through physical activities and sensory modalities.

0 to 1 month

Involuntary behavior
Primarily reflexive
Autistic orientation
No concept of self or others

1 to 4 months

Reflexive behavior, gradually replaced by voluntary movement
Activity centered around body
Initial attempts to repeat and duplicate actions
Much trial-and-error behavior
Attempts to modify behavior to varied stimuli (sucking breast vs. bottle)
Symbiotic orientation
Unable to differentiate self from others
Engages in activity because it is pleasurable

4 to 8 months

Purposeful repetition of actions
Emergence of goal-directed behavior
Discriminates differences in intensity (sounds and sights)
Imitates simple actions
Demonstrates beginnings of object permanence
Anticipates future events (feedings)
Demonstrates awareness that self is separate from others

8 to 12 months

Anticipates event as pleasant or unpleasant
Emergence of intentional behavior
Demonstrates goal-directed behavior
Evidences object permanence
Looks for lost objects
Can imitate larger number of actions
Understands meaning of simple words and commands
Associates gestures and behaviors with symbols
Becomes more independent of mothering figure

Language Development

1 month

Cooing
Makes vowel-like sounds
Makes whimpering sounds when upset
Makes gurgling sounds when content
Smiles in response to adult speech

1 to 4 months

Makes sounds with smiling
Can make vowel sounds
Vocalizes
Babbles

4 to 8 months

Increasing vocalizations
Uses two-syllable words ("booboo")
Able to form two-vowel sounds together ("baba")

8 to 12 months

Speaks first word
Uses sounds to identify objects, persons, and activities
Imitates wide range of word sounds
Can say series of syllables
Understands meaning of prohibitions such as "no"
Responds to own name and those of immediate family members
Evidences discernible inflection of words
Three-word vocabulary
One-word sentence

Psychosexual Development

Oral stage

Body focus — mouth

Developmental task — gratification of basic needs (food, warmth, and comfort) as supplied by primary caretakers

Developmental crisis — weaning; infant is forced to give up pleasures derived from breast or bottle feedings

Common coping skills — sucking, crying, cooing, babbling, thrashing, and other forms of behaviors in response to irritants

Sexual needs — pleasurable bodily sensations are generalized, although focused on the oral needs; derives physical pleasure from holding, cuddling, rocking, and sucking

Play — tactile stimulation provided through caretaking activities

Psychosocial Development

Trust vs. mistrust

Developmental task — develop sense of trust with primary caretaker

Developmental crisis — weaning from breast or bottle

Play — interactions with caretakers set the basis for development of relationships later in life

Role of parents — infants formulate basic attitudes toward life based on experiences with parents; parents can be perceived as reliable, consistent, available, and caring (sense of trust) or as the negative counterpart (sense of mistrust)

Socialization Behavior

0 to 1 month

Smiles indiscriminately

1 to 4 months

Smiles at human face
Is awake greater portion of day
Establishes sleep-awake cycle
Crying becomes differentiated
Recognizes familiar and unfamiliar faces

Prefers gazing at familiar face
"Freezes" in presence of strangers

4 to 8 months

Constrained in presence of strangers
Begins to play with toys
Fear of strangers emerges
Easily frustrated
Flails arms and legs when upset

8 to 12 months

Plays simple games (peek-a-boo)
Cries when scolded
Makes simple requests with gestures
Intense anxiety with separation
Prefers caretaker figures
Recognizes family members

TODDLER (1 TO 3 YEARS)

Physical Characteristics

1. Weight
   a. Toddler gains approximately 5 pounds per year.
   b. Weight gain decelerates considerably.
2. Height
   a. Height increases approximately 3 inches per year.
   b. Body proportions change; arms and legs grow at faster rate than head and trunk.
   c. Lumbar lordosis of spine is less evidenced.
   d. Toddler is achieving a less pudgy appearance.
   e. Legs have a "bowing" appearance (tibial torsion).
3. Head circumference
   a. Anterior fontanel closes by 15 months.
   b. Head circumference increases 1 inch per year.
4. Teeth—first and second molars and cuspids erupt.

Gross Motor Development

15 months

Walks alone with wide-base gait
Creeps up stairs
Can throw objects

18 months

Walks alone with wide-base gait
Begins to run; seldom falls
Climbs up and down stairs
Climbs onto furniture
Plays with pull toys
Can push light furniture around room
Seats self on chair

24 months

Walks with a steady gait
Runs in more controlled manner
Walks up and down stairs using both feet on each step
Jumps crudely
Assists in undressing self
Kicks ball without losing balance

30 months

Can balance momentarily on one foot
Uses both feet for jumping
Jumps down from furniture
Pedals tricycle

36 months

Dresses and undresses self
Pedals tricycle
Walks backward
Walks up and down stairs, alternating feet
Balances momentarily on one foot

Fine Motor Development

15 months

Builds tower of two blocks
Opens boxes
Pokes fingers in holes
Uses spoon but spills contents
Turns pages of book

18 months

Builds tower of three blocks
Scribbles in random fashion
Drinks from cup

24 months

Drinks from cup held in one hand
Uses spoon without spilling
Builds tower of four blocks
Empties contents of jar
Draws vertical line and circular shape

30 months

Holds crayons with fingers
Draws cross figure crudely
Builds tower of six blocks

36 months

Strings large beads
Copies cross and circle
Unbuttons front and side buttons
Builds and balances 10-block tower

Language Development

3 years

Constantly asks questions
Talks whether audience present or not
Uses telegraphic speech (without prepositions, adjectives, adverbs, etc.)
Enunciates the following consonants: d, b, t, k, and y
Omits w from speech
Has vocabulary of 900 words
Uses three-word sentences (subject-verb-object)
States own name
Makes specific sound errors (s, sh, ch, z, th, r, and l)
Pluralizes words
Repeats phrases and words aimlessly

Psychosexual Development

Anal stage

Body focus — anal area
Developmental task — learning to regulate elimination of bowel and bladder
Developmental crisis — toilet training
Common coping skills — temper tantrums, negativism, playing with stool and urine, regressive behaviors such as

thumb sucking, curling hair into knot, crying, irritability, and pouting

Sexual needs—sensations of pleasure are associated with excretory functions; actively explores body

Play—enjoys playing with excreta as evidenced by fecal smearing

Role of parents—to help child achieve continence without overly strict control or overpermissiveness

Psychosocial Development

Autonomy vs. shame/doubt

Developmental task—learning to assert self in the expression of needs, desires, and wants

Developmental crisis—toilet training; child experiences, for the first time, social constraints on behavior by parents

Common coping skills—temper tantrums, crying, physical activity, negativism, breath holding, affection seeking, play, and regression

Play—initiates and seeks play opportunities and activities; seeks attention from caretakers; explores body; enjoys sensations from gross and fine motor movements; plays actively with objects; learns to interact in socially approved ways

Role of parents—serve as socializing agents for basic rules of conduct; impose restrictions for first time on child's behavior; direct focus from primary and immediate gratification of child's needs

PRESCHOOLER (4 TO 6 YEARS)

Physical Characteristics

1. Weight
   a. Preschooler gains less than 2 kg (5 lb) per year.
   b. Mean weight is 18 kg (40 lb).
2. Height
   a. He or she grows 5 to 7 cm (2 to 2½ in) per year.
   b. Mean height is 108 cm (42 in).
3. Posture—lordosis is no longer present.
4. Teeth—preschooler is losing temporary teeth.

Gross Motor Development

4 years
Hops on one foot
Climbs and jumps
Throws ball overhand with increased proficiency

5 years
Jumps rope
Runs with no difficulty
Skips well
Plays catch

6 years
Runs skillfully; can hop and skip
Runs and plays games simultaneously
Able to hit a nail on the head
Begins to ride two-wheel bicycle
Draws a person with a body, arms, and legs
Includes features such as mouth, eyes, nose, and hair

Fine Motor Development

4 years
Uses scissors
Cuts out simple pictures
Copies square

5 years
Hits nail on head with hammer
Ties laces on shoes
Can copy some letters of alphabet
Can print name

6 years
Able to use a fork
Begins to use a knife with suspension

Socialization

Parents are most important figures
Possessive; wants things own way
Able to share with peers and adults
Imitates parents and other adult roles

Sensory

4 years
Very limited space perception
Can identify names of one or two colors

5 years
Can identify at least four colors
Can make distinctions between objects according to weight
Imitates parents and other adult roles

Cognitive Development

Preoperational stage
Child progresses from sensorimotor behavior as a means of learning and interacting with the environment to the formation of symbolic thought.
1. Develops ability to form mental representations for objects and persons
2. Develops concept of time
3. Has egocentric perspective; supplies own meaning for reality

Characteristics of thoughts
Animism: belief that objects have feelings, consciousness, and thoughts as humans do
Artificialism: belief that a powerful agent (natural or supernatural) causes the occurrence of events
Centration: ability to focus on only one aspect of a situation
Participation: belief that events occur to meet the needs and desires of the child
Syncretism: uses a specific explanation for an event as an answer to describe situations that are different in nature from the original one
Juxtaposition: rudimentary form of association and reasoning; connects two events together but does not imply a causal relationship
Transductive: rudimentary form of association and reasoning; associates nonsignificant facts together as a causal relationship
Irreversibility: cannot reverse the process of thinking; cannot backtrack through the content of thoughts from conclusion to beginning

Language Development

4 years

Has vocabulary of 1500 words
Counts to three
Narrates lengthy story
Understands simple questions
Understands basic cause-effect relationships of feelings
Conversation is egocentric
Makes specific sound errors (s, sh, ch, z, th, r, and l)
Uses four-word sentences

5 years

Has 2100-word vocabulary
Uses five-word sentences
Uses prepositions and conjunctions
Uses complete sentences
Understands questions related to time and quantity (how much and when)
Continues specific sound errors
Learns to participate in social conversations
Can name days of week

6 years

Speech sound errors disappear
Understands cause-effect relationships of physical events
Uses language as medium of verbal exchange
Speech resembles adult form in terms of structure
Expands vocabulary according to environmental stimulation

Psychosexual Development

Phallic stage

Body focus—genitals
Developmental task—increased awareness of sex organs and interest in sexuality
Developmental crises—Oedipal and Electra complexes; castration fears; fear of intrusion of body; development of prerequisites for masculine or feminine identity; identification with parent of same sex. In families with only one parent, present resolution of crisis may be more difficult.
Common coping skills—reaction formation; negative feel-

ings toward parent of opposite sex become positive; masturbation during periods of stress and isolation from home

Temperament—amount of jealousy and behaviors vary according to child's past experiences and family environment

Age-specific characteristics

5 *years*—decreased sex play; is modest and evidences less exposure; interested in where babies come from; aware of adult sex organs

6 *years*—sex play is mild, with increased exhibitionism; mutual investigation of sexes.

7 *years*—decreased interest in sex and less exploration; increased interest in opposite sex, with beginning of girl-boy "love" feelings.

Play—dramatic play in which children enact parent roles and same-sex roles

Psychosocial Development

Initiative vs. guilt

Developmental task—development of conscience; increased awareness of self and ability to function in the world

Developmental crisis—modeling appropriate sex roles; learning right and wrong

Common coping skills

Beginning problem-solving skills

Denial

Reaction-formation

Somatization (usually in gastrointestinal system)

Regression

Displacement

Projection

Fantasy

Play—has an active fantasy life; evidences experimentation with new skills in play; increases play activities in which child has control and uses self

Role of parents—supervision and direction are accepted by 5-year-olds; 6-year-olds respond more slowly and negatively to parental requests and directions. Parents are role models for the preschooler, and their attitudes have a great influence on the child's behavior and attitudes.

Plan — provide appropriate play activities and self-care opportunities.

SCHOOL-AGE CHILD

Physical Characteristics

Growth spurt begins. Great variation may be normal. Developmental charts are for reference only. Girls may begin to develop secondary sex characteristics and begin menstruation during this stage. Age of onset of menstruation has decreased in past decade.

Weight — gains 2 to 4 kg (4 to 7 lb) per year

Height — at 8 years of age arms grow longer in proportion to body; height increases at age 9

Teeth — begins to lose baby teeth; has 10 to 11 permanent teeth by 8 years of age and approximately 26 permanent teeth by age 12

Gross Motor Development

6 to 7 years — gross motor activities under control of both cognitive skills and consciousness

8 to 10 years — gradual increase in rhythm, smoothness, and gracefulness of muscular movements; increased interest in perfection of physical skills; strength and endurance also increase

10 to 12 years — high energy level and increased direction and control of physical abilities

Fine Motor Development

Increased improvement of fine motor skills because of increased myelinization of central nervous system

Improved balance and eye-hand coordination

Able to write rather than print words by age 8

Increased ability to express individuality and special interests such as sewing, building models, and playing musical instruments

Exhibits fine motor skills equal to adults by 10 to 12 years of age

Cognitive Development

Concrete operations (7 to 11 years)

Child's thinking becomes increasingly abstract and symbolic in character. Ability to form mental representations is aided by reliance on perceptual senses.

Weighs a variety of alternatives for finding best solutions

Can reverse operations; can trace the sequence of events backward to beginning

Understands concept of past, present, and future

Can tell time

Can classify objects according to classes and subclasses

Understands the concept of height, weight, and volume

Able to focus on more than one aspect of a situation

Language Development

Medium used for verbal exchange

Comprehension of speech may lag behind understanding

Less egocentric in orientation; able to consider another perspective

Understands most abstract vocabulary

Uses all parts of speech, including adjectives, adverbs, conjunctions, and prepositions

Incorporates use of compound and complex sentences

Vocabulary reaches 50,000 words at end of this period

Psychosexual Development

Latency stage

Body focus — sexual concerns become less conscious

Developmental task — gradual integration of previous sexual experiences and reactions. In recent years there has been increased documentation that latency is not a neutral period in the development of sexuality.

Developmental crisis — increased reference to preadolescent sexual concerns, beginning at approximately 10 years of age

Common coping skills — nail biting, dependence, increased problem-solving skills, denial, humor, fantasy, and identification

Parental role—major role in educating child about rules and norms governing sexual behavior and sexuality and in influencing gender-specific behavior

Age-specific characteristics

8 years—high sexual interest; increased activities such as peeping, telling dirty jokes, and wanting more sexual information about birth and sexual lovemaking; girls—increased interest in menstruation

9 years—increased discussion with peers about sexual topics; division of sexes in play activities; relates self to process of reproduction; self-conscious about sexual exposure; interest in dating and relationships with opposite sex in some children

10 years—increasing interest in own body and appearance; many begin to "date" and relate to the opposite sex in group and couple activities

11 to 13 years—concerns about appearance; social pressures to look thin and attractive are a source of stress; misconceptions about intercourse and pregnancy are evident in many children

Psychosocial Development

Industry vs. initiative

Developmental task—learning to develop a sense of adequacy about abilities and competencies as opportunities for social interactions and learning increase; strives to achieve in school

Developmental crisis—in danger of developing a sense of inferiority if does not feel competent in the achievement of tasks

Play—enjoys playing loosely structured activities with peers (e.g., baseball or four square); play tends to be sex-segregated; "rough-and-tumble" play is characteristic of outdoor unstructured play; personal interests, activities, and hobbies develop at this age

Role of family and parents—parents are becoming less significant figures in terms of agents for socialization; association with peers tends to diminish the predominant effect parents have had previously; parents are still perceived and responded to as the primary adult authorities; expectations of teachers, coaches, and religious figures have significant impact on the child's behavior

ADOLESCENT

Physical Characteristics

Adolescence is characterized by rapid growth and initial awkwardness in gross motor activity and by heightened emotionality because of hormonal changes.

1. Somatic changes — girls mature an average of 2 years earlier than boys because of rapid maturation of central nervous system.
2. Height and weight — greater averages in males because of greater velocity of growth spurt and 2-year delay in puberty
3. Dentition
   a. Completed during late adolescence
   b. Eighty percent of adolescents need to have one or more wisdom teeth removed.
4. Puberty
   a. Average age of onset — 12.5 years in females and 15.5 years in males (Table B-2)
   b. Nocturnal emissions commonly reported at 14.5 years (age range — 11.5 to 17.5 years)
   c. Menarche is identification criterion for postpubertal female; average age is 12.5 to 12.8 years

Gross Motor Development and Fine Motor Development

Gradual increases in gross motor and fine motor control are evidenced throughout this period. Both neurologic development and increased practice of skills account for the changes.

Common difficulties associated with physical changes during adolescence are as follows:

1. Skin problems and/or disorders
   a. Eczema
   b. Acne vulgaris
2. Poor posture
   a. Lordosis
   b. Scoliosis
3. Dentition problems
   a. Removal of wisdom teeth
   b. Malocclusion

Table B-2. Changes During Puberty

Male	Female	Both sexes
Thickening and strengthening of pelvic bone structure	Increased diameter of internal pelvis	Increased broadening of body frame
Increased size of scrotum and testicles	Enlargement of breasts, ovaries, and uterus	Darkening and coarsening of pubic hair
Increased sensitivity of genital area	Increased growth of labia	Increased axillary hair
Increased size of penis	Increased size of vagina	Changes in vocal pitch

4. Headaches
5. Weight problems and/or disorders
   a. Juvenile obesity
   b. Anorexia nervosa
   c. Bulimia

Cognitive Development

Formal operations

Ability to think approaches level comparable to adult competencies. Adolescent acquires capacity to reason symbolically about more global and altruistic issues and uses a more systematic approach to problems. Characteristics of thinking include the following:

Takes another perspective into account when processing information

Thinking is not limited by actual circumstances; can apply theoretical concepts to hypothesized or imagined circumstances

Develops an altruistic orientation (fairness and justice)

Develops own value system

Can form deductive and inductive conclusions

Language Development

Uses language as a medium to convey ideas, opinions, and
   values
Incorporates complex structural and grammatical forms
Evident use of slang and peer-accepted terminology

Psychosocial Development

Identity vs. role diffusion

Developmental task—development of a sure sense about
   own unique individuality, based on the needs, desires,
   preferences, values, and belief system that have evolved
   continuously throughout childhood
Developmental crisis—feels a sense of role diffusion; cannot identify accurately what factors are necessary for
   optimal self-growth; is heavily influenced by the opinions and judgments of peers
Play—strenuous and structured physical activities (e.g.,
   football and soccer) tend to be sex-segregated. Heterosex-
   ual relationships evolve, laying the foundation for intimate long-term relationships. Strong, intimate friend-
   ships develop. Cliques appear, which provide strong
   social and emotional support for teenagers. They begin to
   assume adult activities (e.g., vote, drink, and work). Adolescents use fantasy to imagine sexual encounters and
   relationships, and they enhance sexuality by focusing on
   male and female stereotypic activities such as driving fast
   cars, wearing "sexy" clothing, and lifting weights. Ro-
   mance novels have become popular with adolescent girls.
   Activities such as shopping and spending time in clothing and department stores increase.
Coping skills—problem solving; use of defenses (e.g., reaction formation, displacement, identification, suppression,
   rationalization, intellectualization, denial, conversion,
   reaction); use of humor; increased socialization
Role of parents and family—conflicts with parents may
   ensue, arising primarily out of adolescent's need to be
   independent. Parents are influential, subconsciously and
   unconsciously, in the adaptation and use of values and
   beliefs in making decisions
Plan—facilitate and support the social development

APPENDIX C ❖ Immunizations

Just before the beginning of this century, the new science of bacteriology was born. With this new information, the knowledge about infectious agents advanced, and vaccines began to appear that were effective against some diseases. The decline of infectious disease over the last 30 years as a result of the widespread use of immunizations is one of the most dramatic advances in pediatrics. In the 1970s a trend toward declining immunization levels among preschool-age children prompted a major immunization campaign. The success of that campaign was evidenced by immunization figures in 1980. At that time immunization levels of children entering school were as follows: 96% for measles, rubella, diphtheria, and tetanus-pertussis; 95% for poliomyelitis; and 92% for mumps. Many states have legislation requiring specific immunizations before children may enter daycare centers, preschools, and public schools. Such legislation aids in ensuring that the maximal number of children are immunized. A major role of the nurse caring for infants and children is educating parents about immunizations and reviewing the immunization status of each child. Continuing active immunization efforts is necessary to ensure that the rare occurrence of infectious disease that we are currently experiencing in the United States continues.

Some terms must be understood. *Immunity* is the resistance to or protection against a specific disease or infectious agent. There are basically three types of immunity: active, artificial, and passive. *Active immunity* is a long-lasting immunity that results when the body is stimulated to produce its own antibodies. *Artificial immunity* is a type of active immunity wherein antibody production is caused by the introduction of antigens in the form of toxoids and vaccines rather than by a specific disease entity. A *toxoid* is a bacterial toxin that has been chemically treated or heat treated to reduce its virulence without destroying its ability to stimulate the production of antibodies (e.g., the diphtheria and tetanus toxoids). A suspension of the actual microorganisms in weakened or killed form is a vaccine. Typhoid, pertussis, measles, mumps, and rubella are examples of diseases for which there are vaccines. Lastly, *passive immunity* is a form of immediate but transient protection against infectious disease. This type of immunity can be obtained through the administration of preparations of convalescent serum or adult blood products that contain antibodies previously formed against an infectious agent. Passive immunity provides only limited protection against infectious disease.

Age Schedule for Immunizations

The following is a recommended schedule for the immunization of normal or well children (Table C-1). One change in the immunization schedule for children in the United States has been the discontinuation of the smallpox vaccination. The reason for that change is that the risks from receiving the vaccine outweigh the chance of contracting the disease: in 1980, a worldwide eradication of smallpox was announced by the World Health Organization. Recently *Haemophilus b* conjugate vaccine has been added to the immunization schedule.

VARIOUS VACCINES AND TOXOIDS

Diphtheria, Tetanus, and Pertussis

A mixture of all three antigens (diphtheria and tetanus toxoids and pertussis vaccine) and a mineral substance that prolongs and enhances the antigenic properties by delaying absorption comprise the diphtheria, tetanus, and pertussis (DTP) vaccine. Although the diphtheria toxoid does not produce absolute immunity, when given as recommended by the schedule, protective levels of antitoxin continue for 10 years or more. There are three forms of the

Table C-1. Recommended Ages for Immunizations

Age	Immunizations
2 months	DTP, OPV*, HbCV‡
4 months	DTP, OPV, HbCV
6 months	DTP, OPV (OPV is optional), HbCV
12 months	Tuberculin test (depending on the risk of exposure, it may be administered yearly or every other year after this age)
15 months	MMR†, HbCV
15 to 18 months	DTP, OPV, HbCV
4 to 6 years	DTP, OPV
10 to 14 years	MMR
14 to 16 years	Adult tetanus toxoid (repeated every 10 years for lifetime)

*DTP—diphtheria and tetanus toxoids with pertussis vaccine; OPV—oral, attenuated, or weakened poliovirus vaccine.
†MMR—live measles, mumps, and rubella viruses combined in a vaccine.
‡HbCV—*Haemophilus b* conjugate vaccine.

tetanus toxoid: tetanus toxoid, tetanus immune globulin (human), and tetanus antitoxin (usually horse serum).

Poliomyelitis

The Sabin vaccine (OPV), or oral trivalent poliovirus vaccine, is very successful in providing immunity to all three types of poliovirus that cause paralytic poliomyelitis.

Measles, Mumps, Rubella

All three of these live viruses, for measles, mumps, and rubella, are usually combined into one vaccine (MMR). That one vaccine may provide lifelong immunity from each disease. The rubella portion is extremely important in controlling congenital rubella syndrome.

Haemophilus Influenzae Type B

A polysaccharide inactive vaccine. There are three types of this vaccine currently available, all of which appear to be equally effective. (HbOC, PRP-OMP, or PRP-D; refer to American Academy of Pediatrics guidelines for recommendations for vaccine regimen). This vaccine provides protection against the *Haemophilus influenzae* bacteria, which can cause meningitis.

Tuberculin Skin Test

The tuberculin skin test is not an immunization but is a screening device for tuberculosis. The purified protein derivative (PPD) of tuberculin is the most widely used test for tuberculosis. There are two types of PPD: (1) the Mantoux test, which consists of one intradermal injection; and (2) a multiple-puncture test such as the tine test. A positive reaction indicates that the person has been infected by and has developed a sensitivity to the protein of the tuberculin bacillus. Once a positive test is obtained, the individual will continue to react positively and should be monitored through chest x-ray examinations.

Possible Reactions

It is not unusual to have slight reactions to the DTP vaccine. Local reactions (redness and edema) at the infection site are common. Mild to moderate temperature elevations and irritability may occur, but they usually resolve within a few hours. Seizures or neurologic damage rarely occur after the administration of the DTP vaccine. If severe reactions occur, the pertussis portion of the vaccine may be eliminated in the future. Very rarely, vaccine-induced disease occurs; however, this occurrence is usually in immunosuppressed children. Fever and rash have occurred after the administration of the MMR vaccine.

Contraindications

Any time an acute febrile illness is present, immunizations should be postponed. Administration of live virus vaccines is contraindicated, and a physician's consent must be obtained before administering other immunizations in individuals with the following conditions: leukemia, lymphoma, malignancies, immunodeficiency diseases, patients with marked sensitivity to eggs, chicken, or neomycin, patients on immunosuppressive therapy, patients who have recently received immune serum globulin plasma or blood products, or pregnant females. The pertussis vaccine is contraindicated in those patients with a history of a previous reaction to the DTP vaccine.

BIBLIOGRAPHY

ACIP: Measles prevention: recommendation of the immunization practices advisory committee, *Morbid Mortal World Report* 38(9):1, 1989.

American Academy of Pediatrics: *AAP News* 6(11), 1990.

American Academy of Pediatrics: *Report of the Committee on Infectious Diseases,* ed 22, Elk Grove Village, Ill., 1991, AAP.

Centers for Disease Control: Measles—United States, *Morbid Mortal World Report,* 39(13):211, 1990.

Frank J, Loh J: SSPE: But we thought measles was gone, *J Pediatr Nurs* 6(2):87, 1991.

Frenkel LD: Routine immunizations for American children in the 1990's, *Pediatr Clin North Am* 37(3):531, 1990.

Gershon A: Immunization practices in children, *Hosp Pract* 25(9):91, 1990.

Jurgrau A: Why aren't we protecting our children? *RN* 53(11):30, 1990.

U.S. Preventive Services Task Force: Childhood, immunization, *Am Fam Phys* 40(4):115, 1989.

APPENDIX D ❖ Commonly Used Antibiotics

Amoxicillin (Amoxil)
   > 20 kg—250 mg/day q8 hr by mouth (po)
   < 20 kg—20 to 40 mg/kg/day q8 hr po
Ampicillin
   < 25 to 50 mg/kg/day q6 hr po
   > 25 to 50 mg/kg/day q6-8 hr IM or IV
Carbenicillin
   50 to 500 mg/kg/24 hr q4-6 hr IM or IV
   Variability of dose is related to severity of condition.
Cefaclor
   20 to 40 mg/kg q8 hr po
Cephalexin (Keflex)
   25 to 50 mg/kg/day QID po (in severe infections, dosage
     may be doubled)
Chloramphenicol
   50 to 100 mg/kg q6 hr po IV; infants 2 weeks of age or
     younger and children with immature metabolic func-
     tion: 25 mg/kg/day q6 hr po IV
Clindamycin (Cleocin)
   8 to 25 mg/kg/day po
   15 to 40 mg/kg/day TID/QID; IM or IV
Erythromycin
   30 to 50 mg/kg/24 hr po
   Dosage is doubled for more severe infections.
Gentamicin
   Premature infants and neonates < 1 week old—
     2.5 mg/kg/day q12 hr IM or IV
   Infants—7.5 mg/kg/day q8 hr IM or IV

Children—6 to 7.5 mg/kg/day q8 hr IM or IV
Kanamycin (Kantrex)
15 mg/kg/24 hr q8-12 hr IM or IV
Methicillin
100 to 300 mg/kg/day q4-6 hr IM or IV
Oxacillin (Bactocill)
<40 kg—50 to 100 mg/kg/24 hr q6 hr po, IM, or IV
>40 kg—250 mg to 1g/24 hr q4-6 hr po, IM, or IV
Absorption is enhanced through administration of probenecid.
Penicillin G (Benzathine)
Children <12—25,000 to 90,000 units (U)/kg q4-8 hr po
Children >12—400,000 to 600,000 U/kg q6-8 hr po
Penicillin G (Aqueous Penicillin)
<12—25,000 to 100,000 U/kg q6 hr po; 25,000 to 300,000 U/kg q4 hr IM or IV
>12—1.6 to 3.2 million U q6 hr po; 1.2 to 2.4 million IM or IV
Nafcillin (Nafcil)
Neonates—10 mg/kg TID, QID po
Infants or children—25 to 50 mg/kg QID po
Neonates—10 mg/kg BID IM
Infants or children—25 mg/kg BID IM
Children—50 to 100 mg/kg QID IV
Absorption is enhanced through use of probenecid.
Nitrofurantoin (Furadantin)
5 to 7 mg/kg/day QID po (children greater than 1 month old); children 12 years of age or older—50 to 100 mg QID po
Sulfisoxazole (Gantrisin)
Initially 75 mg/kg/24 hr po; 150 mg/kg/day QID po (maintenance)
Ticarcillin
>40 kg—150 to 300 mg/kg/day q3, 4, or 6 hr IV
<40 kg—50 to 100 mg/kg/day up to 150 to 200 mg/kg/day q4-6 hr

BIBLIOGRAPHY

Govoni L, Hayes J: *Drugs and nursing implications*, Norwalk, CT, 1988, Appleton & Lange.
Karch A, Boyd E: *Handbook of drugs and the nursing process*, Philadelphia, 1989, JB Lippincott.

❖ Taking Blood Pressure and Age-Appropriate Cuff Size

1. Determine cuff size (Table E-1).
   a. Width of cuff not less than one half nor greater than two thirds of upper arm length
   b. Width of cuff plus 50% of length extremity
   c. Largest size in which rubber bladder fits comfortably and completely encircles extremity.
2. Position manometer at observer's eye level.
3. Take blood pressure with patient in relaxed environment.
4. Take with patient in supine position.
5. Do not deflate cuff at rate less than 2 to 3 mm Hg/second.
6. Take on three separate occasions (Table E-2).

Table E-1. Age-Appropriate Cuff Size

Cuff name	Width (cm)	Length (cm)
Newborn	2.5-4	5-10
Infant	6-8	12-13.5
Child	9-10	17-22.5
Adult	12-13	22-23.5
Large adult arm	15.5	30
Adult thigh	18	36

From Report on the Task Force on Blood Pressure Control in Children, *Pediatr* 59 (suppl):797, May 1977. Reproduced by permission of *Pediatrics*.

Table E-2. Normal Blood Pressures

Age (years)	Diastolic (mm Hg)	Systolic (mm Hg)
Boys		
3 to 5	> 60	> 95
6 to 10	> 70	> 100
11 to 18	> 80	> 120
Girls		
3 to 5	> 60	> 95
6 to 10	> 70	> 110
11 to 14	> 80	> 120
15 to 18	> 80	> 130

❖ Laboratory
Values

The following are normal laboratory values unless otherwise stated.
1. Red blood cells (RBCs)
   a. Infant (1 to 18 months) — 2.7-5.4
   b. Preschooler — 4.27
   c. School-ager — 4.31
   d. Adolescent — 4.60
2. White blood count (WBC)
   a. Infant — 6000-17,500
   b. Preschooler — 5500-15,500
   c. School-ager — 4500-13,500
   d. Adolescent — 4500-11,000
3. Reticulocyte count
   a. Newborn — 3.2% ± 1.4%
   b. Neonate — 0.6% ± 0.3%
   c. Infant — 0.3% to 2.2%
   d. Remaining ages — 0.5% to 1.5%
4. Platelet count
   a. Newborn — 84,000-478,000/μl
   b. Remaining ages — 150,000-400,000/μl
5. Partial thromboplastin time (PTT)
   a. 60-85 seconds nonactivated
   b. 25-35 seconds activated
6. Prothrombin time (PT)
   a. Newborn — < 17 seconds
   b. Remaining ages — 18-22 seconds

7. Hemoglobin (Hb)
   a. 1 to 3 days old — 14.5-22.5 g/dl
   b. 2 months old — 9.0-14.0 g/dl
   c. 6 to 12 years old — 11.5-15.5 g/dl
   d. 12 to 18 years old (male) — 13.0-16.0 g/dl
   e. 12 to 18 years old (female) — 12.0-16.0 g/dl
8. Hematocrit (Hct)
   a. Newborn — 44% to 75%
   b. Infant — 28% to 42%
   c. 6 to 12 years old — 35% to 45%
   d. 12 to 18 years old (male) — 37% to 49%
   e. 12 to 18 years old (female) — 36% to 46%
9. Bleeding time
   a. Normal time — 2-7 minutes
   b. Borderline time — 7-11 minutes
10. Serum iron concentration — 30-70 µg/g
11. Serum transferrin — 200-400 mg/dl
12. Serum ferritin concentration (abnormal) — < 10-12 µg/L
13. Serum ferritin determination
    a. Male — 20-300 µg/dl
    b. Female — 20-120 µg/dl
14. Serum iron — 50-120 µg/dl
15. Total serum bilirubin
    a. At birth — < 2 mg/dl
    b. Up to 1 month — ≤ 1 mg/dl
16. Bilirubin, direct — 0-0.2 mg/dl
17. Arterial blood gases
    a. Partial pressure of oxygen (P_{O_2}) — 75-100 mm Hg
    b. Partial pressure of carbon dioxide (P_{CO_2})
       (1) Infant — 27-40 mm Hg
       (2) Remaining ages — 35-45 mm Hg
    c. pH
       (1) Premature (cord) — 7.15-7.35
       (2) Premature (48 hours) — 7.35-7.5
       (3) Newborn — 7.27-7.47
       (4) Infant — 7.35-7.45
       (5) Child — 7.35-7.45
18. Serum electrolytes
    a. Sodium (Na^+)
       (1) Premature infant — 132-140 mmol/L
       (2) Infant — 139-146 mmol/L

   (3) Child—138-145 mmol/L
   (4) Adolescent—136-146 mEq/L
  b. Potassium (K^+)
   (1) Infant—4.1-5.3 mEq/L
   (2) Child—3.4-4.7 mmol/L
   (3) Adolescent—3.5-5.1 mmol/L
  c. Chlorine (Cl^-)—98-106 mmol/L
  d. Carbon dioxide (CO_2)
   (1) Infant—27-41 mmol/L
   (2) Child
    (a) Male—35-48 mmol/L
    (b) Female—32-45 mmol/L
19. Serum calcium
  a. Premature infant—6-10 mg/dl
  b. Full-term infant—7.5-11 mg/dl
  c. Child—8.8-10.8 mg/dl
  d. Adolescent—8.4-10.2 mg/dl
20. Blood urea nitrogen (BUN)
  a. Newborn—8-18 mg/dl
  b. Infant or child—5-18 mg/dl
  c. Adolescent—8-17 mg/dl
21. Creatinine
  a. Cord—0.6-1.2 mg/dl
  b. Newborn—0.3-1.0 mg/dl
  c. Infant—0.2-0.4 mg/dl
  d. Child—0.3-0.7 mg/dl
  e. Adolescent—0.5-1.0 mg/dl
22. Serum glutamic-pyruvic transaminase (SGPT)
  a. 6-12 months—16-36 IU
  b. 2-17 years—6-22 IU
23. Serum glutamic-oxaloacetic transaminase (SGOT)
  a. 6-12 months—$\leq$ 40 IU
  b. 2-17 years—10-30 IU
24. Creatine phosphokinase (CPK)
  a. Infant—20-31 U/L
  b. Infancy to adolescence—15-50 U/L
25. Serum uric acid
  a. Female—2.0-6.0 mg/dl
  b. Male—3.0-7.0 mg/dl
26. Serum phosphorus
  a. Premature infant—4.6-8.0 mg/dl
  b. Newborn—5.0-7.8 mg/dl

27. Serum glucose—40-100 mg/dl
28. Serum amylase dehydrogenase; children—45-200 dye U/dl
29. Serum cholesterol
    a. 1-4 years—≤ 210 mg/dl
    b. 5-14 years—≤ 220 mg/dl
    c. 15-20 years—≤ 235 mg/dl
30. Serum lipase
    a. Infant—9-105 U/L
    b. Remaining ages—20-180 U/L
31. Sweat test—negative
32. Albumin in meconium—negative
33. Urinalysis
    a. Specific gravity—1.003-1.035
    b. pH
       (1) Infant—5.0-7.0
       (2) Remaining ages—4.8-7.8
    c. Protein—negative
    d. Blood—negative
    e. Sugar—negative
    f. Ketones—negative
34. Cerebrospinal fluid (CSF)
    a. Specific gravity—1.007-1.009
    b. Glucose
       (1) Infant/child—60-80 mg/dl
       (2) Remaining ages—40-80 mg/dl
    c. Protein
       (1) Newborn—45-100 mg/dl
       (2) Child—10-20 mg/dl
       (3) Adolescent—15-40 mg/dl
    d. pH—7.33-7.42
    e. Cell count
       (1) Neonate—0.5 polymorphonuclear; 0-5 mononuclear; 0-5 RBCs/mm^3
       (2) Remaining ages—0 polymorphonuclear; 0-5 mononuclear; 0-5 RBCs/mm^3

❖ Abbreviations

<	Less than
>	Greater than
ABG	Arterial blood gas values
ADH	Antidiuretic hormone
AGN	Acute glomerulonephritis
AIDS	Acquired immunodeficiency syndrome
ALT	Alanine aminotransferase
ANLL	Acute nonlymphoid leukemia
AOM	Acute otitis media
A/P	Anteroposterior
AP	Apical pulse
ASO	Antistreptolysin O
AST	Aspartate aminotransferase
Ax	Axillary
BID	Twice a day
BMA	Bone marrow aspiration
BPD	Bronchopulmonary dysplasia
BUN	Blood urea nitrogen
C & S	Culture and sensitivity
Ca^+	Calcium
Cal	Calories
CBC	Complete blood count
cc	Cubic centimeter
CDC	Centers for Disease Control
CHF	Congestive heart failure
CID	Cytomegalic inclusion disease

Cl	Chloride
cm	Centimeter
CMV	Cytomegalovirus
CNS	Central nervous system
CO_2	Carbon dioxide
COM	Chronic otitis media
CPK	Creatinine phosphokinase
CPP	Cerebral perfusion pressure
CPR	Cardiopulmonary resuscitation
CSF	Cerebrospinal fluid
CT	Computerized tomography
CUG	Cystourethrogram
CVA	Cerebrovascular accident
CVP	Central venous pressure
d	Day
D5W	5% dextrose in water
DC	Discontinue
DIC	Disseminated intravascular coagulation
dl	Deciliter (100 ml)
DTP	Diphtheria, tetanus, and pertussis
ECG	Electrocardiogram
EEG	Electroencephalogram
EMG	Electromyogram
EP	Erythrocyte protoporphyrin
ESR	Erythrocyte sedimentation rate
ET	Endotracheal
EUG	Excretory urogram
FB	Foreign body
5-FC	5-fluorocytosine
Fe	Iron
FEP	Free erythrocyte porphyrin level
FET	Force-expiration technique
FFP	Fresh frozen plasma
FTT	Failure to thrive
g	Gram
GER	Gastroesophageal reflux
GI	Gastrointestinal
gr	Grain
HAV	Hepatitis A
Hb	Hemoglobin
HBV	Hepatitis B

Hct	Hematocrit
H_2O	Water
HOB	Head of bed
hr	Hour
I & O	Intake and output
ICP	Intracranial pressure
IDDM	Insulin-dependent diabetes mellitus
I/E	Inspiratory/expiratory
IG	Immune globulin
IM	Intramuscular
IQ	Intelligence quotient
ITP	Idiopathic thrombocytopenic purpura
IV	Intravenous
IVFD	Intravenous fast drip
IVP	Intravenous pyelogram
JRA	Juvenile rheumatoid arthritis
K^+	Potassium
KG	Kilogram
L	Liter
lb	Pound
LDH	Lactic dehydrogenase
LOC	Level of consciousness
LP	Lumbar puncture
M^2	Square meter
MAP	Mean arterial pressure
mcg	Microgram
MCH	Mean corpuscular hemoglobin
MCHC	Mean corpuscular hemoglobin concentration
mEq	Milliequivalent
Mg	Magnesium
mg	Milligram
min	Minute
ml	Milliliter
mm^3	Cubic millimeter
MMR	Measles, mumps, and rubella vaccine
mOsm	Milliosmole
MTX	Methotrexate
Na^+	Sodium
NA	Non-hepatitis A
$NaHCO_3$	Sodium bicarbonate
NAS	No added salt

NB	Non-hepatitis B
NG	Nasogastric
NPO	Nothing by mouth
NS	Normal saline
NSAIDs	Nonsteroidal antiinflammatory agents
OPV	Oral poliovirus vaccine
P	Phosphate
PBI	Protein-bound iodine
P_{CO_2}	Partial pressure of carbon dioxide
PDA	Patent ductus arteriosus
PERL	Pupils equal and react to light
PERLA	Pupils equal, react to light and accommodate
PE tubes	Pressure equalizer tubes
PHN	Public health nurse
pl ct	Platelet count
po	Oral; by mouth
PO_2	Partial pressure of oxygen
pr	By rectum
prn	As needed
PROM	Passive range of motion
PT	Prothrombin time
PTT	Partial thromboplastin
q	Every
qd	Daily
QID	Four times a day
qod	Every other day
RBC	Red blood cell; red blood count
RDS	Respiratory distress syndrome
ROM	Range of motion
RSV	Respiratory syncytial virus
SBS	Short bowel syndrome
SGOT	Serum glutamic-oxaloacetic transaminase
SGPT	Serum glutamic-pyruvic transaminase
SIDS	Sudden infant death syndrome
SOB	Shortness of breath
SOM	Serous otitis media
SQ	Subcutaneous
TB	Tuberculosis
TCDB	Turn, cough, and deep breathe
TID	Three times a day

TPN	Total parenteral nutrition
tx	Treat
U	Units
UA	Urinalysis
UGI	Upper gastrointestinal
URI	Upper respiratory infection
UTI	Urinary tract infection
VNA	Visiting Nurses' Association
VS	Vital signs
VSD	Ventricular septal defect
WBC	White blood cell; white blood count
WNL	Within normal limits

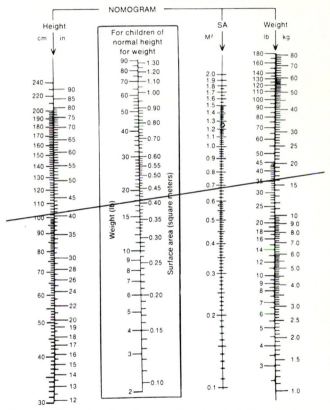

NOMOGRAM

Height
cm | in

For children of
normal height
for weight

SA
M²

Weight
lb | kg

For estimation of surface area: surface area is indicated where a straight line connecting height and weight intersects surface area (SA) column, or if patient is roughly of normal proportion, from weight alone (enclosed area). Line shows SA determination (0.68 M²) for child 41 inches tall who weighs 35 lb.

Nomogram modified from data of E Boyd by CD West. From Behrman RE, Vaughan VC ed: *Nelson textbook of pediatrics*, ed 12, Philadelphia, 1983, WB Saunders.

❖ Index